Mastering the
medical long case
2e

A tribute to my parents and my family.
And to Hanna, with love.

Mastering the medical long case

An introduction to case-based
and problem-based learning
in internal medicine

2e

S Rohan Jayasinghe

MBBS (Honours Class 1) (Sydney), MSpM (UNSW), PhD (UNSW), FRACP
Director of Cardiac Services and Cardiology, Gold Coast Hospital
Professor of Cardiology, Griffith University School of Medicine
Professor and Chair of Medicine, Bond University School of Medicine
Queensland, Australia

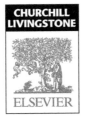

CHURCHILL
LIVINGSTONE

ELSEVIER

Sydney Edinburgh London New York Philadelphia St Louis Toronto

Churchill Livingstone
is an imprint of Elsevier

ELSEVIER

Elsevier Australia. ACN 001 002 357
(a division of Reed International Books Australia Pty Ltd)
Tower 1, 475 Victoria Avenue, Chatswood, NSW 2067

National Library of Australia Cataloguing-in-Publication Data

---

Jayasinghe, S. Rohan.

Mastering the medical long case : an introduction to case
based and problem based learning in internal medicine /
S. Rohan Jayasinghe.

2nd ed.

ISBN: 978 0 7295 3839 8 (pbk.)

Includes index.
Bibliography.

Medical history taking.
Diagnosis--Case studies.
Medicine--Examinations, questions, etc.

616.0751

Publisher: Sophie Kaliniecki
Developmental Editor: Sunalie Silva
Publishing Services Manager: Helena Klijn
Editorial Coordinator: Lauren Allsop
Edited by Kay Waters
Proofread by Pam Dunne
Cover and internal design by Trina McDonald
Index by Michael Ferreira
Typeset by TnQ Books and Journals Pvt. Ltd.
Printed in China by 1010 Printing International Ltd.

Contents

Author's note

This book is meant to be an examination aid and not a therapeutic manual. Clinical medicine as described here is what is practised in most leading teaching hospitals and tertiary referral centres in Australia, and relates to the experience of the author and colleagues. The author disclaims any legal responsibility associated with the application of the modalities of clinical management discussed here. Medicine is changing fast. Although every attempt has been made to provide accurate and complete information consistent with the practice of medicine at the time of publication, information given here may become outdated due to changes in medical science. Readers are advised to refer to therapeutic and clinical manuals for the practical application of the concepts discussed in this book. This book is an examination aid only.

Primum non nocere.
[First do no harm. First principle of medicine.]

It is a great privilege to be invited to write this second edition of *Mastering the medical long case*. This endeavour has enabled this popular textbook to be made more comprehensive and current. The management principles discussed here are in keeping with the latest evidence and trends in modern medicine.

The fundamentals in the introduction I wrote for the first edition still hold true, no matter what developments have taken place in the science and technology of medical practice. The basics of clinical evaluation, beginning with the building of confidence and rapport, followed by thorough history taking and physical examination, cannot be replaced or bypassed. *Mastering the medical long case* is all about perfecting the practice of good and safe medicine. With the advancement of modern therapeutics, a demographic shift is taking place in the patient population. Patients are surviving longer and as a consequence tend to accumulate more diseases along the way. Their lists of medications keep getting longer and they have social, economic and occupational problems that also need addressing. This complexity in the management of patients is fast becoming the norm in clinical medicine, and it is not surprising that many authorities consider the long case the most significant component of their respective examinations. The clinical examinations of the Royal Australasian College of Physicians, undergraduate and postgraduate medical schools and postgraduate training authorities worldwide, have the long case examination or an equivalent in their assessment programs. Particularly with the Royal College of Physicians in Australia, the long case has become a significant parameter by which a physician's competence is measured at the qualifying examination.

With advances in global communication and the rapidity and ease of global travel, developments in medicine seem to spread to all corners of the earth very quickly. Accordingly, medical practice has become more or less uniform all over the world.

During a discussion on the best way to prepare for the long case section of the physician's examination, a reputed specialist at the Prince of Wales Hospital in Sydney (where I trained as a registrar) said that it is all about 'just becoming really good at what you usually do in the wards with managing your patients'. This statement sums up the basic principle behind the required preparation for the medical long case. A very good physician trainee or a medical student needs to be able to assess patients with multiple serious medical problems thoroughly and systematically, analyse the issues involved, identify the problems in their order of priority (both medical and social), organise relevant investigations and formulate a comprehensive management plan. The candidate should do this with every patient they encounter in their daily clinical practice. So carrying out these daily tasks with diligence and curiosity may be all that is necessary to achieve long case mastery. A mere reproduction of this is all that is necessary at the examination to pass with flying colours!

PRACTICAL TIPS

Discuss your patients with your seniors and ask questions when you have any doubts. Do not be a passive participant. Always try to imagine what you would do if you were in charge. Take responsibility in the crucial decisions regarding the management of your patients. Look up the latest journals and publications to keep in touch with the most recent trends in diagnostics and therapeutics, and try to apply these in the care of your patients. Ask what your consultant thinks about the plan of management you propose.

It is important to have worked with many different specialists in order to be experienced and comfortable with the management of patients with various disorders involving different organ systems. Specialties such as renal medicine and cardiology give the candidate or student exposure to the management of quite ill patients with many complicated medical and social problems. Oncology gives an opportunity to participate in making crucial decisions regarding active treatment and best palliation. All specialties have made tremendous progress in therapeutics in recent years, and the only way to learn the application of such modern therapeutics in the management of patients is to work with the relevant teams.

As you can appreciate, the long case is essentially a process of gathering all the relevant information from the patient and bringing this together to understand what is happening with the patient at that precise moment. Once that objective has been achieved, the next step is to decide what needs to be done to tackle the various problems that have been identified. Decision-making is the key to the long case, and the candidate's decisions (preferably judicious, mature and confident) can make the difference between passing or failing the exam.

Be organised

Although it is important to have a commanding knowledge of the various major medical conditions, this in itself is insufficient to be able to handle a long case confidently and competently. As the long case is an interplay between many serious and minor medical conditions, the candidate has to be able to apply his or her knowledge appropriately to understand how the combination of various diseases is affecting the patient. Direct application of the recommended therapy for a condition may not be feasible in the long case setting, due to the presence of complicating factors of other diseases and the potential for adverse reactions with multiple other medications. In addition, there may be psychological, social, financial and cultural issues that further complicate the case. For example, a patient who has ischaemic heart disease as well as asthma may not tolerate beta-blocker therapy well, while a patient who has ischaemic heart disease as well as migraine will not tolerate nitrate therapy well. In such circumstances, candidates should be able to decide on the best combination of medications to treat one condition without exacerbating the other.

Medicine ain't just medicine

In addition to the medical aspects of the long case, importance should be given to the social, financial and psychological aspects. Therapeutic decisions should be tailored to the patient's context and needs. Active therapy, palliation and recruitment of research-based novel therapy may all be applicable in various situations. The candidate should be able to make a rational decision regarding the choice of therapy after taking into account all the important factors. The formulated plan of management should be effective, safe, practical and financially feasible. The candidate has to be able to defend his or her approach when questioned by the examiners. It is not wise to change your plan to any significant extent when challenged, because you are expected to make firm and well-informed decisions from the outset. Remember that the examiners don't necessarily challenge your decision because it is wrong, but because they want to make sure that you are confident, convinced and clinically mature enough to stand by your decision.

The all-important final thrust

Another key aspect in the long case—the 'final thrust' at the examination—is the presentation. A good style of presentation will certainly impress the examiners. Clear organisation of the information, demonstration of empathy and a broad understanding of all areas of concern to the patient are important aspects of a good presentation. Presentation skills are acquired only through constant practice. Learn to speak clearly, at a reasonable speed. Sit relaxed, with your head held high. Maintain eye contact with the examiners at all times. Listen carefully when the examiners speak or ask questions. Do not interrupt examiners, and never criticise an examiner! Some candidates audio- or even video-record their long case presentation, to review and correct mistakes.

MEDICAL STUDENTS

Mastering the medical long case gives medical students an ideal opportunity to see how the various therapeutic concepts discussed in textbooks are put into practice. You may discover that not everything in the textbook is directly applicable to the practical setting, because diseases don't always present as well-demarcated, separate entities. Medical students should try to undertake terms in all medical specialties, to gain experience in dealing with patients suffering from diseases of different organ systems. Try to spend as much time as possible in the wards and participate in the ward rounds, ward meetings and teaching sessions. Talk to patients, allied health professionals and patients' relatives; you will learn a lot and improve your communication skills.

Listening to registrars presenting long cases to consultants will be an enriching educational experience. Establish a good rapport with your registrar and politely request permission to be present when she or he presents a long case. After the case presentation, discuss with the registrar the areas of the case that were unclear to you.

Each long case can be considered a short textbook on the relevant medical conditions. You can learn your medicine by doing long cases. Consider each patient you see in the ward, emergency department and outpatients clinic as a long case. Take the most detailed history you can, do the most detailed but relevant physical examination, and devise the best plan of management after much thought and consideration. Try not to cut corners. Spend time sorting out patients. As you become more experienced with handling the long case, your speed will improve. And if you cultivate a real enthusiasm to learn from the cases you see, you will begin to enjoy them. Good luck with your long cases, both at the examination and in your clinical career!

Rohan Jayasinghe
Surfers Paradise
Summer 2008

Reviewers

I would like to offer my sincere gratitude to the following experts, who kindly reviewed and provided advice, corrections and suggestions on the relevant sections and the long cases of this book. I would also like to thank those whose work was instrumental in the development of the first edition of this book. Responsibility for any errors, omissions and inaccuracies in the information lies with the author.

Dr Balaji Hiremagalur FRACP, MMedStat,
Director of Nephrology
Gold Coast Health Service District
Gold Coast

Dr Jagadeesh Kurtkoti MD
Senior Registrar in Renal Medicine
Gold Coast Hospital
Gold Coast

Dr Vance Manins MBBS, FRACP
Heart Transplant Fellow
Royal Perth Hospital
Perth

Dr Jenny Ng MBBS, FRACP
Consultant Rheumatologist
Gold Coast Hospital
Gold Coast

Dr George Ostapowicz MBBS, FRACP
Senior Gastroenterologist
Head of Gastroenterology
Gold Coast Hospital
Gold Coast

Dr David Platts MBBS, FRACP
Cardiologist
Prince Charles Hospital
Brisbane

Dr Arman Sabet MD
Senior Staff Neurologist
Gold Coast Hospital
Gold Coast

Dr Siva Sivakumaran MBBS, FRACP
Director of Respiratory Medicine
Gold Coast Hospital
Gold Coast

Dr Thomas Titus MBBS, MD, MRCP, PhD
Staff Specialist in Nephrology
Gold Coast Hospital
Gold Coast

Dr Jeremy Wellwood MBBS, FRACP
Director and Senior Haematologist
Gold Coast Hospital
Gold Coast

Acknowledgments

Michael Trikilis, Chief Radiographer, Cardiac Catheterisation Laboratory, Gold Coast Hospital, for coronary angiography images

Michael May and Vivek Kulkarni, echo technicians at the Gold Coast Hospital, for cardiac echo images

Radiology Department at Gold Coast Hospital for abdominal ultrasound images
Radiology Department at Prince Charles Hospital for cardiac MRI images
Radiology Department at Westmead Hospital for radiographic images

I am indebted to Developmental Editor Sunalie Silva and the staff at Elsevier for their tremendous support and facilitation in making this second edition a comprehensive and high quality product.

Part

01

Clinical
assessments

Approach to the long case

TO THE PHYSICIAN TRAINEE

The 'long case' is the main focus of interest in the physician's examination. Candidates at the FRACP examination are given two long cases. It is very important to perform well in the long cases, to secure a comfortable overall pass at the examination. This book introduces the long case to the novice in the field and attempts to correct some flaws in more experienced players. These instructions are aimed mainly at candidates taking postgraduate clinical examinations. However, there is also useful advice and information for medical students preparing for the clinical component of their examinations and for students participating in their clinical rotations. The case discussions in the latter section of this book are also aimed at providing useful guidance to medical students involved in problem-based learning (PBL) and case-based learning (CBL) modules.

The long case is an art that needs mastering. Long case mastery will not only help candidates to pass the examination but will also equip the trainee with the skills and expertise to handle any complicated medical case. These skills are vital to the candidate's future life as a physician. While preparing for the clinical examination, the candidate is expected to acquire as much expertise as possible within a very short time. Such intense learning will not happen at any other time in your career. Therefore, it is important to approach this time of preparation knowing what to do and how to go about doing it. The preparatory period should be well planned and executed, with utmost commitment to your goal. It is important to plan this preparation systematically, so that no aspect of clinical medicine is missed or omitted. It is also important to achieve your peak level of performance at the right time. Peaking too early can lead to exhaustion and a lacklustre performance by the time of the examination, and peaking too late may mean 'missing the boat'.

An ideal way to start preparing is to fully understand what the preparation is for. It is therefore important to become familiar with the examination and what exactly will take place on the day. At the examination the candidate is usually given 1 hour to spend with the patient unobserved by the examiners or the 'bulldog' (the bulldog is a basic trainee registrar from the host hospital assigned to attend to the candidate on the day of the examination). During this period, a detailed history needs to be obtained, and a thorough physical examination performed, focusing particularly on the main system involved. The candidate is usually given a warning 10 minutes before the end of his or her time with the patient. Then another 10 minutes is given as preparation time before the candidate is introduced to the examiners. There are usually two examiners for each candidate on the long case, one being a member of the National Examining Panel (college representative or censor). Occasionally there may be a third member present, acting as an observer. This member of the examining team is usually a new examiner learning the examination process. The 'grilling' is carried out by the two main members of the examining team; later in the day, the 'observer' may swap seats with the college censor to actively participate in the 'grilling' process.

The examinee is expected to present a clear, sufficiently detailed and well-organised long case within 7–10 minutes and develop a comprehensive management plan. The candidate may be interrupted at any time during this period if further clarification is needed on any aspect of the case. The candidate usually spends 25 minutes with the examiners, and after the presentation there should be sufficient time for the examiners to assess the candidate's knowledge. Of course, this is extremely valuable time for the candidate to demonstrate as much knowledge and clinical wisdom as they can. Ideally, if the candidate is confident with the case, they will be able to control the discussion, and this will convey an air of competence.

During the discussion, the candidate should mention the relevant investigations that they would perform. At this point, the examiners will present a radiological imaging study or a blood or serology test result and ask the candidate for an interpretation. Other investigation results—including electrocardiograms, lung function studies, nerve conduction studies, hormonal studies and nuclear medicine scans (but not pathological specimens)—may also be produced.

A practical tip

It is important to have a set approach to the long case, and to use this system repeatedly during practice cases until you have mastered the long case. Candidates should develop a format to address the history and the physical examination, and thereby avoid any 'fatal' mistakes or omissions.

A stack of cards can be very convenient for taking notes when with the patient. This also provides a hard surface to write on, as often there will not be a table available by the bedside. The best technique is to use the cards according to a prepared format. Mnemonics (see p 5) can be used to remember the format even in the stressful circumstances of the practice exams and the real exam. The way you organise the cards is also important. The long case can be divided into sections, and cards organised accordingly; this will make your presentation easier as well as neater. An average case may need about 20 cards, and these should be clearly numbered at the top right-hand corner.

- Card 1 should contain the patient's name, age and the opening statement, which is a concise but sufficiently detailed introductory overview of the case.
- Card 2 should be for the presenting complaint and then associated conditions. Past history, medications, allergies, family history, occupational history and social history should be placed in that order.

The social history has to be very detailed; accordingly, this section comes as a subset of cards, with a separate mnemonic to help remember all aspects of the social history. Another advantage of using cards is that they can be held close to eye level with your head held high, thus facilitating constant eye contact with the examiners. It is important to maintain eye contact. (In fact, some senior examiners expect so much of it that one examiner advised his candidates to learn the long case by heart and stop using written records of the case at all.)

Taking a history

Establishing trust and confidence

The first 20 minutes of the hour with the patient should be spent on history taking. In the exam setting you should try to obtain as much help as you can from the patient by quickly explaining how important the exercise is to you. A strong bonding with the patient can be achieved from the outset by being very courteous and polite. Smile broadly and shake the patient's hand warmly, using both hands. Generate genuine empathy with the patient and be considerate at all times. Try to create an atmosphere of trust and confidence. Establishing a good rapport will ensure that the patient opens up without any hesitation. It is easiest to begin by asking the patient about the medications he or she is currently taking. This may give you a comprehensive overview of the patient's problems and save much valuable time. On some occasions at the real examination, the examiners leave the list of medications with the patient, with instructions to hand it to the candidate only if they request it.

Mnemonics

History and physical examination are the cornerstones of your clinical assessment of the patient. Your whole plan of investigation and management as well projections on the prognosis will be based on what is garnered during your clinical assessment and the case that is built upon this vital information. Therefore, it is essential that your history taking and physical examination be comprehensive, foolproof and watertight—you cannot afford to miss anything! One proven way of ensuring that you don't miss anything is to have a ready-made, comprehensive and complete checklist consisting of everything you need to learn during history taking and physical examination. You will need to memorise this checklist and be able to recall it readily during the examination. Mnemonics are a very useful tool in this regard. This section of the chapter introduces some mnemonics that have been developed for this purpose. Or you might find it easier to develop your own set of mnemonics.

The following mnemonic for history taking is comprehensive and covers almost all aspects of the history:

    P P M A F O S T

P **Presenting complaint** and the details thereof

P **Past history**, intercurrent illnesses and relevant details

    For each disease mentioned in this section of the history, it is important to get the following details:

    1 When, how and who made the diagnosis.

    2 What treatment has been administered and whether there have been any complications or side effects associated with it. For each drug the patient is currently taking, mention the dosage and frequency. The candidate is expected to know the generic name of each drug and should be able to identify the generic names of almost all the commonly used drugs.

    3 What the current level of disease activity is and how the patient is affected by it.

M Medication history

If all the patient's current medications have been mentioned already in the previous section, it will be sufficient just to mention the list of medications again as a brief summary. Some examiners like to hear the list separately. Listing the medications may also provide the candidate with an opportunity to see whether there are any drugs with significant interactions.

A Allergies

F Family history

O Occupational history

S Social history

T Travel history

Relevant in cases with infectious diseases and exotic conditions.

Social history

Many a fatal mistake can be made by not addressing the social history adequately. Therefore it is important to have a separate mnemonic to probe into all the important aspects of the social history. The mnemonic for the social history is:

S E M I G — C H D P — N S — D I P — V A S P

(It is easier to remember this if you break it up into five segments as suggested here and review it many times a day.)

S Smoking history

E Ethanol/alcohol history

M Marriage

Marital status, previous marriages and, if single, reason for not marrying etc.

I Independence

Level of independence with activities of daily living. If the patient needs assistance, find out who the main care provider is and how well they are coping.

G GP

Relationship with the patient's general practitioner, frequency of visits etc.

C Children

Number of children and other relevant details such as ages, gender, who they live with if the patient has a broken relationship with their partner.

H House/home

This should include details such as the number of steps needed to climb to enter or exit the house, the number of steps the patient has to climb inside the house, whether the patient has any disability, how she or he manages at home, and whether the house has been modified to accommodate the patient's needs.

D Driving

Ask whether the patient drives and, if not, how they get around.

P Pets

Whether the patient keeps any pets. This may be important in situations of socially isolated patients and also in patients suspected of having zoonotic infections such as psittacosis.

N Nutrition

Obtain details about the main meals. A detailed dietary history may be necessary in an obese or malnourished patient.

S Sleep

Ask questions to exclude obstructive sleep apnoea, such as whether the patient has been told by their bed partner that they snore, whether the patient feels refreshed in the morning on waking up, any early-morning headaches, early-morning diuresis, daytime somnolence (e.g. falling asleep at the steering wheel of a vehicle while driving). Also ask about insomnia—whether it is initial (difficulty falling asleep, associated with depressive situations) or terminal (waking up too early, associated with anxiety disorders)—or any complaints from the bed partner about distressing leg movements (restless legs syndrome).

D Depression

Ask whether the patient has ever been depressed and, if so, when, why and what treatment they have had. Ask whether the patient is currently depressed—here it may be necessary to enquire into the presence of any vegetative symptoms of depression, such as anorexia, anhedonia (lack of interest in pleasurable activities) or initial insomnia.

I Insight

Check the patient's insight into their medical condition. This also includes enquiring into the patient's knowledge about the disease, about living with it and its prognosis.

P Problem

Ask what the patient's biggest problem currently is, as they perceive it. For example, a patient who is critically ill with infective exacerbation of end-stage emphysema may still be more worried about his disabled wife, who is alone at home, than about his own illness. In such a situation, as much importance should be given to organising adequate care for the wife as to the treatment of the patient's medical condition.

V Visits

If the patient's usual residence is far from the hospital, it is important to ask who visits the patient at the hospital and how often this happens.

A Associations

Ask whether the patient belongs to any relevant association or an organised body (e.g. Multiple Sclerosis Association, Blind Society), where they can obtain information and support.

S Support

Ask who provides the main social support base for the patient while in hospital and when discharged to the community.

P Pastime

Ask what the patient's usual pastime is. This is important particularly in retired or disabled, homebound patients.

Physical examination

On completing the history, an adequately detailed physical examination should be performed, with the main emphasis on the system involved with the patient's current presentation (Fig 1.1). It is wise to spend about 20 minutes on the physical examination. Elements of the physical examination include vital observations of the pulse rate, respiratory rate, temperature and blood pressure (postural pulse and blood pressure if indicated), and the systems-specific examination.

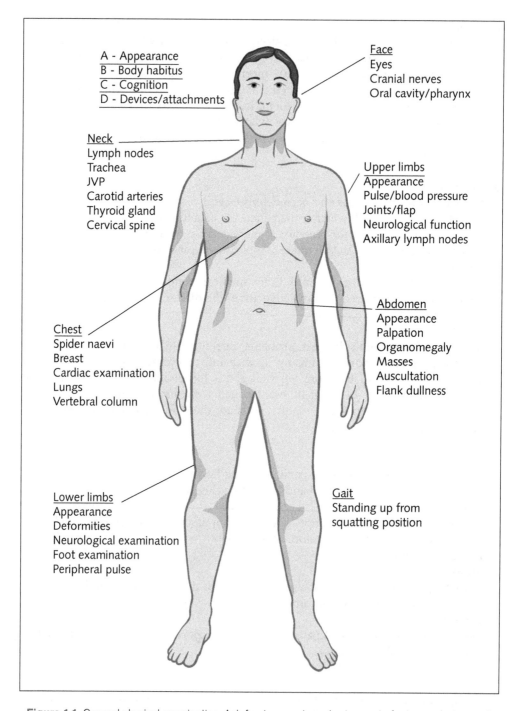

A - Appearance
B - Body habitus
C - Cognition
D - Devices/attachments

Face
Eyes
Cranial nerves
Oral cavity/pharynx

Neck
Lymph nodes
Trachea
JVP
Carotid arteries
Thyroid gland
Cervical spine

Upper limbs
Appearance
Pulse/blood pressure
Joints/flap
Neurological function
Axillary lymph nodes

Chest
Spider naevi
Breast
Cardiac examination
Lungs
Vertebral column

Abdomen
Appearance
Palpation
Organomegaly
Masses
Auscultation
Flank dullness

Lower limbs
Appearance
Deformities
Neurological examination
Foot examination
Peripheral pulse

Gait
Standing up from
squatting position

Figure 1.1 General physical examination. Ask for: temperature chart, report of urine analysis, result of per rectal examination.

Initial components of the examination can easily be remembered as:
A B C D E F G (as easy as that!)

A Appearance

B Body mass index
An estimate would be sufficient, but some patients may be aware of their body weight and height.

C Cognition
It may be necessary to perform a Mini-Mental State Examination, particularly in such cases as suspected dementia, alcoholism, stroke and HIV infection.

D Devices and attachments
Do not forget to mention the intravenous catheters and the infusions running through them, an indwelling catheter, cardiac monitoring device attached to the patient, and any inhalants or continuous positive airway pressure devices lying on the table next to the patient.

The physical examination can be carried out by dividing it into different systems and examining each system separately. Some candidates may find this too time-consuming, particularly when there are significant time limitations. In such circumstances it may be wise to perform the examination from one end of the body to the other and then compartmentalise while writing up. The following is a simple model that is easy to remember.

E Entire body (head to toe)
Head:
- Face—appearance/specific features, such as rashes
- Eyes—neurological and ophthalmological examinations
- Remainder of the cranial nerve examination
- Oral cavity and pharynx

Neck: lymph nodes, trachea, jugular venous pressure, carotid arteries, thyroid gland and the cervical spine

Upper limbs (distal to proximal):
- appearance, deformities
- pulse, blood pressure, joints, flap
- neurological assessment—tone, power, reflexes, coordination, sensation
- axillary lymph nodes

Chest: cardiac examination, lungs, vertebral column, spider naevi, breast etc

Abdomen: appearance, palpation, organomegaly, masses, auscultation, flank dullness

Lower limbs: appearance, deformities, neurological examination (as per upper limb), foot examination, peripheral pulse

F Functionality
Assess limb movements and the ability to perform different functional tasks based on the clinical assessment thus far. This may involve assessment of muscle strength, neurological function and joint mobility. Check coordination if relevant.

G Gait
Study the patient's gait and observe them standing up from a squatting position, to assess proximal weakness.

Gait disorders
- *Wide-based gait* (ataxic-drunkard)—cerebellar disorders
- *Shuffling gait* (marche petit pas)—Parkinson's disease
- *Steppage gait* (high-stepping)—peripheral neuropathy, foot drop
- *Circumduction*—hemiparesis
- *Trendelenburg gait*—hip joint pain
- *Scissor gait*—lower limb spasticity

Remember to ask (the bulldog) for the results of the urine analysis and the per rectal examination, and for the temperature chart.

Presentation

In the presentation, the candidate can start off with the vital observations and go on to describe different systems, commencing with the main system involved. It is important to mention relevant negatives and the absence of signs that would be expected to have been present in the classic setting. If no abnormality was found in a certain system and the system is not involved in the presenting pathology, it may be adequate just to mention that the examination of the particular system was 'unremarkable'. This may leave more time for the discussion.

If the history is very detailed and time is running short, it may be necessary to complete the latter part of the history while examining the patient. The mnemonics mentioned above may help in such a situation, and can be used as a checklist.

The last 20 minutes should be spent on clerical pursuits. It is important to arrange the presentation appropriately, to decide on which components to mention and what to withhold, and to prepare strong opening and closing statements. A comprehensive list of differential diagnoses should be thought of and relevant investigations should be decided on. When mentioning a particular test, it is vital to mention what is being looked for (e.g. 'I would like to see the full blood count—looking for a polymorpho-nuclear leucocytosis').

Discussion

Introduction

Much time and mental energy should go into preparing a suitable opening statement (Fig 1.2). This should be concise but detailed enough to give the examiners a broad overview of what is about to be presented. It should demonstrate the clinical maturity of the candidate, and a good opening statement can always put the examiners at ease and give vital points to the candidate. It is important to maintain full eye contact with the examiners during the opening statement and this can be achieved only by learn-ing the statement by heart. A rambling and overly detailed opening statement will bore the examiners and give the impression that the candidate has not identified the crux of the case.

The 10 minutes of preparation time, before being introduced to the examiners, should be spent on revising the case and learning by heart the opening (introductory) and closing statements.

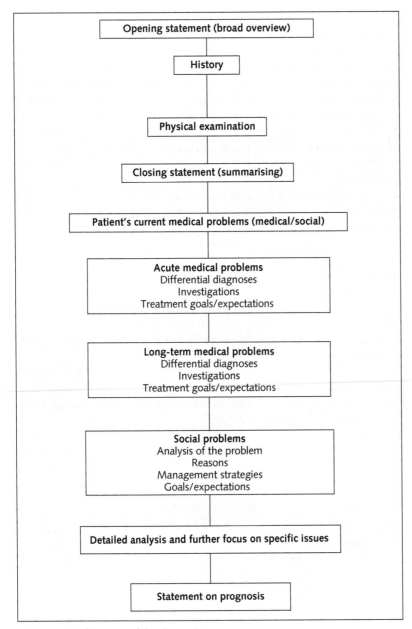

Figure 1.2 Structure of the discussion

Closing statement

The closing statement is a recapitulation of the essential aspects of the case. This must be concise but sufficiently detailed, like the opening statement. The difference between the opening and the closing statements is that the former is an anticipatory statement, and the latter a conclusive statement with indications of diagnostic possibilities and management options. After the closing statement comes the 'main issues' section.

The issue(s)

Most cases may have a single extremely important issue, which is the 'main plot', and identification of this issue is consistent with the expected level of maturity of the candidate at the examination. There may then be significant other issues that need to be identified. These can be discussed under two major headings: **acute issues** and **long-term issues**. Each of these can be further analysed under two subheadings: **social issues** and **medical issues**. Candidates should also mention how many problems they have identified before coming up with the list (e.g. 'I have identified two acute medical problems and a social problem. There is also a long-term medical problem that needs addressing.').

Management plan

After describing the issues that matter, a broad management plan should be introduced. The problems identified can be expanded under the medical and social subheadings according to the following compartmentalisation:

- The main 'problem'
- Possible differential diagnoses
- Relevant investigations and the expected results
- Proposed treatment or management:
  - Medical
  - Social

With regard to investigations, the candidate is expected to propose the most judicious investigation appropriate to the clinical setting, and to avoid giving long lists of non-specific investigations. When suggesting an invasive investigation, the candidate should be able to justify the risks involved in view of the benefits expected. The candidate should be aware of the costs involved with different investigations, and all decisions should be cost-effective in the general setting.

The candidate's treatment plan should be comprehensive, and he or she is expected to make decisions with confidence and the competence of a general physician, with a

MEDICAL

Problem	Differential diagnoses	Investigations	Expected results	Treatment
1. 2. 3.				

SOCIAL

Problem	Management plan
1. 2.	

Figure 1.3 Layout of the management plan

sound knowledge of all specialties of internal medicine. The candidate should be capable of defending the plan of management based on the most up-to-date evidence. It therefore pays to be thorough with the current treatment guidelines and pathways developed and introduced by various authorities (e.g. National Heart Foundation), reputed institutions and hospitals (e.g. Mayo Clinic). I cannot over-emphasise the importance of being familiar with the latest results of major randomised controlled multi-centre trials and other ground-breaking large-scale studies that define the practice of contemporary evidence-based medicine.

It is very important to emphasise a team approach to the management of issues in the broader sense, with the participation of the relevant specialists, the patient's general practitioner (GP) and allied health workers, such as disease educators, social worker, occupational therapist, physiotherapist, speech pathologist and, of course, a diversional therapist as required. If the patient's management problem is discharge planning and post-discharge care, it is important to demonstrate a sound knowledge of the community resources available for such patients. Here the family conference and liaison with the GP are important concepts.

Contemporary medicine attaches great significance to after-care and follow-up of patients. Candidates need to have a wide appreciation of the different chronic disease management programs and ambulatory care programs available for the ongoing care of patients in the community setting. The candidate is also required to provide plans on how to educate the patient, develop satisfactory insight into their condition and ensure good compliance with the management plan.

TO THE MEDICAL STUDENT

This book aims to provide an introduction for medical students entering and progressing through the clinical years of their training. *Clinical integration* involves putting together the subject matter learnt in the preclinical stages (also called *basic science information*) in the context of the patient. This programs your thinking to exercise clinical rationalising based on the background knowledge gained in the preclinical learning. Essentially it is an exercise for the student to start thinking like a doctor.

This book aims to aid the system of *problem-based learning* (PBL) and *case-based learning* (CBL) that has become the cornerstone of teaching in many medical schools. It provides the basic clinical information required to approach the more commonly encountered clinical challenges in internal medicine. Students are introduced to thinking in a systematic manner when approaching a patient. When you have become proficient in obtaining a general history and performing a good general physical examination (as discussed earlier in this chapter), you will then be ready to take on the more specialised clinical scenarios discussed in this book.

The physician plays the role of detective, gathering all the vital clues and evidence to build the case at hand. The clues are gathered during your history and physical examination. Therefore it is important that you have a clear idea of what you are looking for when taking the history and performing the physical examination. Once you have obtained a detailed history and have performed a thorough physical examination, you are then ready to put your thoughts together, to *build the case*. This involves coming up with a set of *differential diagnoses* based on the evidence you have gathered and your clinical reasoning. Then you should think of the investigations you need to order or refer the patient to, for the purpose of proving or excluding the various differential diagnoses. Based on the results of the investigations, you can reorganise your list of differential diagnoses and rank them from the most likely to the least likely. If you can identify a single diagnosis as the absolute based on the evidence at hand, it becomes your *definitive diagnosis.*

Now you are ready to come up with your *plan of management.* This needs to be comprehensive and should include *direct therapeutics* (pharmacological, interventional or surgical) and *supportive measures* (patient education, psychosocial aid, physiotherapy, rehabilitation etc). You should know what outcomes to expect from the different therapeutic decisions you make. Optimal monitoring of the patient's response to treatment is very important.

Once the patient is treated for the acute condition, you should think of ongoing management once discharged from the care of the acute care provider. This involves building a *long-term management plan* in the setting of ambulatory care (outpatient follow-up), general practice and community care.

Remember: clinical medicine can only be learnt at the patient's bedside! Only practice will make you a good clinician. Proactively participating in ward rounds, spending time with the resident staff, performing clinical duties under the supervision of junior medical staff, and participating in departmental clinical and teaching meetings are some activities that will help you immensely and facilitate your efforts to make the most of what is available for learning in the teaching hospital setting.

So, in summary, when approaching the patient (see box on p 15) you should be alert to the important clues with diagnostic, prognostic and management implications. Look for these initially during the clinical assessment (history and physical examination). Once you have completed your clinical assessment, you must develop a list of differential diagnoses. The next step in the clinical work-up is to decide on and perform the relevant investigations. The investigations are aimed at proving or excluding the differential diagnoses in order to narrow them down to a definitive diagnosis. Investigations need to be relevant and cost effective. (Medical students and inexperienced junior doctors are notorious for blindly ordering all the tests in the book.) Once you have arrived at the definitive diagnosis, the next step is to plan the management. Management has two main arms: treating the presenting complaints, and preventing recurrences or future clinical events.

Case vignettes and long case discussions

The clinical vignettes in the coming chapters are there to stimulate your thoughts. Once you have gained a good insight into the vignette you may find answers to some of your questions in the text that follows. Some questions may require further more specialised and detailed research. The text sets the stage and guides you through this learning exercise.

The case discussions in the third part of the book will give you an in-depth appreciation of how advanced clinical reasoning is done. Although this is aimed at medical registrars, these cases will give you a solid foundation upon which to build your clinical career.

Approach to the patient

1 Ensure that the patient is clinically and haemodynamically stable. If the patient is unstable (e.g. desaturating, hypotensive), you might first be required to provide acute care to stabilise the situation.

2 When you are sure the patient is stable, introduce yourself and establish the necessary confidence and trust. Build a rapport with the patient.

3 Obtain essential clues by observing the patient's surroundings (immediate environment).

4 Obtain a detailed history, with particular focus on the presenting complaint. Ensure that the patient is well oriented and of satisfactory mental status. This will have a major bearing on the accuracy of the information you expect to gather. If the patient is not of sound mental state, the history may need to be obtained from a second party who is privy to the patient's health status, such as the wife, husband, partner, parent, sibling or even the GP.

5 Perform a detailed physical examination with a particular focus on the system related to the presenting complaint.

6 Decide on a list of differential diagnoses.

7 Based on clinical reasoning, try to arrive at a definitive diagnosis.

8 Decide on the most relevant and useful investigations.

9 Order or perform the said investigations.

10 Decide on the plan of management, based on the clinical assessment as well as the results of the investigations.

11 Decide on the long-term management and means of preventing future clinical events.

12 Identify and address the patient's psychological, social and occupational needs.

13 Provide patient education—a very important aspect of total medical care.

SYMPTOMS ASSESSMENT

Symptoms assessment is where it all begins: the patient presents with symptoms. As the clinician you decide on your path of assessment according to what the patient complains of as symptoms. It is therefore extremely important for the clinician to be thorough in understanding and evaluating symptoms. The questions asked and the information focused on in analysing the patient's symptoms help the clinician to establish a roadmap of enquiry. Your subsequent progression to the cascade of steps in your clinical evaluation, such as physical examination, investigational testing, formation of the list of differential diagnoses and making a definitive diagnosis, are all based on the information you obtain during the taking of the history. Therefore, the foundation of your clinical involvement with every patient is the history you take of their presenting symptoms.

It is useful to have a 'ready-to-use' aid in the form of a checklist for approaching the various symptoms a candidate might encounter in the long case. Below are discussed the commonly encountered symptoms, together with the relevant issues that need to be investigated. When encountering each problem, ask for details as described.

PAIN

Ascertain:

1   The nature of the onset and the events surrounding the onset (gradual or sudden). If the pain was of sudden onset, what was the patient doing at the time?
2   Precipitating factors
3   Exact location and radiation
4   Severity and character
5   Factors that exacerbate or relieve the pain
6   Duration, diurnal pattern, temporal pattern, progression
7   What the patient has done so far in addressing the pain (e.g. doctors involved, medication taken), including non-pharmacological means that have been tried, such as acupuncture, chiropractic and physiotherapy.

Back pain

Back pain is very common. In addition to the following salient clinical features, it is important to enquire into the occupational and functional difficulties associated with the symptom. Clinical features to concentrate on include:

1 The points listed above under 'Pain'
2 Neurological symptoms in the lower limbs
3 Bladder and bowel function abnormalities
4 Radicular pain.

The differential diagnoses that need to be considered can be grouped under six broad subheadings for ease of comprehension and memorising:

- *Traumatic injury*
- *Mechanical*—muscular, postural, spondylosis (prolapse of the vertebral disc), spinal stenosis, diffuse idiopathic skeletal hyperostosis (DISH), spondylolisthesis, fibromyalgia
- *Inflammatory*—ankylosing spondylitis, sacroiliitis due to any seronegative arthropathy, septic arthritis of the sacroiliac joint (more common in the young male adult)
- *Metabolic*—osteoporosis-associated pathological fracture, osteomalacia, Paget's disease of bone, renal osteodystrophy
- *Neoplasia*—metastatic cancer, multiple myeloma, primary bone tumour
- *Referred pain*

Acute disc prolapse

Acute disc prolapse is a particularly common disorder, and so it is important to be able to identify features that suggest this diagnosis. The onset of pain is usually associated with such activities as lifting. The patient presents with lower back pain, muscular spasms and at times lancinating pain, paraesthesias and weakness of the lower limbs due to neurological involvement.

Basic steps in management include bed rest during the acute stage when the pain is excruciating, analgesia according to the pain ladder concept, and muscle relaxants. The patient should be advised to mobilise as pain permits. If pain persists unabated beyond 6–10 weeks, or there is significant neurological deficit, neurosurgical review is indicated. Surgical therapy involves microdiscectomy or hemilaminectomy. If there is bladder or bowel involvement, it should be considered a neurosurgical emergency and acted on promptly.

Spinal canal stenosis presents with spinal claudication—that is, pain and paraesthesias, particularly in the buttocks, on walking and relieved by rest. The management should essentially include a neurosurgical review.

Headache

Vital elements of the clinical assessment include:

1 The factors listed above, under 'Pain'
2 Associated other symptoms, such as:
   - *neck stiffness and photophobia*—suggesting meningitis
   - *gastrointestinal symptoms, transient neurological deficit*—suggesting migraine
   - *jaw claudication*—suggesting temporal arteritis
   - *purulent nasal discharge and facial tenderness*—suggesting chronic sinusitis
   - *eye irritation*—suggesting cluster headache
   - *early-morning exacerbation*—could suggest increased intracranial pressure, chronic renal failure with azotaemia or obstructive sleep apnoea.

Chest pain

This is a very common presentation and can indicate a medical emergency. It is therefore important to distinguish the more serious, time-critical and potentially life-threatening differential diagnoses from those that are not so serious. The precise location of the pain, associated other symptoms, its severity, haemodynamic stability and oxygenation as well as the patient's background history (age, coronary risk factor profile etc) may provide vital clues to the seriousness of the current presentation.

Differential diagnoses of chest pain:
- acute myocardial infarction
- angina
- pulmonary embolus
- pneumothorax
- dissection of the thoracic aorta
- pericarditis
- pneumonia
- pleurisy
- oesophagitis
- oesophageal spasm
- gastritis
- peptic ulcer disease
- mediastinitis
- costochondritis
- musculoskeletal pain.

DYSPNOEA

This common symptom could be due to a cardiovascular pathology, pulmonary pathology, chest wall pathology or even hysteria. It is important to distinguish between the possible causes, because the management strategies are very different for each of the possible diagnoses. The vital information in association with dyspnoea includes:

1. Onset and progression
2. Association with rest or exertion. Quantify the level of effort tolerance by asking the patient how far they can walk on flat ground before getting breathless (dyspnoea distance).
3. Presence of orthopnoea or paroxysmal nocturnal dyspnoea
4. Relieving factors and exacerbating factors
5. Previous and current level of exercise performance
6. Duration
7. What the patient has done so far in addressing the symptom
8. Other associated symptoms—angina, cough, fever, pleuritic chest pain.

Differential diagnoses that need to be considered in a dyspnoeic patient are:
- pulmonary oedema
- pulmonary congestion
- chronic airway limitation
- asthma
- pulmonary embolism
- interstitial lung disease
- pneumonia

- *Pneumocystis carinii* pneumonia in the immunocompromised
- essential pulmonary hypertension in the young female patient
- anxiety disorder.

Auscultation for crepitations (rales) is an important next step in the clinical assessment of the dyspnoeic patient.

Crepitations

Define the character of the crepitations—fine, medium or coarse. Describe the distribution and also identify other associated sounds such as wheezing and bronchial breath sounds.

Common differential diagnoses include:

- pulmonary fibrosis / interstitial lung disease (fine crepitations)
- bronchiectasis (coarse crepitations)
- pulmonary congestion / pulmonary oedema (may associate with wheezing)
- atelectasis (basal).

FEVER

Fever is a common symptom that can indicate many different types of pathology. A thorough initial evaluation therefore is invaluable. Features of the presentation that need to be focused on include:

1 Onset and duration
2 Temporal pattern and variation
3 Any new medications taken prior to the onset of fever
4 Associated other features, such as:
- cough, sputum production, chest pain and dyspnoea—suggesting pulmonary sepsis
- previously known valve pathology, palpitations, intravenous drug use, recent invasive procedures such as dental work—suggesting infective endocarditis
- diarrhoea, nausea, vomiting, abdominal pain—suggesting gastrointestinal sepsis
- headache, neck stiffness, photophobia—suggesting central nervous system sepsis (encephalitis, cerebritis or meningitis)
- joint pain, skin lesions—suggesting a vasculitis or connective tissue disease
- previous or existing intravenous devices and inflamed cannula sites.

Pyrexia of unknown origin

Pyrexia of unknown origin (PUO) by definition is a fever that has persisted for more than 3 weeks without an identifiable cause, despite extensive investigation. Some possible causes include:

- sub-acute bacterial endocarditis
- concealed abscess (e.g. subphrenic, pelvic, dental)
- malignancy (melanoma, lymphoma, sarcoma)
- connective tissue disorders
- HIV
- parasitic infestations
- osteomyelitis
- tuberculosis
- glandular fever / Epstein Barr virus
- exotic infections such as Lyme disease, Ross River virus etc in the traveller.

JOINT PAIN/STIFFNESS

In the clinical assessment it is important first to establish whether the presentation is that of a *monarthritis* or *polyarthritis*. Then check the distribution and the symmetry or asymmetry thereof. Other information that is useful includes:

1 Location and the exact joints involved
2 Onset, duration, diurnal pattern
3 Duration of pain and stiffness each day
4 Functional impairment
5 Precipitating and relieving factors and medications consumed so far
6 Progression over time and space
7 Associated other features, such as rash, weight loss, ocular symptoms, oral symptoms, genital symptoms
8 Muscle ache, headache, fevers.

Arthritis

Differential diagnoses that need to be considered include:
* rheumatoid arthritis
* osteoarthritis
* gouty arthritis / crystal arthropathy
* seronegative arthropathy
* mechanical trauma
* polymyalgia rheumatica.

FALLS

Falls could be due to general debility, neurological deficit, visual impairment or musculo-skeletal pathologies. Vital information about the symptoms includes:

1 Onset, duration, frequency
2 Exact causative associations with the falls, such as leg weakness, visual impairment, tripping over and difficulty with steps
3 Functional status and mobility, currently and prior to the onset of falls
4 Association with micturition, standing and coughing
5 Other symptoms such as presyncope, syncope and vertigo
6 Time of the fall, what the patient was doing immediately before the fall, position/posture before the fall
7 Any difficulty with balance and coordination
8 Possible precipitating conditions, especially in the elderly, such as urinary tract infection, sedative hypnotic medications, tricyclic antidepressants, Parkinson's disease, alcohol consumption and stroke
9 Palpitations
10 Any injury sustained due to the fall
11 Use of assisting devices, such as a walking frame or stick.

Falls associated with syncope/presyncope

Differential diagnoses that need to be considered are:
* bradyarrhythmias
* complete heart block
* tachyarrhythmias (especially sustained ventricular tachycardia)

- vasovagal syncope
- micturition syncope
- cough syncope
- postural hypotension
- drug effects
- pulmonary embolism
- cataplexy
- stroke, especially in the brainstem region.

DIZZINESS

It is important to question the patient closely to ascertain exactly what they mean by 'dizziness'. If the features of the presentation include imbalance associated with a sensation of the surrounding environment rotating or moving, it may be indicative of vertigo. However, if the patient complains of blacking out, impending blackout or loss of consciousness, it may in fact indicate presyncope or syncope. An eyewitness account would be invaluable in this setting (asking about associated fitting, incontinence, presence of arterial pulse etc). Differential diagnoses include:

- *Vertigo*—benign positional vertigo, tinnitus, labyrinthitis, acoustic neuroma
- *Syncope*—neurocardiogenic shock, severe bradycardia, ventricular tachycardia, vasovagal attack, postural hypotension, carotid body hypersensitivity, micturition syncope, ischaemia in the vertebrobasilar system, migraine, grand mal epilepsy.

SPECIFIC DISEASES AND CONDITIONS

There are some disease conditions that are often encountered in the long case. Examiners expect candidates to be very thorough with these conditions because they are common in the candidates' clinical practice. These 'bread-and-butter' conditions include:

- alcoholic liver disease
- anaemia
- asthma
- chronic airway limitation
- chronic corticosteroid use
- congestive heart failure
- diabetes mellitus
- diarrhoea
- HIV infection
- inflammatory bowel disease
- ischaemic heart disease
- multiple sclerosis
- renal transplantation
- stroke
- rheumatoid arthritis.

In each condition encountered in the long case setting, four questions need to be addressed:

1 What do you ask in the history?
2 What signs do you look for in the physical examination?

3 What investigations do you order?

4 What is the optimal management?

When the candidate can competently address these four issues, with almost all types of conditions one could expect to find in a long case, he or she is ready to comfortably pass the examination. Most conditions commonly presenting as long cases are covered in the following chapters. They are discussed under the relevant specialties for convenience of reference, but remember that in the long case these conditions do not present as separate entities. Those conditions not discussed here will be dealt with in the discussion sections of some of the sample long cases that follow (in Section 3).

Cardiac conditions are very commonly encountered in the long case setting. Given that cardiac disease is the most common morbidity in the world's adult population, a cardiac condition could be encountered as the main pathology or an associated condition in the long case setting. Common cardiology long cases the candidate should be well versed in are: heart failure, ischaemic heart disease, arrhythmias and hypertension. Also important are valve disease and associated clinical decision-making processes, including timing of surgery if indicated in the patient with a cardiac valvular pathology.

HYPERTENSION

Case vignette
A 57-year-old man is admitted to hospital with severe chest pain. The pain is of sudden onset, tearing in character and radiating to the back. He is diaphoretic and anxious. On examination his pulse is regular at 110 bpm. His heart sounds are normal and the chest is clear. His blood pressure in the right arm is 190/100 mmHg and in the left arm 170/70 mmHg.
1 What are the possible differential diagnoses in this case?
2 What constitutes your detailed clinical assessment of this man (in addition to what is provided in the vignette)?
3 What investigations would you request?
4 Outline your detailed plan of management, with relevant reasoning.

Approach to the patient
Hypertension is a common finding in patients seen in the examination (see box over leaf for causes of hypertension), but rarely is it the major problem in management. Nevertheless, some thorough and accessible knowledge of hypertension can impress the examiners. *Hypertension* is practically defined as blood pressure readings above 140/90 mmHg on three separate occasions a week apart. However, the lowest blood pressure within

the limits of tolerance is desirable. In the diabetic patient, the optimal blood pressure is 125/75 mmHg. Patients with hypertension should be investigated for other cardiovascular risk factors, because the identification and management of the full continuum of cardiovascular risk is of paramount importance.

Causes of hypertension

- Primary/idiopathic (95% of cases)
- Obesity
- Obstructive sleep apnoea
- Alcoholism
- Renal artery stenosis
- Parenchymal renal disease
- Renal tumours
- Gestational
- Pre-eclampsia
- Congenital adrenal hyperplasia
- Hypothyroidism
- Hyperthyroidism
- Acromegaly
- Conn's syndrome (primary hyperaldosteronism)
- Cushing's syndrome
- Phaeochromocytoma
- Polycythaemia vera
- Acute intermittent porphyria
- Raised intracranial pressure
- Medication-induced (oral contraceptives, corticosteroids, cyclosporin)

History

Ask:
- how high the blood pressure was when first diagnosed and what treatment the patient has had so far
- who monitors the blood pressure, how often it is checked and what the usual level of control is
- about other vascular risk factors and any known end-organ damage.

Bi-occipital headache is the classic symptom of severe hypertension. Nocturia is an early symptom of the malignant phase.

Examination

Check the blood pressure and look for a postural drop. If the blood pressure is very high, check the other arm and repeat the measurement at the end of the physical examination for confirmation.

Examine the optic fundus for features of hypertensive retinopathy (see Fig 3.1 and box) and, if present, describe your findings according to the Keith-Wagener-Barker classification (see box overleaf). An apical heave and a loud aortic component of the second heart sound are signs that suggest left ventricular hypertrophy due to long-standing high blood pressure. Examine for a renal bruit, adrenal masses, polycystic kidneys, bitemporal hemianopia or acromegalic body habitus and cushingoid body habitus to exclude a secondary cause for the hypertension (see box overleaf).

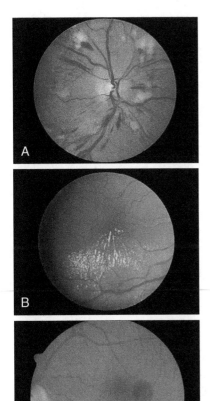

Figure 3.1 Hypertensive retinopathy
(A) Flame haemorrhages and cotton wool spots
(B) Macular exudates ('star') (C) Haemorrhage from a macroaneurysm (reprinted from Batterby M, Bowling B 2005 *Ophthalmology: an illustrated colour text,* 2nd edn. Elsevier, p 56, figs 1–3)

Features of hypertensive retinopathy

- *None*—no detectable abnormality
- *Mild*—focal and generalised arteriolar narrowing; copper and silver wiring of arterioles; arteriovenous (AV) nipping
- *Moderate*—blot, dot or flame-shaped haemorrhages, cottonwool spots, microaneurysm, yellow and white exudates
- *Severe*—papilloedema (in addition to haemorrhages and exudates)

Retinopathy is indicative of increased risk of stroke, myocardial infarctions and death. Odds increase with worsening severity of retinopathy.

Keith-Wagener-Barker classification of hypertensive retinopathy

- *Grade 1*—Mild/focal constriction and sclerosis of the arterioles
- *Grade 2*—Moderate to severe constriction and sclerosis of arterioles with enhanced reflexivity and AV nipping
- *Grade 3*—Above changes together with retinal haemorrhages/cottonwool exudates
- *Grade 4*—Above changes together with papilloedema

Causes of secondary hypertension

- Obesity
- Alcohol excess
- Renal parenchymal disease
- Renal artery stenosis
- Acromegaly
- Hyperaldosteronism
- Cushing's disease
- Phaeochromocytoma
- Renin-secreting tumour

Clinical issues of significance in a patient with high blood pressure are:

1 Is the blood pressure actually high? This raises the question of measurement error and, more particularly, 'white coat' hypertension (persistent 'white coat' hypertension has also been described as a sentinel marker of possible constant hypertension and therefore should not be ignored). In patients with poorly controlled hypertension (or in whom the diagnosis is uncertain), consider the need for 24-hour ambulatory blood pressure monitoring. Blood pressure monitored overnight should show a drop during the first half of the night. Blunting or absence of this 'nocturnal dip' is associated with enhanced cardiovascular risk.

2 How much target organ damage is present and how does this influence the prognosis?

3 Is there an underlying renal or endocrine cause amenable to treatment other than lowering blood pressure?

4 What other cardiovascular risk factors are present?

Investigations

Investigations that should be requested in a patient with hypertension are:

1 Electrolyte profile and renal function indices—looking for evidence of renal failure. Abnormal renal function indices should prompt further investigations to rule out parenchymal renal disease.

2 Electrocardiogram (ECG)—looking for left ventricular hypertrophy by voltage as well as strain criteria and evidence of ischaemic heart disease

3   Chest X-ray—to exclude cardiomegaly, left ventricular hypertrophy and congestive cardiac failure (X-ray is capable of detecting only quite gross and irreversible left ventricular damage)

4   Echocardiogram—to assess left ventricular wall thickness and chamber size and any evidence of diastolic dysfunction (especially if there is clinical evidence of left ventricular hypertrophy or heart failure) (Fig 3.2)

5   Urine analysis—looking for proteinuria. A positive urine analysis for proteinuria should be followed up with a 24-hour urine collection to quantify the proteinuria and to assess creatinine clearance. Proteinuria of more than 2 g per day is much more likely to reflect primary renal disease and usually indicates a need for renal biopsy. Calculate the albumin-to-creatinine ratio (ACR), which is an important cardiovascular risk marker.

6   Fasting blood sugar levels and lipid profile—to assess the presence of other significant cardiovascular risk factors.

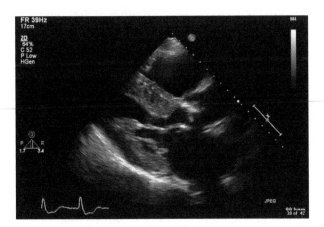

Figure 3.2 Echocardiogram of left ventricular hypertrophy

Creatinine clearance needs to be checked to clarify renal function but does not really help to distinguish between primary renal disease causing high blood pressure and renal impairment secondary to hypertensive nephrosclerosis. If there is no significant proteinuria or renal failure, a trial of effective blood pressure lowering for 6 months can be given. Deterioration of renal function at any stage is an indication for investigation. The additional investigations in this setting include a renal ultrasound (looking for renal shrinkage suggesting chronic renal failure or renovascular disease, or enlarged kidneys suggesting conditions such as polycystic kidney disease), a DTPA scan (to assess renal perfusion) and a renal arterial Doppler study (to exclude renal artery stenosis). If clinical evidence indicates renal artery stenosis, further study with computed tomography (CT) or magnetic resonance (MR) angiography is indicated.

The major endocrine investigation is the aldosterone/renin ratio, to detect primary hyperaldosteronism. This is now believed to account for 10–15% of people presenting with essential hypertension, but this does not mean that they all need adrenalectomy.

Other endocrine investigations include: serum renin index (to exclude renin hyper-secretion) and 24-hour urinary cortisol (to screen for Cushing's syndrome).

If there is suspicion (tachycardia, palpitations, sweating, anxiety, postural hypoten-sion) of phaeochromocytoma, perform serum catecholamine level, urinary metaneph-rines and urinary vanillylmandelic acid level.

Management

It is not wise to commence treatment at the first diagnosis itself unless there is malig-nant hypertension, end-organ damage (see box) or significant other vascular risk fac-tors, or comorbidity. (Treat with antihypertensive agents if the diastolic pressure is > 100 mmHg, or systolic > 200 mmHg, or systolic pressure > 160 mmHg together with end-organ damage. The presence of other cardiovascular risk factors would be another indication for treatment.) Observation for 3−6 months with recommen-dation of non-pharmacological methods such as progressive muscle relaxation, weight reduction (if relevant), reduction of alcohol consumption, salt restriction and regular physical exercise would suffice initially. It is important to advise the patient against smoking. If present, hyperlipidaemia and diabetes should be treated. If the blood pressure remains elevated (>140/90 mmHg) despite adequate lifestyle modification (or due to failure of lifestyle modification), pharmacotherapy should be initiated.

End-organ damage due to hypertension

- Myocardial infarction
- Left ventricular hypertrophy
- Cardiac failure
- Stroke
- Hypertensive nephropathy
- Hypertensive retinopathy
- Arteriosclerosis

Selection of the appropriate antihypertensive agent should be guided by several factors, including: the patient's comorbidities, age, sex, ethnic background and drug allergies. Initially an attempt should be directed at monotherapy, and the commonly used agents are thiazide diuretics, beta-blockers, calcium channel blockers, angiotensin-converting enzyme (ACE) inhibitors and angiotensin II receptor blocker (ARB). If monotherapy is inadequate, combination therapy can be considered. An ACE inhibitor with a diuretic, or a beta-blocker with a diuretic, are two such combinations. There are combination pills containing an ACE inhibitor or an ARB together with a thiazide diuretic that can be prescribed. Hypertension that is not well controlled with conventional agents even with up titration and combination warrants further investigation and the addition of potent, less commonly used agents such alpha receptor blockers, centrally acting agents or arterial vasodilators.

Comorbidities that can influence the choice of therapy

- *Diabetes mellitus*—ACE inhibitors are the most suitable agents. Where ACE inhibitors are not tolerated, the other options to consider include ARBs and calcium channel blockers. Beta-adrenergic receptor blockers and thiazide diuretics can interfere with glycaemic control. ACE inhibitors and ARBs have significant and useful synergy in severe high blood pressure and diabetic nephropathy.
- *Gout*—beta-blockers, ACE inhibitors, calcium channel blockers and alpha-blockers are suitable. Thiazide diuretics can exacerbate gout.
- *Dyslipidaemia*—ACE inhibitors, calcium channel blockers and alpha-blockers are recommended. Beta-blockers may be less desirable due to their adverse effects on the lipid profile.
- *Ischaemic heart disease*—diuretics, beta-blockers, calcium channel blockers, ACE inhibitors and ARBs are suitable because of their protective properties in coronary vascular disease.
- *Congestive cardiac failure*—ideal agents include beta-blockers, ACE inhibitors, ARBs and diuretics, which also have proven value in the management of cardiac failure.
- *Peripheral vascular disease*—calcium channel blockers, alpha-adrenergic receptor blockers and diuretics are desirable agents. Beta-blockers are contraindicated.
- *Pregnancy*—for mild hypertension in pregnant patients, methyldopa and the alpha- and beta-adrenergic receptor blocking agent labetolol are good choices. In preeclampsia, nifedipine is a suitable agent; however, urgent delivery of the baby is an absolute requirement. Severe hypertension in the pregnant patient can be managed with intravenous (IV) hydralazine.

Adverse effects of some antihypertensive agents

It is important to have a commanding knowledge of the properties and adverse effects of the commonly used antihypertensive agents. Below is a list of adverse effects seen with different classes of antihypertensive agents, together with some important properties of selected agents.

- *Thiazide diuretics*—hypercholesterolaemia, hyperglycaemia, thrombocytopenia and gout
- *Beta-blockers*—bradycardia, postural hypotension, depression and cold peripheries. Agents with intrinsic sympathomimetic activity, such as pindolol, rarely cause bradycardia. The cardioselective agent atenolol is less lipid-soluble, and therefore has minimal central nervous system side effects.
- *ACE inhibitors*—angio-oedema, cough, postural hypotension, hyperkalaemia, progression of renal failure and first-dose hypotension. First-dose hypotension is a rarity but is seen particularly in patients on low-sodium diets and high-dose diuretics.
- *Angiotensin II receptor blockers*—similar to ACE inhibitors but cough is less common
- *Calcium channel blockers*—headaches, sweating, palpitations and ankle oedema
- *Alpha-blockers*—first-dose hypotension. Long-acting alpha-blockers such as doxazocin have less first-dose hypotension effect.
- *Vasodilators*—minoxidil is an agent used in resistant hypertension. It is one of the most potent antihypertensive drugs available. Minoxidil can cause sodium and water retention, leading to ankle oedema and, in the rare case, pericardial effusion. Another undesirable side effect of minoxidil is hypertrichosis.

Hydralazine has its use in pregnancy and sometimes in cardiac failure. Hydralazine can cause drug-induced lupus. Nitroprusside is another vasodilator agent that is used in hypertensive crises and dissection of the aorta.

ISCHAEMIC HEART DISEASE AND ACUTE MYOCARDIAL INFARCTION

Sometimes examiners like to test candidates' knowledge of the management of common acute medical conditions. No condition is more common than acute myocardial infarction in the physician trainee's case repertoire, and the candidate is expected to be thoroughly familiar with the management of this condition.

Case vignette

A 45-year-old man presents with retrosternal chest tightness of 3 hours' duration. The pain is dull in nature, 7/10 in severity and radiating along the left arm. The onset was at rest. He also complains of progressive dyspnoea and associated nausea. He denies any cardiovascular risk factors apart from a strong family history. On examination his pulse rate is 100 bpm, low in volume and regular. His blood pressure is 90/60 mmHg. There are fine crepitations bibasally in the lung fields. The ECG shows deep T wave inversions in leads I, III and aVF.

1   **What further investigations would you order and what is your immediate plan of management?**

Upon stabilisation the patient is admitted to the coronary care unit (CCU). His Killip class is 2 (see box). He is managed on aspirin, metoprolol 12.5 mg twice daily and IV heparin. While in CCU his blood pressure drops to 70/40 mmHg and pulse rate to 40 bpm. His pain is progressive and the ECG shows further deepening of the T wave inversions and new ST depression in the said leads, and also in leads aVR, V_1 and V_2.

2   **How would you manage him in this instance?**

He is commenced on an IV glycoprotein IIb/IIIa inhibitor and referred for early catheterisation. Catheterisation reveals occlusion of the posterior descending branch of the right coronary artery, which is successfully reopened by balloon angioplasty and stenting. On day 2 he develops fever and pleuritic chest pains.

3   **What are your differential diagnoses and planned management?**

On day 3 he develops acute pulmonary oedema and cardiogenic shock. Auscultation reveals a new harsh pansystolic murmur audible all over the precordium.

4   **What are your possible differential diagnoses and proposed investigations and management?**

5   **This man's cholesterol profile on admission showed isolated hypertriglyceridaemia. Discuss your management options.**

Killip classification of post myocardial infarction prognosis

- *Class 1*—No evidence of heart failure (6% mortality)
- *Class 2*—Third heart sound, basal crepitations (17% mortality)
- *Class 3*—Pulmonary oedema (30–40% mortality)
- *Class 4*—Cardiogenic shock (60–80% mortality)

(Adapted from Killip T, Kimball J T 1967 Treatment of myocardial infarction in coronary care unit. A two-year experience with 250 patients. *American Journal of Cardiology* 20:457)

Approach to the patient

History
Ask about:
- the onset of symptoms and associated symptoms
- the relationship between the pain and trigger factors such as physical exertion and emotional stress
- details of the pain—severity, exact location, radiation, factors that exacerbate or relieve the pain
- descriptive characteristics of the pain—such as sharp, dull or heavy feeling
- whether there is a pleuritic nature to the pain
- coronary risk factors
- the patient's past history, especially cardiovascular history
- whether the patient has experienced similar pain in the past.

Examination
First and foremost, check the vital signs and establish haemodynamic stability. If the patient is having an acute episode of coronary ischaemia (or other emergency such as pneumothorax, pulmonary embolus) they may become rapidly unstable, with haemodynamic compromise or cardiopulmonary arrest.

Once the patient is stable, perform a detailed cardiovascular examination. Look in the fundus for hypertensive or diabetic changes. Listen to the heart for additional sounds such as the third and fourth heart sounds. Listen to the lung bases for crepitation of congestion.

Management
In any acute myocardial infarction the first priority is to assess the patient's clinical stability and assess the requirement for, and urgency associated with, coronary revascularisation. Remember: patients presenting with an infarction could present with acute pulmonary oedema, cardiogenic shock, malignant ventricular tachyarrhythmias or severe bradycardia. Once the patient's haemodynamic stability and cardiac rhythm stability are established, perform an urgent ECG to confirm the diagnosis and identify the nature of the infarction—whether it is an ST segment elevation infarction (STEMI) or a non-ST segment elevation infarction (non-STEMI).

STEMI

If the infarction is a STEMI, urgent reperfusion therapy is needed. Acute reperfusion therapy could be primary percutaneous transluminal coronary angioplasty (primary PTCA) with insertion of a stent or thrombolysis. If the centre offers a primary angioplasty service and the patient fulfils the criteria (see box), urgent transfer to the cardiac catheterisation laboratory should take place. Patients presenting in the first 4–6 hours of onset of chest pain are considered suitable for primary PTCA. Previous coronary artery bypass grafts, peripheral vascular disease, untreatable terminal illness and dementia are exclusion criteria for this procedure.

If primary PTCA is not an option, the patient should be thrombolysed with the relevant thrombolytic agent. If the patient presents within the first hour after the onset of chest pain, thrombolysis would be a preferred option (the 'golden hour' phenomenon). Usually a recombinant tissue plasminogen activator (rTPA) or an analogue is given to the patient immediately. Streptokinase is an alternative for patients over the age of 65 or those with evidence of an inferior myocardial infarction presenting after 4 hours of the onset of chest pain. Those who have been treated with streptokinase previously should not be given streptokinase again, due to the heightened risk of an allergic reaction.

The ECG criteria for primary PTCA and thrombolysis are similar (see box), but thrombolysis may be useful up to 12 hours or even 24 hours after the onset of chest pain.

Criteria for primary PTCA or thrombolysis

- ST segment elevation of more than 1 mm in more than two contiguous limb leads

or

- ST segment elevation of more than 2 mm in more than two contiguous precordial leads

or

- new left bundle branch block.

If the decision is made to administer thrombolytics, the patient should not have any contraindications (e.g. risk of haemorrhage or allergy) to such therapy. If thrombolytic therapy has not been effective and the patient is a strong candidate for reperfusion therapy, attempts should be made to organise urgent rescue angioplasty.

Non-STEMI

If a non-STEMI, the patient should be managed initially with anticoagulation and antiplatelet therapy. The patient should subsequently be referred for early coronary catheterisation.

All patients presenting with myocardial infarction (STEMI or non-STEMI) or acute coronary syndrome (unstable angina or non-STEMI) should be considered for anti-ischaemia therapy. The routinely used agents include oral or IV beta-blockers, as guided by the pulse rate and blood pressure, and aspirin. Patients treated with primary PTCA and stenting are given clopidogrel in addition to aspirin. If the patient complains

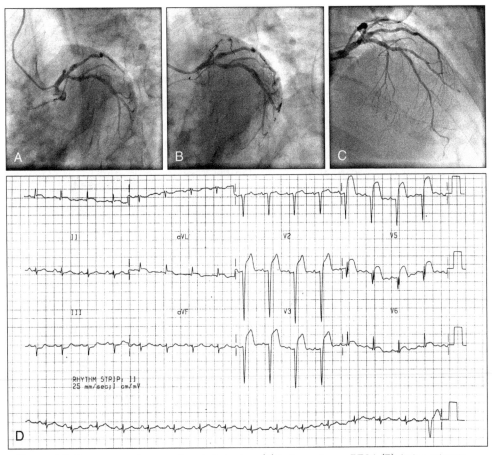

Figure 3.3 Coronary angiogram of occluded artery (A) before primary PTCA (B) during primary PTCA (C) after primary PTCA; (D) ECG showing ST segment elevation in the antroseptal and lateral leads, indicating complete occlusion of the LAD artery

of angina, oral, topical or IV nitrates and/or morphine should be administered. An ACE inhibitor should be commenced within the first 24 hours of the infarction if the blood pressure permits. Angiotensin II receptor blockers are also useful in this setting. Patients with post-infarction heart failure benefit from aldosterone antagonist eplerenone. Unless the patient has been treated with primary PTCA or streptokinase, they should be anticoagulated with unfractionated or fractionated heparin. According to current evidence, all patients presenting with coronary ischaemia benefit from statin therapy regardless of the baseline fasting cholesterol level.

Patients with acute coronary syndrome benefit from IV antiplatelet therapy in the way of platelet glycoprotein IIb/IIIa inhibitor agents such as tirofiban or eptifibatide in addition to heparin.

The patient should be admitted to the CCU for continuous ECG monitoring. Serial cardiac enzymes or troponin levels should monitored. Patients who sustain right ventricular damage may become profoundly hypotensive. They need IV volume infusion as the first line of therapy. Those in cardiogenic shock require inotropic therapy in the form of IV dobutamine or dopamine to support cardiac function and haemodynamic stability.

Post-infarct ventricular fibrillation

Ventricular fibrillation within the first 24 hours of an infarction indicates a more favourable prognosis than those occurring afterwards. Episodes of ventricular fibrillation after the first 24 hours signify a guarded prognosis, and consideration should be given to the implantation of a cardiac defibrillator. Inferior or posterior myocardial infarctions can damage the AV node or the cardiac conduction system, leading to heart block. These patients need urgent insertion of a temporary pacemaker. Some may recover their nodal and conduction function as the oedema and inflammation associated with the acute event settles, but others who sustain permanent damage need insertion of a permanent pacemaker (PPM). Complete heart block in a patient who suffers an anterior myocardial infarction signifies a bad prognosis due to the extensive area of myocardial damage.

Follow-up

Follow-up management includes a transthoracic echocardiogram to assess the ejection fraction and to look for segmental left ventricular wall motion abnormalities, valvular defects, ventricular septal defect, ventricular thrombus and ventricular aneurysms. Ejection fraction can also be assessed by performing a nuclear gated heart pool scan. Patients who have an ejection fraction of less than 40% after an infarction are at high risk (30%) of sudden cardiac death over the next 5 years. These patients qualify to be treated with a prophylactic implanted cardiac defibrillator (ICD) usually 40 days after the infarction, according to current evidence.

Patients suffering from post-infarct angina need early coronary angiography to define the coronary anatomy before deciding on definitive therapy. Stable patients should have an exercise stress study, looking for reversible ischaemia. This may take the form of a stress echocardiography, stress ECG or nuclear medicine perfusion study. The presence of reversible ischaemia or ischaemia associated with stress are indications for coronary angiography. Definitive treatment with angioplasty, with or without stenting of the involved artery, or coronary artery bypass grafting, should be decided upon as guided by the coronary anatomy.

Prior to discharge, patients should be recruited to a post-myocardial infarction rehabilitation program and modification of cardiovascular risk factors should be encouraged. Some patients may need counselling and significant reassurance to help them recover from the acute event. Others may need advice on lifestyle and occupational issues, relevant information and education, counselling on sexual matters, dietary advice, help with giving up smoking and partner counselling.

CONGESTIVE CARDIAC FAILURE

Case vignette

A 38-year-old woman is admitted with progressive dyspnoea of 1 week's duration, orthopnoea and paroxysmal nocturnal dyspnoea. She has been otherwise well. She has no other history of significance and she is not on any regular medications. On examination her pulse rate is 90 bpm, regular and low in volume. Her jugular venous pressure (JVP) is elevated to the mandibular angle and there are diffuse fine crepitations in the lung fields bilaterally. In the precordium there is an S3 gallop. She has bipedal pitting oedema.

1   **Discuss the possible differential diagnoses and your diagnostic work-up.**
2   **Describe your management goals and detailed plan of management.**
3   **An echocardiogram reveals a dilated left ventricle with global hypokinesis. Her estimated ejection fraction is 35%. Discuss the management and prognostic implications of this additional information.**
4   **Discuss how you would address the psychosocial implications of this woman's illness and the support you would organise.**
5   **In the event of her not responding convincingly to maximal medical management, describe the advanced and/or novel therapeutics that could be considered.**

Approach to the patient

History

A discussion of cardiac failure should focus on all features relevant to the condition. The candidate should be able to assess the severity of the disease accurately. Ask about the patient's exercise tolerance and interpret the severity of heart failure according to the New York Heart Association (NYHA) classification (see box). Ask about:
- orthopnoea (ask how many pillows the patient uses)
- paroxysmal nocturnal dyspnoea
- whether the patient has a known history of ischaemic heart disease or hypertension. If not, ask whether the patient has angina.

NYHA functional classification of patients with heart failure
- *Class I*—no limitation of physical activity. Ordinary physical activity does not cause undue fatigue, palpitation or dyspnoea.
- *Class II*—slight limitation of physical activity. Comfortable at rest, but ordinary physical activity causes undue fatigue, palpitation or dyspnoea.
- *Class III*
  - *IIIA*—marked limitation of physical activity. Comfortable at rest, but less than ordinary activity causes undue fatigue, palpitations or dyspnoea.
  - *IIIB*—marked limitation of physical activity. Comfortable at rest, but minimal exertion causes undue fatigue, palpitations or dyspnoea.
- *Class IV*—unable to carry out any physical activity without symptoms or discomfort. Symptoms of cardiac failure present at rest. If any physical activity is undertaken, discomfort is increased.

The patient may complain of anorexia, which may be due to hepatic congestion. Ask about the various medications she or he has been treated with and any adverse effects associated with therapy.

Look for agents that can precipitate heart failure, such as NSAIDs, rosiglitazone, diltiazem and verapamil. Obtain a detailed social history, enquiring into the level of support available at home and how the patient copes with their physical limitations. Ask whether the patient has a scale at home and whether their body weight is monitored regularly. Enquire about the heart failure care plan and compliance thereof.

Examination

In the physical examination, look for the presence of tachypnoea and tachycardia. The patient may be hypertensive or hypotensive. Assess the JVP and quantify the elevation. Ascertain the character of the arterial pulse, which is usually thready and weak. Patients with severe cardiac failure may demonstrate Cheyne-Stokes respiration. Feel the apex beat, looking for a lateral shift or a heave. Auscultation may reveal an S3 gallop. Listen for murmurs that would suggest a valvular pathology such as aortic stenosis, aortic regurgitation and/or mitral regurgitation and tricuspid regurgitation. Left ventricular enlargement may lead to mitral annular dilatation, which may cause functional mitral regurgitation with a pansystolic murmur.

Listen to the lung fields for crepitations and percuss for stony dullness of an effusion. Examine the abdomen for tender hepatomegaly and ascites. Severe tricuspid regurgitation with congestion may cause pulsatile hepatomegaly. Check for peripheral oedema and define its distribution.

Investigations in the setting of acute and chronic cardiac failure and the many different therapeutic options available are popular topics used by examiners to test the candidate's knowledge. Never forget the socioeconomic aspects of cardiac failure and the important management goals of improving the patient's quality of life and preventing recurrent hospital admissions.

Pathogenic causes

Remember that congestive heart failure is a clinical presentation that has an underlying cause. Therefore, in approaching congestive cardiac failure, first consider possible pathogenic causes (see box).

Causes of congestive cardiac failure

1 Ischaemic heart disease
2 Chronic systemic hypertension
3 Cardiomyopathy
4 Valvular heart disease (especially aortic regurgitation, aortic stenosis and mitral regurgitation)
5 Ventricular septal defect
6 Viral myocarditis
7 Toxic myocarditis
8 Infiltrative disorders
9 High output status (anaemia, thyrotoxicosis, pregnancy, arteriovenous fistula, beriberi)
10 Medications with negative inotropic properties (beta-blockers, verapamil)

One of the most common causes of cardiac failure is ischaemic heart disease. Cardiac failure in ischaemic heart disease could be due to a massive infarction and associated ventricular wall damage, severe mitral regurgitation, acute interventricular septal rupture or ischaemic cardiomyopathy secondary to multiple previous infarctions. Severe hypertension can lead to systolic heart failure as well as diastolic heart failure secondary to left ventricular hypertrophy. Valvular heart disease, particularly severe mitral and aortic valvular disease, can lead to congestive systolic or diastolic failure.

Acute bacterial endocarditis can cause damage to the valve leaflets and may lead to cardiac failure. Dilated cardiomyopathy, idiopathic or due to numerous causes (e.g. viral myocarditis, chronic alcohol abuse, cardiotoxic chemotherapeutic agents such as anthracyclines or other cardiotoxins), can cause cardiac failure. The causes of high-output cardiac failure are severe anaemia, beriberi, Paget's disease, thyrotoxicosis and arteriovenous fistulae.

Investigations

Your battery of investigations should be aimed at confirming your clinical diagnosis, assessing the severity and identifying the underlying cause. The most important investigations in a patient with cardiac failure are:

1 Full blood count—looking for anaemia
2 Electrolyte profile and renal function indices—hyponatraemia is common in severe congestive cardiac failure. A low cardiac output can lead to inadequate renal perfusion and thus to prerenal renal failure. Renal effect of diuretic therapy and associated volume depletion/dehydration are important factors of concern.
3 Plasma B-type natriuretic peptide (BNP) levels
4 Levels of serum markers of cardiac damage—such as troponin I or T and the MB fraction of the enzyme creatinine kinase (CKMB)
5 Urine analysis—looking for protein, blood, white cells and organisms
6 Arterial blood gases—to assess the level of oxygenation and the acid–base status, particularly in the severely dyspnoeic and those in pulmonary oedema
7 Electrocardiogram—looking for evidence of acute ischaemia, previous ischaemic cardiac damage, arrhythmias and left ventricular hypertrophy. Severe left ventricular hypertrophy can cause diastolic cardiac failure. The most common cause of left ventricular hypertrophy is chronic hypertension. Left ventricular hypertrophy together with asymmetrical septal hypertrophy is seen in hypertrophic obstructive cardiomyopathy. Patients in significant cardiac failure have a propensity to develop arrhythmias, particularly ventricular tachycardia, which can progress to ventricular fibrillation.
8 Chest X-ray—looking for cardiomegaly as well as pulmonary congestion
9 Transthoracic echocardiogram—looking for wall motion abnormalities and valvular lesions. The echocardiogram will quantify the ejection fraction and the dynamic ventricular chamber and wall dimensions.
10 Thyroid function tests—hyperthyroidism can lead to high-output cardiac failure. Hypothyroidism causes low-output cardiac failure as well as diastolic cardiac failure due to pericardial effusion.
11 Serum vitamin B_1 levels in potentially malnourished patients—to exclude beriberi (remember: this is very rare in our society!)
12 Renal arterial Doppler study—to exclude renal artery stenosis in the patient who suffers from recurrent episodes of unexplained pulmonary oedema (flash pulmonary oedema).

Management

Acute decompensated cardiac failure

1 Acute decompensated cardiac failure or pulmonary oedema is a medical emergency. Vital observations should be made first: respiratory rate, pulse rate, blood pressure and arterial oxygen saturations via pulse oximetry. The primary objectives are reestablishment and maintenance of haemodynamic stability and adequate tissue oxygenation.

2 Sit the patient bolt upright immediately and give supplementary oxygen via a facial mask at a rate of 6 L/min. If the patient is still desaturating, try giving 100% oxygen via a non-rebreather mask (great caution should be exercised when giving supplementary oxygen to patients with a history of chronic fixed airways disease). Those refractory to oxygen supplementation alone may respond to continuous positive airway pressure (CPAP) or bilevel positive airways pressure (BIPAP)—non-invasive ventilation.

3 Vascular access should be established with at least one wide-bore cannula in each arm. Give IV frusemide 80–120 mg, while monitoring the urine output. Administer subcutaneous or IV morphine at an initial dose of 2.5–5 mg. This has an anxiolytic effect as well as the capacity to reduce the preload by vasodilatation. Intravenous or topical nitrate therapy should also be given. This reduces the preload as well as the afterload in addition to facilitating coronary perfusion. Refractory fluid overload may require IV infusion of frusemide at the rate of 5–10 mg/h. Glyceryl trinitrate infusion helps reduce preload and thus improve symptoms. However, the patient should have a satisfactory blood pressure.

4 The patient needs insertion of an indwelling urinary catheter and close nursing supervision.

5 The following investigations should be performed immediately: a 12-lead ECG, mobile chest X-ray, arterial blood gases, full blood count, serum electrolyte profile, together with renal function indices and markers of myocardial damage. The patient needs an urgent echocardiogram to ascertain the cardiac anatomy, function and in particular the ejection fraction and cardiac filling pressures. Some patients may benefit from a right heart catheter (Swan-Ganz catheter) to continuously monitor right heart pressures. This information helps in the fluid balancing act.

6 Once clinically stable, the patient's anti-failure therapy should be optimised, as discussed below. The patient should be placed on salt and fluid restriction (e.g. 1000–2000 mL/day) while maintaining a strict fluid balance, and should be weighed daily.

7 Nesiritide (a recombinant BNP) is an arterial and venous vasodilator. This agent has some proven benefit in the treatment of decompensated heart failure and fluid overload. Nesiritide should not be given if the patient is in shock or is very hypotensive.

8 Those with clinical signs of severe pump failure and hypotension may benefit from inotrope therapy. Dobutamine, dopamine and adrenaline are commonly used. These help rapid symptomatic improvement but can trigger malignant ventricular arrhythmias and in fact increase mortality rates. Intraaortic balloon pump is also a useful therapeutic option in this situation.

9 Levosimenden is a calcium sensitiser that has shown benefit in the treatment of acute decompensated heart failure. It improves cardiac output and decreases pulmonary capillary wedge pressure. This is an expensive drug that has proven survival benefits to the patient.

BNP level and cardiac failure

Elevated plasma BNP level has diagnostic and prognostic value, as it helps to distinguish between cardiac failure and other causes of acute dyspnoea.
- BNP > 500 ng/L—diagnostic of severe heart failure
- BNP < 100 ng/L—heart failure is unlikely
- BNP 100–500 ng/L in a dyspnoeic patient—may also suggest right heart failure, pulmonary embolism or chronic renal failure.

Long-term management of cardiac failure

Below is an outline of the fundamental principles in the pharmacological management of systolic cardiac failure.

1 If the patient is haemodynamically stable, beta-blocker therapy should be considered first. Carvedilol has alpha- as well as beta-adrenoreceptor-blocking qualities. It is indicated in symptomatic cardiac failure with a severity consistent with Class II–III according to the NYHA classification (see box, p 35). This drug has to be started at a low dose and the dose gradually increased over a few weeks while observing the level of tolerance and efficacy. It can be commenced in hospital and followed up after discharge. Bisoprolol and metoprolol (long acting) have also shown benefit to patients in randomised controlled trials. Bisoprolol has cardiac beta receptor selectivity and as such can be given to patients with asthma or emphysema. It is better tolerated by patients with low blood pressure due to its lack of alpha receptor blocking activity.

2 ACE inhibitor therapy for symptomatic as well as asymptomatic congestive cardiac failure has been very beneficial, particularly in patients with an ejection fraction of less than 40%. When commencing therapy, short-acting ACE inhibitors such as captopril 6.25 mg given three times a day are preferred over long-acting, once-daily preparations such as perindopril or lisinopril. If short-acting preparations are used at the beginning, adverse effects of therapy can be better managed by stopping the drug promptly. When the patient demonstrates good tolerance, switch to a long-acting preparation for ease of administration and better compliance. All patients treated with ACE inhibitors should be monitored for hyperkalaemia and progression of renal failure.

3 Angiotensin II receptor inhibitors can be used for symptomatic cardiac failure where there is ACE inhibitor intolerance. Both agents demonstrate equal efficacy.

4 Diuretic therapy should be commenced. Loop diuretics are preferred for their strong diuretic action, which facilitates afterload reduction. These agents can also lead to vasodilatation and thus cause preload reduction and relieve pulmonary congestion.

5 When there is inadequate response to the loop diuretic alone, consider combination diuretic therapy, with the addition of a thiazide or spironolactone

for the potent effect of sequential diuresis. When patients are on combination diuretic therapy, electrolyte imbalances and deterioration of renal function indices should be watched for.

6   Oral or transdermal nitrate therapy, for preload reduction and the relief of cardiac ischaemia.

7   Hydralazine combined with isosorbide dinitrate is a proven alternative for the ACE inhibitor-intolerant, symptomatic patient.

8   Digoxin is useful in persistent congestive cardiac failure despite ACE inhibitor therapy. This is of benefit to patients in sinus rhythm as well as those in atrial fibrillation.

9   Oral anticoagulation is indicated for patients with a history of previous thrombo-embolism, chronic or paroxysmal atrial fibrillation or a left ventricular thrombus.

10   Aldosterone receptor antagonists such as spironolactone (and eplerenone) administered long term have been shown to minimise the aldosterone-mediated myocardial fibrosis in patients with chronic congestive cardiac failure; a cardiac failure patient has high levels of aldosterone in the circulation as a compensatory response.

11   Intravenous diuretics and IV inotropic (dobutamine) therapy may be useful in refractory fluid retention and refractory cardiac failure.

12   Cardiac resynchronisation with biventricular pacing is beneficial to the patient in sinus rhythm, in particular those who have a prolonged QRS complex in the ECG (> 120 ms). The case for cardiac resynchronisation can be further proved if there is echo evidence of dyssynchrony.

13   An implanted cardiac defibrillator has been shown to be protective for patients who suffer from recurrent symptomatic sustained ventricular tachycardia and episodes of ventricular fibrillation.

14   Highly specialised centres offer left ventricular assist devices (LVADs) that can be implanted to assist the pump function of the left ventricle. These battery-operated devices can be used as bridging therapy prior to cardiac transplantation and in selected groups of patients as destination (definitive) therapy. In very refractory cases, cardiac transplantation should be considered.

Diastolic cardiac failure

Diastolic cardiac failure is an entirely different clinical phenomenon. It is the most common cause of heart failure in the elderly (> 75-year age group). Common causes of diastolic failure are:

1   chronic ischaemic heart disease
2   left ventricular hypertrophy due to chronic hypertension
3   persistent or recurrent tachyarrhythmias
4   diabetes mellitus
5   restrictive cardiomyopathy, which could be due to amyloidosis, haemochromatosis or sarcoidosis
6   hypertrophic obstructive cardiomyopathy
7   constrictive pericarditis
8   pericardial effusion.

   Clinical assessment is paramount in these patients. Physical examination should show evidence of pulmonary congestion, elevated JVP and an S4 gallop on auscultation.

Investigations

Investigations that should be requested are:

1   Chest X-ray—there may be no evidence of cardiomegaly.
2   If the chest X-ray suggests calcific pericarditis, a CT scan or a magnetic resonance imaging (MRI) scan of the chest would be useful to confirm the diagnosis of constrictive pericarditis.
3   Full blood count, electrolyte profile, renal function indices and serum BNP levels.
4   Echocardiography—may show left ventricular hypertrophy and also quantify the ventricular chamber dimensions and wall thickness.
5   Cardiac catheterisation—may further help, by chamber pressure assessment, in diagnosing as well as distinguishing between restrictive cardiac pathology and constrictive pericarditis.
6   Stress electrocardiography, nuclear medicine stress perfusion scanning or stress echocardiography—should be done to exclude cardiac ischaemia.
7   Right ventricular cardiac biopsy—if amyloidosis, haemochromatosis or sarcoidosis is suspected as the causative mechanism.

Management

1   Judicious diuretic, beta-blocker and topical nitrate therapy, commencing with small initial doses.
2   If in atrial fibrillation, the ventricular rate should be controlled to facilitate adequate diastolic filling of the ventricle, which already has a compromised filling capacity.
3   Strict control of hypertension to prevent further progression of the disease.
4   Beta-blocker or verapamil therapy in hypertrophic obstructive cardiomyopathy.

General management of cardiac failure

In all cardiac failure patients, consider vaccination against *Pneumococcus* as well as influenza virus. The candidate will be expected to formulate a working plan, in collaboration with the community resources available, to optimally manage and maintain the patient on discharge. Patient education, nutrition, physical activity, fluid balance, weight monitoring and early recognition of decompensation are important aspects of such a plan. Consideration should be given to a shared-care plan, in association with the patient's general practitioner. Ambulatory care provision by a multidisciplinary heart failure team offers significant clinical and prognostic benefits to all heart failure patients.

ATRIAL FIBRILLATION

Case vignette

An 86-year-old woman is admitted with palpitations and dyspnoea on minimal exertion. She also complains of retrosternal heaviness. She has a history of hypertension and diverticular disease. She has had several previous admissions with falls and per rectal bleeding. She is managed on amlodipine 5 mg daily. She is an independently living widow. On examination her pulse rate is 120 bpm with an irregularly irregular rhythm. Her blood pressure is 150/95 mmHg. The ECG shows atrial fibrillation and voltage evidence of left ventricular hypertrophy.

1 **What is your main concern about this woman's current clinical status?**
2 **Discuss your management options and the pros and cons thereof.**
3 **Describe how you would explain your proposed management to this woman.**
4 **Describe the issues of importance when planning her discharge.**

Approach to the patient

Atrial fibrillation (AF) is the most common arrhythmia seen in clinical practice and is highly likely to be encountered in the long case setting. Studies have demonstrated a 1% prevalence of AF among adults. Prevalence increases with age and with structural heart disease. Atrial fibrillation can double mortality and increase the risk of stroke five-fold. Patients may present initially with palpitations, angina, presyncope and fatigue. Atrial fibrillation with a rapid ventricular response can cause clinical instability and the patient may develop coronary ischaemia or heart failure.

History

Ask about:

- any past history of rheumatic heart disease, valvular disease and surgery, diabetes, thyroid disorders and previous attempts at direct current (DC) cardioversion
- previous history of strokes
- the patient's insight into this chronic disorder and the potential risks associated with it
- warfarin therapy—how the INR is monitored, associated bleeding complications, and whether the patient keeps a record of daily warfarin doses and the INR
- drug interactions and/or side effects in the past
- alcohol consumption.

Establish the patient's coronary risk factor profile. Based on the clinical assessment, calculate the patient's CHADS2 score (see box). The higher the CHADS2 score, the more compelling the case for treating the patient with warfarin to prevent embolic stroke.

CHADS2 score

Score:
- 1 point each for the presence of any of the following factors:
  - age > 75 years
  - history of hypertension
  - history of diabetes mellitus
  - history of congestive cardiac failure
- 2 points for:
  - previous history of ischaemic stroke or transient ischaemic attack (TIA).

CHADS2 scores:

0 Can be managed with aspirin alone for the prevention of ischaemic stroke.

1, 2 May benefit from either form of therapy, and so treatment should be based on the overall clinical risk.

> 3 Strong indication for warfarinisation.

Examination

Physical examination may reveal an irregularly irregular pulse. Establish the quality of peripheral pulse and the rate. Check the blood pressure for hypertension. Look for signs of hyperthyroidism. Listen to the precordium for a mitral murmur. Look for signs of congestive cardiac failure. Check for evidence of amiodarone toxicity, such as slate-brown skin discolouration, pulmonary fibrosis and hypo- or hyperthyroidism.

Investigations

1 12-lead ECG—looking for the absence of P waves, the ventricular rate, evidence of coronary ischaemia or Wolff-Parkinson-White syndrome
2 Echocardiogram—looking for mitral valve disease, left ventricular hypertrophy, left atrial dimensions (in chronic AF, the left atrium remains significantly dilated and this is an indication of the persistent nature of AF) and spontaneous echo contrast. A transoesophageal echo (TOE) may be required if the AF is subacute and consideration is given for DC cardioversion. This imaging modality is required to visualise any thrombi in the left atrial appendage.
3 Loop recorder or Holter monitor—may be required to diagnose paroxysmal AF in patients in sinus rhythm
4 Thyroid function tests—to exclude hyperthyroidism
  Those who experience angina with rapid AF may require coronary angiography.

Causes of secondary atrial fibrillation

- Chronic hypertension
- Mitral valve disease
- Ischaemic heart disease
- Hyperthyroidism
- Cardiomyopathy
- Wolff-Parkinson-White syndrome
- Rheumatic heart disease

Management

Management of AF has two primary objectives: rate control and/or rhythm control. The secondary objectives include symptom management and stroke prevention. The relative prognostic merit of rhythm control over rate control as definitive therapy is still being debated and pivotal trials thus far have failed to deliver a verdict.

Rate control

Those who are at high risk of embolic stroke due to left atrial thrombus are best treated with rate control and anticoagulation. The stroke risk is high if the patient is over the age of 65, in the presence of coronary risk factors, mitral disease or if AF has been present for more than 48 hours. The ideal agent in this setting is warfarin and the INR should be maintained at 2–3. Those below 65 years of age with no additional risk features may be managed with aspirin alone.

Risk factors for AF-associated stroke

Risk factors include:
- Age > 65 years
- Previous stroke or TIA
- Hypertension
- Diabetes
- Known ischaemic heart disease
- Valvular disease
- Dilated LA on echocardiography (and spontaneous echo contrast)
- Left atrial appendage thrombus demonstrated on TOE
- History of rheumatic heart disease
- Left ventricular failure.

Rapid ventricular response in the setting of atrial fibrillation (rapid AF) contributes to most presenting symptoms. AF with rapid ventricular response can precipitate coronary ischaemia, congestive heart failure and pulmonary oedema. Chronic rapid AF may lead to tachycardia-induced cardiomyopathy and heart failure.

More rapid rate control is achieved with IV digoxin, verapamil, diltiazem or a beta-blocker such as propanolol. Intravenous amiodarone is also useful in combination for rate control; however, inadvertent pharmacological cardioversion could happen.

Oral agents are preferred over IV agents, given the side effects of hypotension and severe bradycardia that could be encountered with the latter. Long-term rate control is achieved by oral administration of the same agents as mentioned above. If the patient is experiencing severe symptoms or is haemodynamically unstable, consider urgent direct current (DC) cardioversion, preferably upon the exclusion of left atrial thrombus by TOE.

Amiodarone can increase serum digoxin levels and therefore caution should be exercised when using these two agents in combination. Those who are refractory to pharmacological rate control or intolerant of the same may benefit from radiofrequency ablation of the AV node with the implantation of a PPM.

Rhythm control

There is no convincing evidence to support the benefits of rhythm control over rate control in patients with AF. One study showed a worse outcome for mortality and stroke risk in patients who underwent cardioversion. This may be attributed to lower usage of warfarin in this patient population. However, rhythm control may help alleviate symptoms, and reduce the number of drugs the patient has to take and also the inconvenience of monitoring INR. It is reasonable to cardiovert AF without TOE or anticoagulation if done within 48 hours after the onset.

After 48 hours, safe practice guidelines dictate that the patient be anticoagulated (with INR maintained at 2–3) for about 3 weeks prior to cardioversion and for about 4 weeks after. However, if a TOE can be performed to exclude any suggestion of a thrombus, cardioversion can take place safely without preprocedure anticoagulation. Direct current cardioversion with a starting shock of 200 J is the most efficient and rapid means of achieving rhythm control. The shock should be synchronised to avoid precipiting ventricular fibrillation (VF).

Pharmacological rhythm control can be achieved and maintained with agents such as flecainide, sotalol, amiodarone, procainamide and quinidine. With their usage, pro-arrhythmia and QTc prolongation should be watched for. Amiodarone has very complex and unpredictable pharmacokinetics and a long list of adverse effects (see box). Flecainide should not be used to treat patients with known heart disease. Patients with ischaemic heart disease may benefit from the beta-blocker effect of sotalol.

Amiodarone side effects

- Hyperthyroidism/hypothyroidism
- Hepatotoxicity
- Photosensitivity
- Pulmonary fibrosis
- Skin and corneal deposition
- Bradycardia/hypotension
- Malignant arrhythmias
- Polyneuropathy
- Phlebitis (with IV infusion)

Non-pharmacological rhythm control can be achieved with surgical 'maze' procedure or percutaneous isolation and ablation of pulmonary veins. Careful patient selection and operator expertise are essential.

HEART TRANSPLANTATION

Indications:
- NYHA Class IV heart failure—end-stage heart failure due to multiple causes that is not responding to maximal medical therapy. Usually if the life expectancy is less than 1 year without transplantation.
- VO_2 max < 12 mL/kg/min in cardiopulmonary functional capacity testing
- Intractable severe ischaemia not amenable to revascularisation
- Recurrent uncontrollable ventricular arrhythmias.
  Common aetiologies:
- Dilated cardiomyopathy, ischaemic cardiomyopathy. However, most forms of heart failure can result in being listed for heart transplantation.
- Myopathies with cardiac involvement such as Becker's muscular dystrophy

Contraindications:
- Age > 65 years. However, this cut-off may be altered in certain instances. Clinically suitable patients aged 65–70 years are evaluated on an individual basis.
- Fixed pulmonary vascular resistance > 5 Wood units (or trans-pulmonary gradient > 15 mmHg).
- BMI > 30
- Active systemic infection
- Active systemic disease such as collagen vascular disease
- Diabetes mellitus with significant end-organ damage
- Irreversible renal dysfunction (e GFR < 40). Occasionally patients with double organ failure may be considered for a combined heart–kidney transplant if required.
- Recent pulmonary embolism (< 6 weeks)
- Unhealed peptic ulcer
- Active malignancy. Patients with malignancies who have demonstrated a 3–5 year disease-free interval may be considered, depending on the tumour type and the evaluating program.
- An ongoing history of substance abuse (e.g. alcohol, drugs, tobacco)
- Psychosocial instability
- Inability to comply with medical follow-up and obligatory care.

Pre-transplantation work-up

1 General evaluation:
- History and examination including height and weight
- Rectal examination
- Faecal occult blood test in patients > 50 years
- CT scan of head, chest and abdomen in all patients > 60 years and smokers > 50 years
- Females—clear PAP smear within last year and mammogram if > 45 years
- DEXA scan
- Prostate-specific antigen (PSA) in males > 50 years

2 Cardiac assessment:
- ECG
- Gated blood pool scan (within 3 months of referral)
- Echocardiogram
- 24-hour Holter monitor
- Carotid duplex in all patients with ischaemic heart disease and all patients > 50 years
- Right heart catheter. Measure pulmonary vascular resistance (PVR), trans-pulmonary gradient (TPG = mean pulmonary artery pressure (PAP) – mean pulmonary capillary wedge pressure (PCWP)) and cardiac output.
- Coronary angiography where indicated
- Endomyocardial biopsy > 5 specimens (in carefully selected cases)

3 Haematology:
- Blood group
- FBE/ESR, platelets, coagulation studies, serum protein electrophoretogram (EPG)

4 Biochemistry:
  - Urea and electrolytes (U&Es), creatinine, glucose, liver function tests (LFTs), serum urate, Mg, Ca, phosphate, creatine kinase (CK), creatine kinase myocardial bound (CKMB)
  - Fasting cholesterol, triglycerides, HDL and LDL
  - 24-hour urine for total protein and creatinine clearance, urine EPG
  - Thyroid function tests (TFTs)
5 Microbiology:
  - Urine microscopy and culture
  - Methicillin-resistant *Staphylococcus aureus* (MRSA) screen
  - Mantoux test
6 Immunology:
  - Immunoglobulin levels and protein electrophoresis
  - Autoantibodies: include antinuclear factor, anti DS-DNA, rheumatoid factor
7 Serology:
  - HBsAg, surface antibody and core antibody, Hepatitis C and HIV 1 & 2
  - Cytomegalovirus (CMV), Epstein-Barr virus (EBV)
  - Herpes simplex, herpes zoster, *Toxoplasma*
8 Respiratory:
  - Forced expiratory volume (FEV$_1$), vital capacity and carbon monoxide diffusion (DLCO) are required as a minimum
  - Sleep study—in all patients with suspected sleep apnoea or pulmonary hypertension
9 Dental:
  - Orthopantomogram (OPG)
  - Examination
10 Radiology:
  - Chest radiography
  - DEXA scan (bone mineral density)
  - CT scans as above
11 Referrals (should be made to):
  - Social worker
  - Physiotherapist
  - Occupational therapist
  - Nutritionist
  - Transplant nurse
  - Transplant coordinator

Post-transplantation management

1 *Endomyocardial biopsies*
  These are performed to assess for allograft rejection. They may be performed as frequently as every week for the first month, with the frequency decreasing over time. Commonly around 15 heart biopsies are performed in the first year after a heart transplant.
  Extra heart biopsies may be performed whenever clinically indicated. Common indications that may suggest acute rejection include:
  - hypotension
  - shortness of breath
  - arrhythmias, particularly supraventricular arrhythmias (especially AF or atrial flutter)

- unexplained fever
- reduced left ventricular ejection fraction
- oedema
- unexplained poor health.

2 *Surveillance and investigations*

Follow-up visits are frequent for the first month because regulation of immunosuppression is being adjusted during this time. The frequency of visits gradually diminishes until the patient is generally seen on a 6-monthly or annual basis. Certain centres perform coronary angiography annually after transplantation, to monitor the patient for the development of coronary allograft vasculopathy (CAV). Alternatively, dobutamine stress echocardiography is performed to screen for CAV, particularly in the later years. This is particularly the case as often the patients have a degree of renal impairment precluding the use of contrast agents used during coronary angiography. However, intravascular ultrasound (IVUS) is the most accurate way to detect CAV, although this is not a routine test and is performed in only a few centres.

3 *Immunosuppressant therapy*

The cornerstone of immunosuppression is triple therapy with cyclosporin, mycophenolate mofetil and prednisolone. Alternative agents include azathioprine, sirolimus and tacrolimus. Basiliximab (Simulect®), an interleukin-2 receptor antibody, may be used early (days 1 and 4).

It is also important to recognise that there are numerous significant drug interactions to be aware of, especially with the immunosuppressant medications.

Complications

1 *Sepsis*

Infection is a significant problem in transplant patients. Preventive measures should be instituted. During the early post-transplant course, bacterial infections are of primary concern. Fungal infections can appear, particularly among inpatients, diabetics or those over-immunosuppressed. Prophylaxis for *Pneumocystis carinii* is universally administered, as is therapy for CMV infection. Maintain vigilance for other uncommon infectious processes including *Listeria, Legionella, Chlamydia* and *Nocardia* infections.

2 *Rejection*

Hyperacute rejection can occur immediately after blood flow is restored to the allograft. Thereafter, rejection can be classified as either *acute cellular rejection* (common form) or *acute vascular/humoral* rejection (less common) and chronic rejection.

Rejection is monitored for by regular endomyocardial biopsies. Endomyocardial biopsies can be classified as: Grade 0 (none), Grade 1R (mild), Grade 2R (moderate), or Grade 3R (severe) (International Society for Heart Lung Transplantation (ISHLT) Revised 2004 classification).

Depending on severity, rejection can usually be treated with pulsed IV methyl prednisolone for 3 days followed by a weaning dose of increased oral prednisolone (usually starting at 60 mg). Alternatively, anti-thymocyte globulin may be required in severe cases.

3 *Late graft failure*

Allograft vascular disease is the main cause of late graft failure and death. It is also called *chronic rejection*. The coronary arteries develop a progressive concentric intimal hyperplasia. This is seen along the full length of the coronary artery, unlike the discrete stenoses seen with plaque disease in native coronaries. This hyperplasia can develop as early as 3 months after transplantation. The cause of the process is unclear but there are both immunological (humoral) and non-immunological mechanisms involved. CMV infection and recurrent rejection episodes are thought to be associated with the cause. Current research indicates that the initial ischaemia/reperfusion injury of the allograft coupled with repeated rejection episodes might contribute to the process. Statins may help with prevention. Often the only effective therapy is retransplantation. The process can sometimes (but rarely) be treated by stenting or surgical grafting of the diseased vessels.

4 *Malignancy*

Malignancy is also a significant problem in heart transplant patients, particularly in the later stages. Heart transplant patients are at increased risk of both solid organ tumours and lymphoproliferative tumours. Skin cancers are a frequent problem (squamous cell carcinomas especially but also basal cell carcinomas and melanomas).

5 *Hypertension*

This is a common problem after cardiac transplantation, both early and late. Prednisolone and cyclosporin are common early causes, with later renal impairment a common exacerbating factor. It is important to treat hypertension, as some transplant candidates may not have been exposed to significant blood pressure elevations for some time and it can result in hypertensive encephalopathy.

6 *Dyslipidaemia*

This is also a common problem following heart transplantation and exacerbates the development of transplant CAV. It is multifactorial in aetiology, with immunosuppressants, renal impairment and loop diuretics all contributing to its development. Heart transplant patients are usually treated with a statin on a routine basis to manage this condition.

7 *Renal impairment*

Renal dysfunction, both early and late, can be a significant cause of morbidity and mortality for heart transplant patients. Again it is multifactorial in aetiology. However, it is commonly due to calcineurin inhibitors ('cyclosporin kidney').

8 *Diabetes*

Up to one-third of post heart transplant patients may have or develop diabetes. This may be brought on or exacerbated by steroids and immunosuppressant therapy (cyclosporin and tacrolimus).

9 *Osteoporosis*

This is frequently a major longer-term cause of significant morbidity for the heart transplant patient. Long-term steroid use, renal impairment and calcineurin inhibitors are common causes. As such, these patients are often managed on calcium, vitamin D, weight-bearing exercises and bisphosphonates.

10 *Arrhythmias*

These are relatively common after heart transplantation. It is important to recognise that atrial arrhythmias (AF and atrial flutter) are often markers of acute rejection and usually dictate the performance of an endomyocardial biopsy.

Some patients may have a persistent bradycardia after a heart transplant (due to sinus node dysfunction) and may require a PPM (around 15% require a PPM).

11 *Psychological disturbance*

Psychological disturbances from steroid therapy can occur in the immediate post-transplant period. These disturbances may be predicted from the pretransplantation psychiatric evaluation and thereby averted. Post heart transplant patients may require therapy with antidepressant medications.

12 *Vaccination precautions*

Heart transplant patients are immunosuppressed and therefore should not be given live attenuated vaccinations, as these could lead to fulminant infection. Patients should only be given killed vaccines or toxoid vaccines.

Survival rates

Overall survival rates after heart transplantation are 80% at 1 year and 50% at 10 years (ISHLT data 1992–2001).

Respiratory medicine

ASTHMA

Asthma is commonly encountered in the long case, and a thorough grasp of the principles of asthma management is essential.

> **Definition**
>
> **Asthma:** reversible, inflammatory airways disease. Inflammation could be mediated by eosinophils or other cells (lymphocytes and neutrophils).

Case vignette

A 28-year-old female patient has been admitted with fever, chills and rigors. She also has a productive cough and pleuritic chest pains. She has been recently diagnosed with asthma.

She smokes 5–10 cigarettes a day. She works in a bakery and describes symptoms of rhinorrhoea and wheezing while at work and after work. She has been prescribed an inhaler by her GP, but has not been compliant. On examination her temperature is 38°C and respiratory rate 20. Her oxygen saturation is 88% on room air. There are diffuse polyphonic wheezes in the lung fields, with bronchial breath sounds in the left mid to lower zone. Her sputum mug shows rusty purulent sputum.

1 Discuss her clinical picture in light of her background history.
2 Describe your immediate plan of management.
3 Draw up an asthma management plan for this woman.
4 Discuss the steps you would take to improve her compliance with medications.

Approach to the patient

History

Symptoms of chronic cough, especially nocturnal cough, wheezing and complaints of chest tightness, can be clues to consider asthma in the list of differential diagnoses in the dyspnoeic patient. In the known asthmatic, there are some questions that should invariably be asked.

Ask about:

- the current asthma management regimen, and frequency of bronchodilator use. Check whether the patient is using a bronchodilator at an unusually high frequency.
- what the known precipitants of asthma attacks are and how often the patient experiences exacerbations
- whether the patient has ever been hospitalised or treated in the intensive care unit for exacerbation of asthma
- whether the patient has a nocturnal cough
- whether the patient monitors their airway function with a peak flow meter at home. If they do monitor the peak flow, ask how often it is performed and the usual and most recent readings.
- the variability of the peak flow meter readings before and after bronchodilator therapy. Persistent variability is indicative of poor disease control.
- seasonal variation of symptoms and association with exercise
- whether an allergist has been consulted or special tests for allergy (skin prick test and radioallergosorbent (RAST) test) have been performed
- corticosteroid use—how often the patient is prescribed oral steroids, the maximum dose and the minimum dose ever, and the side-effect profile the patient has experienced
- how this chronic condition has affected the patient's day-to-day life and occupational activities.

Examination

The patient who has had poorly managed asthma since childhood may show evidence of stunted growth. Observe for evidence of dyspnoea and tachypnoea. Notice whether the patient is using accessory muscles for breathing. Check whether the patient has the fine tremor induced by beta agonist therapy. Feel for tracheal tug. Look for evidence of cyanosis. Do not forget to look for evidence of chronic systemic steroid use, such as easy bruising, ecchymoses, cushingoid body habitus and cutaneous striae. Listen to the lung fields for polyphonic wheezes. Perform forced expiratory timing.

Management

The candidate should formulate an ideal 'asthma management plan' for every poorly controlled or newly diagnosed asthmatic patient. Two of the most common causes of poor asthma control are non-compliance with medications and poor inhaler technique. Therefore it is important to ascertain the patient's level of drug compliance and to ask about the inhaler devices used. Elements of a good asthma management plan are as follows:

1 Ascertain the current level of asthma control. The plan should be aimed at addressing the current severity of the disease.

2   If control is very poor, with frequent exacerbations and frequent bronchodilator use (daily or several times a day), a course of oral corticosteroids together with high-dose inhaled steroids should be commenced. Oral steroids should be tapered and stopped as soon as disease control is achieved.

3   When the level of disease control is suboptimal despite maximum inhaled corticosteroid therapy, an inhaled long-acting beta$_2$ adrenergic receptor agonist such as salmeterol or oxymeterol should be commenced. Combined preparations of inhaled steroids and long-acting bronchodilators are becoming increasingly popular due to their convenience of use, thus improving compliance.

4   Short-acting bronchodilators should be used only in paroxysmal exacerbations of the disease.

5   In special situations, when the level of control is still poor, leukotriene inhibitors and theophylline should be considered as possible additions to the regimen. Leukotriene inhibitors have shown particular benefit in exercise-induced asthma and aspirin-sensitive asthma.

The patient should be given a good insight into his/her disease condition and taught the proper techniques for using an inhaler device. Referral to an asthma educator would be a wise step. Particularly in young and relatively young, active patients, it is important to make an assessment of how the disease affects their day-to-day lives as well as occupational, educational and social activities.

6   Provide the patient with an asthma self-management plan (see box). Such plans have shown benefit to the adult patient with asthma. The plan should include instructions to the patient on how to self-adjust medications according to the symptoms.

7   All asthmatics should be immunised against seasonal influenza and pneumococcal pneumonia.

Asthma self-management plan

One objective of the asthma action plan is to educate and empower the patient to assume some control over the management of this chronic condition. The plan should be able to educate the patient on how to recognise worsening of symptoms and signs of impending danger. The plan should be in writing and individualised to the patient. It should carry the following information:

- the patient's peak flow readings when stable, when symptomatic, during exacerbations and also when there is a danger of very severe exacerbations
- preventer and reliever medication dose requirements during the abovementioned stages
- instructions on self-adjusted dose increments during exacerbations (up to a maximum dose) and dose decrements when feeling better
- clear instructions on seeking urgent medical help when in danger
- contact details of the doctor and the pharmacist in case the patient needs further assistance.

Candidates should be familiar with the different inhaler devices, as some patients know their inhaler device or the medication in it only by its colour and shape (Fig 4.1).

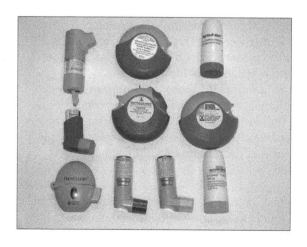

Figure 4.1 Different inhaled therapy devices currently used in the management of asthma and COPD (courtesy Ron Breene, pulmonary educator, Gold Coast Hospital)

Therefore, during the preparation period the candidate should consult the hospital asthma educator or the asthma nurse consultant for further information on the various inhaler devices and become familiar with the proper techniques for use. Candidates should be able to interpret formal lung function study reports quickly and accurately.

Drugs used in asthma

Asthma medications are broadly classified into two categories based on their clinical effects. The first category is the group of medications that improve symptoms (relievers) and the second category prevent exacerbations (preventers).

- *Relievers*—are short-acting beta$_2$ agonists such as salbutamol, terbutaline, and long-acting beta$_2$ agonists such as efemeterol. Tiotropium and ipratropium bromide are inhaled anticholinergic bronchodilator agents with a slower onset of action. Theophylline, which is capable of relaxing bronchial smooth muscle, is also used to treat severe and acute exacerbations of asthma. However, due to its wide adverse effects profile (nausea, diarrhoea, arrhythmias) it is rarely used these days.
- *Preventers*—include inhaled corticosteroids such as beclomethasone, budesonide, fluticasone and ciclesonide. Other preventers are leukotriene receptor blockers (montelukast) and cromoglycates (mast cell stabilisers).
  - *Inhaled corticosteroids* have proven benefits in reducing exacerbations, reducing mortality and recurrent hospital admissions. These agents are known to improve overall quality of life in chronic asthmatics. However, long-term high-dose therapy with topical corticosteroids can bring about systemic adverse effects such as cataracts, osteoporosis, glaucoma and cutaneous fragility.
  - *Leukotriene inhibitors* such as montelukast have particular use in the treatment of aspirin-induced asthma and in preventing exercise-induced asthma. They can be combined with inhaled steroids when adequate control is not achieved with single-agent therapy.

– *Cromones* such as nedocromil sodium and sodium cromoglycate are capable of preventing early and late bronchoconstrictor reactions to allergen exposure and therefore have particular use in seasonal allergic asthma. They have shown benefit in the prevention of exercise-induced asthma. Nedocromil is useful in the treatment of asthma-associated cough.

Occupational asthma

Occupational asthma is a common occupational morbidity and is quite likely to be encountered in the long case setting. It is a diagnosis in cases of adult-onset asthma.

Approach to the patient

Ask about the patient's occupation, precise onset of symptoms, diurnal patterns of symptoms and occupational exposure related rhinitis or rhinoconjunctivitis in the past. The patient may report improvement in symptoms outside the workplace. Ask about cigarette smoking, which is known to exacerbate the condition. Most cases of occupational asthma are due to immunoglobulin E (IgE)-mediated immunological response. This form of occupational asthma has a characteristic latency prior to the onset of symptoms after exposure.

Investigations

Occupational asthma is usually investigated by performing serial lung function measurements before and after exposure (at work and away from work on repeated occasions). Serial measurement of peak expiratory flow rate (PEFR) may provide useful information but lack diagnostic accuracy. Referral to an immunologist for blood or skin prick testing for specific IgE may enhance definitive diagnosis.

Management

Early and adequate management of occupational asthma is of prime importance, because failure to control the disease early can lead to a very poor prognosis. The management plan should involve an occupational health physician. Respiratory protective gear, when used properly, helps reduce the risk of occupational asthma but does not prevent its onset. Complete avoidance of allergen exposure is an important first step. Medical management is similar to that of standard asthma management. Remember to discuss the patient's job and financial issues and also possible worker's compensation claims (if relevant in the jurisdiction).

High-risk occupations associated with asthma

- Nurse
- Sawmill worker
- Painter
- Crop duster
- Animal handler

- Bird handler
- Chemical worker
- Baker
- Builder
- Welder

Chronic severe asthma

A minority of patients may have recalcitrant disease with hallmark features of frequent severe exacerbations requiring hospitalisation, significant associated morbidity, resistance to commonly used anti-asthma agents and significant steroid dependency. In addition to high mortality rates this patient group suffers from significant drug adverse effects and places a major (disproportionate) burden on the healthcare budget. It is important to ensure that these patients are properly worked up and investigated to exclude non-compliance or missed other diagnoses that could be contributing to the situation.

The management objectives in the patient group are reduction in the number of hospitalisations, steroid weaning and restoration of productivity. Some may respond to very high-dose inhaled steroids such as fluticasone or very high-dose long-acting beta agonists. Other agents that could be used in this setting include cyclosporine, gold and methotrexate. The efficacy of the latter is variable and fraught with significant adverse effects.

CHRONIC OBSTRUCTIVE PULMONARY DISEASE (COPD)

Chronic obstructive pulmonary disease (COPD) or chronic airflow limitation (CAL) is an extremely common long case pathology.

Definition

Chronic obstructive pulmonary disease: irreversible airways disease that incorporates chronic bronchitis, emphysema and chronic asthma with fixed airflow obstruction.

Approach to the patient

History

In the history of patients with known or suspected chronic airflow limitation, enquire about current or previous smoking, occupational exposure to fumes, dust and gases, environmental exposure to such agents and any family history of lung disease. The smoking history (including marijuana) has to be comprehensive and detailed. Also ask about chronic sputum production, wheezing, dyspnoea and the level of effort tolerance.

Cardiac disease is common in this patient cohort, and therefore it is important to enquire extensively into this and obtain details.

Examination

Look for tar-stained fingernails, cyanosis, pursed-lip breathing, barrel-shaped chest, subcostal retraction, decreased breath sounds and wheezing on unforced expiration. Particular attention should be focused on excluding a fixed wheeze, which could suggest the presence of a bronchial tumour. Look for evidence of cor pulmonale: elevated JVP, peripheral oedema, parasternal heave and a loud P_2.

Smoking-associated comorbidities in patients with smoking-related lung damage (COPD)

- Ischaemic heart disease
- Peripheral vascular disease
- Recurrent respiratory sepsis
- Lung carcinoma
- Carcinoma of head and neck
- Carcinoma of the bladder
- Carcinoma of the oesophagus
- Carcinoma of the colon
- Renal carcinoma
- Peptic ulcer disease
- Sexual dysfunction in men
- Osteoporosis in women
- Secondary polycythaemia
- Depression/anxiety
- Tobacco–alcohol amblyopia

Investigations

Ask for the chest X-ray, looking for evidence of hyperinflation, flattened diaphragmatic shadows, decreased peripheral lung markings and the absence or presence of other lung pathology (lung malignancy in smokers). It should be remembered that only severe emphysema can reliably be diagnosed in a plain chest X-ray.

Other investigations of value include:

1 Spirometry or formal lung function studies, with readings before and after bronchodilator therapy—looking for reversibility of the obstructive airway picture. The total lung capacity would be increased and the vital capacity and carbon dioxide diffusion (DLCO) would be decreased. Patient develops dyspnoea on minimal exertion when forced expiratory volume in 1 second (FEV_1) drops to 30% of predicted. Forced expiratory time (FET) is a simple bedside test that can be used to assess lung function. FET of over 6 seconds indicates severe airflow limitation.

2 Arterial oxygen saturations and arterial blood gases performed on room air— looking for hypoxaemia, carbon dioxide retention and acid–base imbalance.

57

3 Haemoglobin level—looking for elevated levels, particularly if arterial partial pressure of oxygen is less than 55 mmHg.

4 Full blood count—looking for erythrocytosis/polycythaemia and elevation of the white cell count if an infection is present. A haematocrit of > 52% in males and > 45% in females is diagnostic of erythrocytosis. A packed cell volume (PCV) of > 55% is very significant and an indication for long-term oxygen therapy.

5 Formal lung function tests—including carbon monoxide diffusion capacity (particularly if the severity of the dyspnoea is out of proportion to the FEV_1) and lung volumes. Most patients benefit from a trial of steroids to assess steroid responsiveness with FEV_1/forced vital capacity (FVC) measured before and after.

6 High-resolution CT of the lung—to look for dilated terminal airways typical of emphysema and to exclude other parenchymal lung pathology.

7 A sleep study—warranted if obstructive sleep apnoea is suspected (this should be considered if there is polycythaemia or cor pulmonale despite daytime arterial oxygen partial pressure being maintained above 60 mmHg).

8 Alpha$_1$-antitrypsin levels—especially in patients under 40 years of age with a positive family history of emphysema.

9 Sputum microscopy—in infective exacerbations, sputum may contain neutrophils and pathogenic bacteria. Most frequently associated organisms are *Moraxella catarrhalis*, *Haemophilus influenzae* and *Streptococcus pneumoniae*.

10 A trial of steroids is indicated, to assess the patient's steroid responsiveness. FEV_1/FVC is measured before and after the challenge, looking for an improvement of significance.

Management of chronic airflow limitation

Candidates should formulate a suitable plan for the optimal management of the patient's condition. A sound and practical plan of action would be very useful. The main objective of the optimal management plan is to improve the patient's activity levels and overall quality of life. This is achieved by treating symptoms, preventing exacerbations and preserving lung functions. Recruit the patient into a pulmonary rehabilitation program and encourage them to undertake light exercise. This helps improve morbidity, quality of life and mortality.

Formulate a collaborative management plan with the participation of the patient's general practitioner, community nursing sister and other community resources, with the main objective of preventing recurrent hospital admissions due to exacerbations. Physical rehabilitation and progressive exercising should be a major part of the long-term management plan.

The following are the integral components of the plan:

1 Instructions on the different medications and how to use them. Don't forget to stress the need for good compliance.

2 If the patient is suffering from frequent severe exacerbations, they should be commenced on oral corticosteroids. Start treatment with prednisolone 30 mg and plan to decrease the dose according to the clinical improvement. (IV hydrocortisone is indicated in very severe exacerbation of chronic airway limitation, and the decision to use this should be guided by the clinical findings.)

3 Commence twice-daily inhaled steroids using a spacer or an Accuhaler® device. These devices have better efficacy in the delivery of medication to the airways.

4 Twice-daily inhaled long-acting bronchodilator therapy should be considered if there is only suboptimal response to inhaled steroids alone. Combined formulations of inhaled steroids and a long-acting beta$_2$ receptor agonist are more appealing to patients due to the convenience of their use.

5 Ipratropium bromide or tiotropium (Spiriva®) via a metered dose inhaler and a spacer device four times a day has also been shown to be beneficial to these patients. Some patients may benefit from theophylline therapy, an agent rarely used these days.

6 Short-acting bronchodilator via a metered dose inhaler should be prescribed, to be taken only as needed.

7 Phosphodiesterase 4 inhibitors such as cilomilast and roflumilast given systemically are also known to control the inflammatory process. There is emerging evidence of its clinical benefits to patients with COPD.

8 Acute exacerbation may warrant antibiotic therapy. One example is the combination of IV ceftriaxone 1 g once daily with oral roxithromycin 150 mg twice daily. Other agents to consider are penicillin, ampicillin, azithromycin and clarithromycin.

   On recovery, the patient should be given oral antibiotics (for example, roxithromycin or amoxycillin) at discharge, with instructions to take prophylactically on identification of the earliest signs of an infective exacerbation (patient should be instructed to be on the alert for such symptoms as any unusual cough, sputum production, fever, dyspnoea or malaise). Also instruct the patient to see their general practitioner with a view to recommencing oral corticosteroid therapy in such circumstances. Rotating different agents may be useful in preventing antibiotic resistance.

9 Advice on and help in stopping smoking (topical nicotine patches or effective anti-craving agents such as bupropion hydrochloride) and avoiding airborne hazards. Varenicline is a novel agent that has shown promise in assisting smoking cessation.

10 Patient education should be provided on the condition and its current severity, contributory lifestyle factors that need modification, and how to slow progression of the disease and prevent complications.

11 Assess the patient's need for oxygen supplementation at home (see box overleaf).

12 If the patient remains significantly dyspnoeic and incapacitated despite all the above measures, or if the patient has giant pulmonary bullae, consider lung volume reduction surgery (bullectomy).

13 If the patient has cor pulmonale, referral to a cardiologist and further investigation (echo/right heart catheterisation) is indicated. Therapy includes loop diuretics, oxygen, optimising airway therapy and rehabilitation.

14 In resistant patients younger than 55 years, consideration should be given to lung transplantation. This process should be triggered with the patient being referred to a centre that has a lung transplantation program and expertise for screening and work-up thereof.

15 All patients should be advised on appropriate nutrition and regular vaccination against *Pneumococcus* and influenza virus.

16 Alpha$_1$-antitrypsin (AAT) deficiency is treated with smoking cessation, with drugs such as tamoxifen or danazol that are known to increase endogenous (hepatic) production of AAT. Administration of purified AAT by IV infusion or inhalation is another means of therapy.

Criteria for home oxygen supplementation

The presence of any one of the following criteria qualifies the patient for home oxygen. Prescribe domiciliary oxygen for at least 19 hours a day.

- PaO_2 of < 55 mmHg or arterial oxygen saturations of $< 88\%$ at rest
- Resting PaO_2 of 56–59 mmHg with cor pulmonale
- PaO_2 of < 55 mmHg or arterial oxygen saturations of $< 88\%$ on exertion or while asleep
- P-pulmonale (of > 3 mm) and evidence of right ventricular hypertrophy on ECG
- Echocardiographic evidence of right ventricular hypertrophy/strain together with pulmonary hypertension
- PCV of > 0.55

BRONCHIECTASIS

Bronchiectasis is defined as abnormal and permanent dilatation of bronchi with associated pooling of secretions, often leading to recurrent or persistent sepsis.

Approach to the patient

History

In the history of a patient with known or suspected bronchiectasis, ask about symptoms of recurrent cough, purulent sputum, dyspnoea, wheeze, haemoptysis and pleuritic chest pain. Check how often the patient experiences exacerbations and how such exacerbations present (usually there is an increase in the volume of sputum and its degree of purulence, with associated fevers and worsening dyspnoea). Ask how the episodes of exacerbation are managed (usually with multiple oral and parenteral antibiotics together with vigorous chest physiotherapy) and enquire about any chronic prophylactic antibiotic use (e.g. oral fluoroquinolones and inhaled aminoglycosides). Record the date of the most recent exacerbation. Ask about recurrent hospital admissions—frequency and average duration of stay on each occasion. Some respiratory physicians admit patients with bronchiectasis regularly for a prophylactic course of IV antibiotics to keep pathogenic bacterial colonies under adequate control.

Enquire about regular chest physiotherapy (self or by partner), forced expiratory techniques (huffing) and postural drainage. Gain insight into the volume of sputum production.

Ask about complications such as massive haemoptysis (due to bronchoarterial fistulae that need management with embolisation of the relevant segment of the bronchial artery). Significant weight loss is a bad prognostic sign in these patients. Ask about any recent weight loss and about general nutrition and appetite.

Ask how the disease is affecting the patient's social, occupational and family life. Enquiry into housing, social and economic problems is of great importance. Check about domestic and housing conditions. Ask about any depression associated with the chronic illness and assess the adequacy of the patient's coping skills and supportive resources. Patient motivation and supportive social or family networks are essential factors in the management of patients with bronchiectasis.

Examiners may be interested in the aetiology of the patient's condition. Ask about childhood illnesses such as measles and whooping cough, any past history of severe viral (adenovirus/influenza virus) or bacterial (*Staphylococcus aureus*, *Klebsiella* sp., anaerobic organisms and tuberculosis) respiratory tract sepsis that could be associated with the onset of symptoms.

The family history may give clues to the aetiology of the disease. Ask about cystic fibrosis and immunodeficiency, including HIV infection. Complaints of recurrent sinusitis and cutaneous sepsis should alert the candidate to the possibility of hypogammaglobulinaemia. Ask about any past history of foreign body aspiration, toxic gas inhalation and aspiration of caustic material, including acidic gastric content.

Check for features of primary ciliary dyskinesia such as recurrent upper respiratory tract infections, otitis media and infertility. Significant asthmatic symptoms should alert candidates to the possibility of allergic bronchopulmonary aspergillosis as a causative factor.

Obtain a detailed history of alcohol consumption, looking for clues of possible recurrent aspiration. A history of pulmonary fibrosis and interstitial lung disease may suggest traction bronchiectasis.

Examination

In the physical examination, look for signs of weight loss, wasting and cachexia. Examine the sputum mug and the temperature chart. Observe for a productive cough, tachypnoea and reduced chest expansion. Look for central or peripheral cyanosis and finger and/or toe clubbing. Some may even have hypertrophic pulmonary osteoarthropathy (HPOA) with tenderness in the wrists and ankles. Percussion of the thorax may show areas of dullness due to consolidation or severe atelectasis. Auscultate for coarse crepitations and wheezing. Check for features of right heart failure due to cor pulmonale and for signs of pulmonary hypertension. Check for hepatosplenomegaly and peripheral oedema. Do not miss situs inversus and dextrocardia with a right-sided apex beat, if present (Kartagener's syndrome—a form of primary ciliary dyskinesis). Look at the sputum mug and estimate sputum volumes, and check the smell.

Investigations

Investigations of bronchiectasis include:

1 Chest X-ray—looking for cystic air spaces, presence of air-fluid levels in the dilated bronchi, thickened bronchial walls with peribronchial cuffing, with the appearance of 'tramlines' and 'ring shadows'.
2 High-resolution CT scan of the chest—to confirm and better define the above features.
3 Formal lung function tests—looking for a reversible obstructive, restrictive or mixed picture.
4 Sputum microscopy and culture, including prolonged cultures in special media for fungi and tubercle bacilli. Organisms that commonly colonise these patients include *Pseudomonas aeruginosa*, *Burkholderia cepacia* (in cystic fibrosis), *Haemophilus influenzae*, *Escherichia coli* and *Staphylococcus aureus*. Bronchial washings too may be of use.
5 Full blood count—may show anaemia due to chronic disease or chronic recurrent haemoptysis. *Eosinophilia* should alert the candidate to allergic bronchopulmonary aspergillosis. ESR and C-reactive protein (CRP) may be elevated. Hypoalbuminaemia, if present, is a bad prognostic sign.

6 Renal function indices—presence of renal failure should signal the diagnosis of possible secondary amyloidosis. Amyloidosis secondary to chronic inflammation usually presents with renal failure and/or hepatosplenomegaly. Cardiac involvement is a rarity.

Where the aetiology is not clear, the following tests may be considered:

7 Fibreoptic bronchoscopy—looking for obstructive lesions
8 Sweat chloride levels—looking for evidence of cystic fibrosis
9 Serum immunoglobulin assay—looking for hypogammaglobulinaemia
10 Sperm assay or respiratory mucosal biopsy—looking for abnormalities of ciliary motility
11 Skin tests and serology for aspergillosis.

Management

The main objectives in the management of bronchiectasis are:

1 to facilitate the clearance of pooled secretions
2 to prevent and treat exacerbations early
3 to control symptoms (especially wheeze and dyspnoea)
4 to ensure good nutrition.

Management consists of the following:

1 Regular twice-daily chest physiotherapy (teach the patient how to self-administer physiotherapy) and training on techniques of postural drainage and forced expiration (huffing).
2 Aerosolised recombinant DNAse to further facilitate clearance of secretions (only in cystic fibrosis). Nebulised NaCl or mucolytics such as N-acetyl cysteine may be of use.
3 Chronic or periodic prophylactic/maintenance antibiotics (see box), depending on the culprit organisms. Patients are managed with single or combination antibiotic therapy. Some patients infected with *Pseudomonas* sp. benefit from nebulised aminoglycosides.
4 Patients with bronchoconstriction benefit from regular bronchodilator therapy. Some patients may benefit from inhaled steroids.
5 Localised disease can be treated successfully with lung resection surgery.
6 Associated right heart failure can be treated with diuretics and, where there is persistent hypoxia, with chronic oxygen supplementation. Severe right heart failure is managed with heart–lung transplantation in suitable candidates.
7 Allergic bronchopulmonary aspergillosis is treated with high-dose steroids, and hypogammaglobulinaemia is treated with regular infusion of normal immunoglobulins.
8 Nutritional dietary supplements, availability of community-based healthcare resources and psychological counselling where necessary.

Antibiotic use in bronchiectasis
- Route
  - Oral, inhaled, parenteral
- Mild to moderate exacerbation:
  - Can be managed as outpatients with oral agents

- Agents—amoxycillin, tetracycline, co-trimoxazole, azithromycin, cephalothin
  - Duration 7–10 days
- Moderate to severe exacerbation:
  - Need IV antibiotics
  - Agents—ticarcillin, with gentamicin or tobramycin, ceftriaxone, ciprofloxacin
  - Nebulised tobramycin is gaining favour as maintenance therapy
- *Mycobacterium avium* complex (MAC) infections:
  - Combinations of 3–4 drugs, such as clarithromycin, rifampicin, ethambutol, streptomycin, to be continued until the patient's culture results are negative for 1 year
- Bronchiectasis secondary to cystic fibrosis:
  - Treat with anti-*Pseudomonas* agents such as tobramycin

CYSTIC FIBROSIS

Cystic fibrosis is the most common cause of bronchiectasis in many parts of the Western world. Therefore, most facts discussed under 'bronchiectasis' apply to cystic fibrosis too. This is an autosomal recessive disorder with an incidence of 1 in 2000 and a carrier frequency of 1 in 25 among Caucasians. In most cases, causative mutation is localised to the cystic fibrosis transmembrane conductance regulator (CFTR) gene in the long arm of chromosome 7, but many more genetic mutations associated with cystic fibrosis have been described, making regular genetic testing difficult and inaccurate. In the past, this disease was associated with childhood fatality. With novel management modalities, patients seem to survive well into adulthood and are now commonly encountered in the practice of internal medicine.

Case vignette

A 25-year-old male with known cystic fibrosis presents with sudden-onset severe pleuritic chest pain of the left side. He also complains of severe dyspnoea. He denies any exacerbation of cough, fever or haemoptysis. On examination he is tachypnoeic and is in evident distress. Breath sounds are significantly decreased in the left upper and mid zones of the lung fields. There are coarse crepitations audible elsewhere.

1 Describe your differential diagnoses to this acute presentation.
2 What investigations would you require?
3 Explain in detail your approach to his management.
4 He has recently married and is keen on having children. On a separate occasion, how would you discuss this matter with him?

Approach to the patient

History

Ask about:

- details of the initial diagnosis, such as age, first presenting symptoms and diagnostic investigations
- current respiratory symptoms of productive cough, wheeze, fever, dyspnoea and haemoptysis. The patient may have had episodes of spontaneous pneumothorax and epistaxis due to nasal polyps.
- details about recurrent exacerbations of respiratory tract infections, multiple hospital admissions and the various forms of antibiotic therapy
- regular physiotherapy, techniques of forced expiration and postural drainage
- sino-nasal symptoms such as nasal obstruction, worsening nasal discharge, facial pain and cough
- gastrointestinal features of steatorrhoea, intestinal obstruction due to meconium ileus equivalent syndrome, and right upper quadrant pain and/or jaundice due to cholesterol gallstones
- nutrition, appetite and weight loss—malnutrition and weight loss are bad prognostic signs of the disease
- regular pancreatic enzyme supplementation and any side effects of this therapy
- heat intolerance and heat exhaustion in hot weather.

A minority of patients suffer from diabetes mellitus, of which the details should be obtained.

It is important to get a detailed family history.

Women suffering from cystic fibrosis are able to conceive but male patients are usually infertile. Ask about any plans for reproduction, genetic counselling and screening, and the coping strategies of the male patient with infertility. Be ready to discuss the ethical issues surrounding facilitated reproduction in cystic fibrosis.

Examination

Look for wasting, cachexia, stunted growth and features of malnutrition. Check the patient's weight. Some patients may have permanent vascular access devices for long-term antibiotic therapy. Observe the temperature chart and the sputum mug. Look for tachypnoea, cyanosis, finger and toe clubbing and hypertrophic pulmonary osteoarthropathy. Perform a detailed examination of the respiratory system as described under 'bronchiectasis'. Perform a detailed abdominal examination, looking for tenderness (particularly in the right upper or lower quadrant) and features of intestinal obstruction (distension, high-pitched bowel sounds or absent bowel sounds). Look for signs of right heart failure due to cor pulmonale.

Investigations

Investigations in cystic fibrosis include initial diagnostic tests and tests to diagnose and monitor the recurrent and persistent complications:

1 Sweat test—a sweat Cl level of > 70 mmol/L is consistent with cystic fibrosis in adults
2 Genetic tests for the most common mutations
3 Chest X-ray—looking for bronchiectasis, pneumonia and pneumothorax

4 Formal lung function tests or spirometry
5 Sputum microscopy and culture. Blood cultures in the febrile patient. Discovery of *Aspergillus* sp. or *Pseudomonas* sp. in the sputum often suggests colonisation rather than infection.
6 Supine and erect abdominal X-rays—looking for air-fluid levels and dilated loops of small intestine suggesting intestinal obstruction
7 Abdominal ultrasonography—to exclude cholelithiasis, where relevant
8 Full blood count—looking for anaemia of chronic disease or megaloblastic anaemia of malabsorption
9 Liver function tests—rarely these patients develop cirrhosis
10 Renal function indices—looking for nephrotoxic effects of aminoglycosides.

Management

1 Regular chest physiotherapy, forced expiration and postural drainage
2 Regular oral or inhaled aerosolised antibiotics for maintenance and the treatment of minor exacerbations. Intravenous antibiotics for severe exacerbations as guided by the results of the microbiological tests.
3 Recombinant DNAse to facilitate the clearance of respiratory secretions
4 Bronchodilator therapy
5 Oral replacement of pancreatic enzyme supplements and lipid-soluble vitamins
6 Dietary advice and monitoring to ensure adequate nutrition and prevent weight loss
7 Meconium ileus equivalent can be treated with enemas of hypertonic radiocontrast agents.
8 Consideration should be given to lung transplantation in end-stage lung disease with respiratory failure. Patients with severe cor pulmonale may need combined heart–lung transplantation.
9 Psychological and social support as necessary. The young patient with a chronic disorder and relatively short life expectancy may suffer from significant emotional distress.

PNEUMONIA

Approach to the patient

History
Ask the patient about:
- presenting symptoms such as fevers, rigors, chills, cough, dyspnoea and pleurisy
- the appearance of the sputum—if available, ask to have a look at the patient's sputum mug. Mucopurulent sputum is associated with bacterial pneumonia.
- other associated symptoms such as fatigue, nausea, vomiting, diarrhoea (sometimes may be associated with the antibiotic therapy)
- comorbidities such as COPD, asthma, immunocompromised status (HIV, splenectomy, chemotherapy, corticosteroid use)
- risk factors such as occupational exposure, diabetes, alcoholism (aspiration) and smoking.

Examination

Check the patient's temperature and also request the temperature chart to ascertain the nature and periodicity of the temperature spikes. Check respiratory rate and pulse rate. Tachypnoea and tachycardia should not be missed. On auscultation note crackles (rales and rhonchi) and bronchial breath sounds. Stony dullness with absent breath sounds may indicate pleural effusion.

Investigations

1   Arterial blood gases, full blood count (looking for leucocytosis and the differential count) and the electrolyte profile, together with renal function indices
2   AP and lateral chest X-ray—looking for consolidation, infiltrates, cavitations, effusion. Distinguish between lobar pneumonia (confined to a lung lobe) and bronchopneumonia (with a diffuse patchy appearance)
3   Sputum microscopy (Gram stain) and culture
4   Atypical serology/viral serology (polymerase chain reaction (PCR) could be useful for atypical bacteria and viruses)
5   Blood culture results
6   Urine results for *Legionella* and pneumococcal antigen
7   Viral cultures and enzyme immunoassay (EIA) or immunofluorescence for viruses

---

Pathogens associated with pneumonia

- *Streptococcus pneumoniae* is the most commonly identified pathogen in most community-acquired pneumonia cases. *Chlamydophila pneumoniae* and *Mycoplasma pneumoniae* are common atypical pathogens of community-acquired pneumonia.
- *Haemophilus* should be considered in patients with chronic lung disease, alcoholic patients and elderly patients.
- If the pneumonia was preceded by influenza virus infection, *Staphylococcus aureus* should be considered a likely pathogen. The latter has a more aggressive clinical course, with potential pulmonary necrosis and toxic shock.
- Diagnosis of influenza pneumonia and *Legionella* pneumonia is of significance due to the potential for epidemic outbreaks.
- If aspiration is a possibility, *Klebsiella* and anaerobic agents should be considered high on the list of pathogenic agents.
- Common pathogens associated with nosocomial pneumonia include *Staphylococcus*, *Pseudomonas* and Gram-negative bacteria.

Management

It is important to identify the features that place a patient with pneumonia at high risk, such as advanced age, confusion, hypotension, tachypnoea and elevated serum urea levels (see box). Such features warrant more aggressive therapy and supportive management (i.e. hospitalisation).

Features indicative of high risk in pneumonia patients
- Advanced age
- Presence of comorbidities (heart failure, renal failure etc)
- Tachypnoea/hypoxia
- Tachycardia
- Severe hypotension
- Confusion
- High fever (> 39°C)
- Acidosis

1 Antibiotics remain the cornerstone of pneumonia therapy. Bacterial community-acquired pneumonia can be treated with an oral macrolide such as clarithromycin or azithromycin or with a fluoroquinolone if the patient is young and stable. Mild to moderate pneumonia requiring hospitalisation can be treated with an IV third-generation cephalosporin such as ceftriaxone.

2 Patients with severe community-acquired bacterial pneumonia requiring hospitalisation may be treated with an extended-spectrum penicillin such as piperacillin/tazobactam together with an aminoglycoside.

3 Atypical pneumonias respond to macrolides or quinolones.

4 Gram-negative agents need treatment with more potent agents such as fourth-generation cephalosporins such as cefepime, or carbapenems such as meropenem.

5 In addition to antibiotic therapy, patients require antipyrexial agents, oxygen therapy (if hypoxic), analgesics and chest therapy.

6 Pneumonia prevention should be discussed in detail. Older individuals (over 50), patients with comorbidities, immunocompromised patients and healthcare workers should have pneumococcal vaccine and the annual influenza immunisation. *Haemophilus* vaccine is indicated for patients with sickle cell disease, those who have had splenectomy and those with leukaemias or HIV.

Complications of pneumonia
- Lung abscess
- Acute respiratory distress syndrome and respiratory failure
- Septicaemia
- Pleural effusion
- Empyema
- Lung collapse
- Haemoptysis

Common neurological conditions seen in the long case are stroke, multiple sclerosis, epilepsy and myasthenia gravis. Any one of these conditions can be the main problem of the case. But many other neurological conditions, such as Parkinson's disease, other movement disorders, peripheral neuropathy, migraine, vertigo, tinnitus and myelopathy, can be present as an associated problem. It is important to look at the case as a whole when encountering these features, because another medical condition or a medication may be the causative factor of the neurological deficit. In such situations, treating the possible precipitating condition or changing the medication may resolve the neurological problem. An example is a patient with a background history of hepatitis C presenting with peripheral neuropathy. The neuropathy is sometimes caused by hepatitis C-associated cryoglobulinaemia. So it is important to contextualise the neurological symptoms and signs, in the interplay of multiple diseases and medications in the long case.

COGNITIVE IMPAIRMENT

It is unusual to encounter a significantly demented patient in the long case examination. However, there have been instances where patients with progressive dementia, but who could still hold a reasonably rational conversation, have been presented at the examination. The objective of such long cases is to assess the candidate's ability to identify the problem of progressive intellectual deterioration and the candidate's knowledge and skills in handling the issues involved, such as remedying any correctable causes, attempting to slow down the deterioration where possible, and preparing for the optimal care of the patient medically and socially in anticipation of the inevitable total dementia.

The candidate should try to identify the broad pattern of cognitive impairment and the type of dementia. The following is a very basic introduction to such classification:

1 *Subcortical dementia*—prominent features include impaired concentration, attention and, later, memory
2 *Alzheimer's type*—prominent features include memory loss, especially short-term memory and language, impairment of visuospatial skills and behavioural change
3 *Frontotemporal*—prominent features include change of personality, disinhibition, impaired language skills and frontal lobe syndrome.

Approach to the patient

Candidates should be able to perform a very quick assessment of the patient's cognitive function, and a formal 'mini mental' test is a useful tool for this. Because this is a standardised and quantitative test, it can provide an objective assessment (though not always very accurate) that would be acceptable to the examiners. A good method to employ here is to memorise the mnemonic, which incorporates the important components of the mini mental test:

O R A — R L C

O   **Orientation**—year/season/month/date/day, country/state/city/hospital/floor (10 points)

R   **Registration**—three words: window, basketball, tree (4 points)

A   **Attention**—serial sevens, or counting backwards from 100 by sevens, or spelling WORLD backwards (5 points)

R   **Recall**—the three words above (3 points)

L   **Language skills**—repeating a phrase such as West Register Street, naming two objects, reading a sentence, writing a sentence and obeying a three-stage command (8 points)

C   **Construction**—copying two intersecting pentagons (1 point).

The maximum score is 30. A score of < 25 may suggest dementia.

In addition to the above assessment, look for features that may give clues to possible intellectual impairment. General demeanor, the response to your initial introduction, smell of urine and extrapyramidal facies are some such important clues. Check for the frontal reflexes.

Investigations

In patients with suspected dementia, a standard dementia screen is warranted. This battery of tests includes:

1   CT or MRI of the head
2   Full blood count with vitamin B_{12} and folate levels
3   Thyroid function tests
4   Midstream urine for microscopy and culture
5   Venereal disease research laboratory test for syphilis
6   Vasculitic and connective tissue disease screen
7   Electroencephalogram (EEG)
8   HIV serology in the young demented.

STROKE AND TRANSIENT ISCHAEMIC ATTACK

Approach to the patient

When approaching a stroke patient, the candidate should be well versed in the basic principles of stroke management.

History

The history must be very detailed and accurately describe the neurological symptoms. Ask about:

* how the patient manages with the neurological deficit
* whether the patient suffers from any predisposing vascular risk factors, such as hypertension, diabetes mellitus, hypercholesterolaemia and smoking

- any history of atrial fibrillation, palpitations, migraine, manipulation of the neck (a precipitating cause for dissection of the carotid or vertebral artery)
- any recent cardiac investigations such as coronary angiography
- recent cessation of anticoagulant therapy for some reason in patients with atrial fibrillation.

In the young stroke patient, consider the possibility of patent foramen ovale and paradoxical embolus.

Also obtain history regarding other thrombotic events (DVT, PE, miscarriages) in the patient or first-degree family members. Ask about alcohol consumption and recent falls that may have caused an intracranial haemorrhage.

Enquire about premorbid as well as the current level of independence and mobility. If the patient is incapacitated, ask about the social support available at home. Ask about the patient's mood.

Differential diagnosis of stroke

- Seizure
- Migraine
- Severe hypoglycaemia
- Traumatic nerve damage
- Intoxication

Examination

Never forget to look for poorly controlled hypertension, fundoscopic changes of hypertension and diabetes, carotid bruits, orbital bruits (commonly heard in the side opposite the carotid occlusion, due to increased contralateral flow), atrial fibrillation, cardiac murmurs and evidence of peripheral vascular disease.

Check the blood pressure in both arms (a difference of more than 20 mmHg systolic may suggest subclavian stenosis and a steal phenomenon). Look for complications such as pressure sores, limb contractures and disuse atrophy of the weak limbs.

See whether the patient has a percutaneous gastrostomy (PEG) feeding tube inserted and, if present, inspect for cellulitis or pus around the insertion site. Check the patient's temperature and look at the temperature chart for any evidence of fevers. Check for DVT in the lower limbs if a peripheral embolic cause is suspected, especially in the younger patient.

With the history and the physical examination, the candidate should be able to accurately characterise the exact neurological deficit and localise the area of the brain involved.

Management

Depending on the type and severity, transient ischaemic attack may be managed at home if timely investigation and adequate treatment can be arranged. Stroke with residual neurological deficit needs to be managed in hospital. Essential therapeutic goals in a stroke patient are early rehabilitation, the prevention of secondary complications such as DVT, aspiration pneumonia, urinary tract infections, limb contractures and pressure sores, prevention of recurrent stroke, and identifying/treating stroke risk factors. Rehabilitation should be planned according to the deficits identified on the examination.

Younger stroke patients (aged under 40 years) should be screened for unusual causes, such as illicit drug use (cocaine), vasculitic disorders, subacute bacterial endocarditis, patent foramen ovale or cardiac septal defects with a right-to-left shunt, paroxysmal atrial fibrillation or atrial flutter, thrombophilia, and inherited disorders such as CADASIL (see box) and homocystinuria. Some patients can develop a 'post-stroke dementia', and therefore the patient's cognitive function should be assessed.

Conditions associated with stroke (ischaemic and haemorrhagic)

- Atherosclerosis of the carotid or vertebrobasilar arterial systems
- Hypertension (lacunar infarcts due to arteriosclerosis of small penetrating arteries of the brain)
- Atrial fibrillation leading to thromboembolism
- Left ventricular aneurysm with mural thrombus
- Spontaneous/traumatic intracranial haemorrhage
- Amyloid angiopathy
- Cerebral autosomal-dominant arteriopathy with subcortical infarcts and leucoencephalopathy (CADASIL)
- Vasculitis
- Connective tissue disorders (e.g. systemic lupus erythmatosus (SLE))
- Narcotic use (e.g. cocaine, amphetamines)
- Bacterial endocarditis (septic emboli/mycotic aneurysm rupture)
- Thrombophilia (e.g. factor C/S deficiency, factor V gene mutation)
- Hypercoagulable states (e.g. polycythaemia, thrombotic thrombocytopenic purpura)
- Cerebral venous thrombosis
- Dissection of extracranial arteries
- Intracranial neoplasms (primary/secondary)
- Cerebral vascular malformations
- Subclavian steal syndrome

Investigations

The following investigations should be considered for the stroke patient, as guided by the clinical assessment:

1 Urine analysis and blood sugar levels—to exclude diabetes mellitus or a precipitating urinary tract infection
2 Full blood count—looking at haemoglobin levels (to exclude polycythaemia), white cell count (to exclude sepsis as a precipitating cause) and platelet count (rarely, essential thrombocythaemia can contribute to stroke)
3 Coagulation profile
4 ESR—to exclude any inflammatory arteritic/vasculitic process
5 Chest X-ray—for cardiomegaly/neoplasms/aspiration
6 ECG—for acute myocardial infarction and AF and troponin levels

7 Fasting blood lipid profile
8 CT or MRI of the head—looking for ischaemic infarcts, haemorrhage or mass lesions
9 Doppler scan of the carotid arteries—and, if the duplex ultrasonography suggests significant carotid stenosis, consider obtaining another confirmatory imaging study such as carotid CT angiography, carotid digital subtraction angiography or MR angiography. If the diagnosis is confirmed, discuss possibility of interventions such as carotid endarterectomy or stent placement in suitable patients.
10 If the patient is in AF, ask for the results of the transoesophageal echocardiogram (TOE)—looking for thrombus or spontaneous echo contrast in the left atrial appendage. This may also show up any atheromatous plaques in the ascending aorta and the arch of aorta that may have contributed to the stroke.
11 In the younger stroke patient, consider also the following investigations:
   • drug screen—looking for narcotic agents
   • vasculitic screen—if there are features of vasculitis
   • blood cultures and cardiac imaging—if endocarditis is suspected
   • cardiac event monitor—looking for paroxysmal AF
   • thrombophilic screen, and transthoracic echocardiogram with bubble study—looking for patent foramen ovale (PFO) (Fig 5.1) or septal defect.

If there is evidence of right-to-left shunt, particularly when right-sided pressures become high (as in Valsalva manoeuvre), a follow-up TOE is indicated to better characterise this shunt with a view to closing it (Fig 5.2).

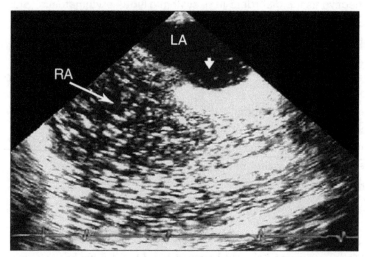

Figure 5.1 Transoesophageal echocardiogram showing a dense echo contrast inside the right atrium (RA), revealing a small PFO with more than five bubbles in the left atrium (LA) (reprinted from Drighil A, El Mosalami H, Albadaoui N et al 2007 Patent foramen ovale: a new disease? *International Journal of Cardiology* 122:9)

Management: stroke

The goals of stroke management are: 1) to determine and address the causative factors (secondary prevention), and 2) to restore functionality.
1 *Control blood pressure*—Initial steps are adequate and cautious control of the blood pressure (aggressive lowering of blood pressure in ischaemic stroke can worsen the neurological damage) and serum glucose level, and-antiplatelet therapy

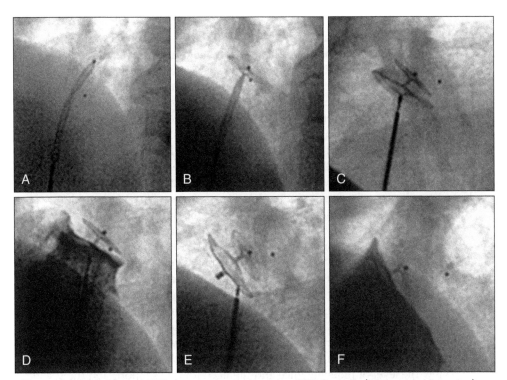

Figure 5.2 Percutaneous PFO closure using an Amplatzer PFO Occluder (left cranial oblique view). (A) The constrained Amplatzer PFO Occluder is advanced within the Amplatzer delivery sheath, which is positioned across the PFO in the left atrium. (B) The left atrial disc is deployed by withdrawing the delivery sheath and then gently pulling against the interatrial septum. (C) Further retention of the delivery sheath under tension of the left atrial disc against the interatrial septum allows for release of the right atrial disc. The device has reassumed its double disc shape connected by a thin waist passing across the PFO. (D) A right atrial contrast injection by hand through the delivery sheath opacifies the right side of the interatrial septum, confirming a correct position of the device. Note the nearly horizontal orientation of the Amplatzer PFO Occluder and the indentation of the septum by the lower part of the disc. This results from the tension of the delivery cable on the device. (E) Release of the device from its delivery cable by counter-clockwise rotation. The device assumes the more perpendicular position of the interatrial septum. (F) Control right atrial angiography by hand injection through the sheath delineating the right atrial septum and correct device position. The left atrial septum can be visualised during the levo-phase (reprinted from Adrouny Z A, Griswold H E 1963 Hemodynamics of mitral valve disease as altered by systemic hypertension. *American Journal of Cardiology* 11:3).

in the form of aspirin, clopidogrel or aspirin/sustained-release dipyridamole combination. Dipyridamole can cause side effects of headache, which may complicate the initial stroke symptoms. The popular approach is to use aspirin during the first few days post ischaemic stroke. This can later be changed to aspirin/sustained-release dipyridamole combination. Clopidogrel may be used in aspirin-intolerant patients. There is also an important role for 'statin' cholesterol-lowering agents and ACE inhibitors in the setting of acute stroke.

2   *Anticoagulation*—If the patient is in AF, there is high suspicion of cardioembolic event or there is carotid/vertebral dissection, anticoagulation with heparin or enoxaparin should be considered. This carries with it a risk of secondary haemorrhagic transformation of the ischaemic infarct, particularly within the first 2 weeks of the event and in cases involving a large vascular territory. For patients

with AF, especially in the setting of a large stroke, it is wise to observe for a few days and repeat the cranial CT prior to commencing anticoagulation therapy.

3   *Treat the cause and give supportive therapy*—Other steps in the general management of the stroke patient include treatment of the specific cause, if one is found (e.g. polycythaemia, vasculitis), and supportive therapy using adequate hydration, prophylactic anticoagulation, pressure care, and antispasmodics such as baclofen (use this agent with caution, as it can lower the seizure threshold in susceptible individuals) to relieve painful muscle spasms. Botulinum toxin is useful in relieving the painful spastic contractures that develop later. The immobilised patient is predisposed to DVT; therefore, prophylactic measures should be initiated. Compression stockings, low-dose subcutaneous unfractionated or fractionated heparin and passive limb movement are some such measures. Vigilance for pressure sores and implementation of preventive measures are also essential. Prophylactic measures are: change of posture at least at 2-hourly intervals, use of a waterbed, pressure-controllable mattress, and good nursing care.

4   *Definitive therapy*—Definitive therapy in the form of carotid endarterectomy or carotid stenting should be considered if there is more than 70% atherosclerotic stenosis of the carotid artery and the stroke is consistent with the arterial lesion in that distribution.

5   *Team approach*—A team approach to management of the patient is essential. Early physiotherapy to prevent limb contracture and facilitate mobilisation, speech pathology review for optimisation of feeding (this may include video-telemetric swallowing assessment) and for rehabilitation of speech, occupational therapy to review the level of independence and the need for any support, and the social worker's involvement to assess the financial issues and social support for the patient and the family, are all important aspects of the management. It is wise to get the discharge planner involved early and to consider a family conference if indicated.

6   *Treat depression*—Stroke victims often become clinically depressed, and this will have a negative effect on the rehabilitation process, where the patient's active participation is highly desired. Consideration should therefore be given to commencing an antidepressant with minimal anticholinergic effects if indicated. An agent such as citalopram is suitable.

7   *Monitor temperature*—Patients should be monitored closely for temperature spikes. Pneumonia (aspiration) is common among stroke victims and has been identified as a major cause of mortality.

8   *Feeding*—Oral feeding should be suspended until the possibility of aspiration is formally excluded. If the patient is unable to tolerate oral feeding for more than 5 days, a decision should be made regarding the insertion of a percutaneous gastrostomy feeding tube, as impaired bulbar muscle function may be permanent.

9   *Rehabilitation*—Remember, rehabilitation is the key issue in the stroke patient!

EPILEPSY

Classification of the patient's seizure type has diagnostic, prognostic and therapeutic significance. It is important to study the different seizure classification systems used in common clinical practice, such as the one defined by the International League against Epilepsy (see box). It is not uncommon for patients to be suffering from a combination of seizure types. Presentation of a simple partial seizure can take many forms. However, there is uniformity in the features of a single patient.

Classification of seizures

Partial seizure

Simple partial (consciousness not impaired)

With motor symptoms:

- Focal motor without march
- Focal motor with march (Jacksonian)
- Versive
- Postural
- Phonatory (vocalisation or arrest of speech)

With somatosensory or special sensory symptoms:

- Somatosensory
- Visual
- Auditory
- Olfactory
- Gustatory
- Vertiginous

With autonomic symptoms or signs (including epigastric, pallor, sweating, etc)

With psychic symptoms (disturbance of higher cerebral function)—usually occur with impairment of consciousness and classified as complex partial:

- Dysphasic
- Cognitive
- Dysmnesic (déjà vu, jamais vu)
- Affective (anxiety)
- Illusions
- Hallucinations

Complex partial (with impairment of consciousness)

- Simple partial onset followed by impairment of consciousness
- Impairment of consciousness at onset
- With impairment of consciousness only
- With automatisms
- Partial seizures (simple or complex) evolving to secondarily generalised seizures

Generalised seizure

Non-convulsive (absence)

- Typical (3/sec spike and slow wave complexes on EEG)
- Atypical (< 3/sec spike and slow wave complexes on EEG)

Convulsive

- Myclonic seizures
- Clonic seizures
- Tonic seizures

- Tonic–clonic seizures
- Atonic ('drop attacks')

Unclassified seizure

(Adapted from Commission on Classification and Terminology of the International League against Epilepsy 1981 Proposal for revised clinical and electroencephalographic classification of epileptic seizures. *Epilepsia* 22:489)

Approach to the patient

History

Ask about:

- prodromal signs—such as déjà vu and jamais vu
- auras—such as pungent smells, anxiety and abdominal discomfort
- events occurring during the first few seconds of each seizure—this is of utmost importance. Often, seizures start focally and then generalise within a few seconds. This will enable the clinician to determine the type of seizure (focal onset versus general onset).
- jerky limb movements or staring
- impairment or loss of consciousness
- automatisms—such as lip smacking, chewing
- how eyewitnesses describe the episodes—observers may report automatisms and loss or impairment of consciousness
- whether the patient is aware or unaware of the events that take place during a complex partial seizure. Progression of simple partial seizures to complex partial seizures is common. In complex partial seizures, the person demonstrates impairment of consciousness together with automatisms. Generalised seizures always cause impairment of consciousness together with tonic–clonic activity (grand mal seizures), myoclonic jerks or absence (petit mal seizures). The patient may know of observer reports to this effect.
- postdromal features—such as Todd's paralysis and excessive drowsiness. Such postictal paresis can last from hours to days. The features of Todd's palsy can also include hemianopic visual loss or sensory impairment and always involve the contralateral side to the side of seizure focus. In complex partial seizures, postdromal features include severe headaches and confusion.
- family history of epilepsy—some epilepsy syndromes, such as juvenile myoclonic epilepsy (JME) are hereditary
- possible precipitants of seizures—such as flickering lights, sleep deprivation. Controlling modifiable seizure triggers helps give better seizure control.
- relevant past history—such as head injuries, febrile seizure as a child, brain surgery, intracranial tumour, stroke, encephalitis or meningitis
- consumption of extraneous agents and conditions that can lower seizure threshold—such as alcohol, recreational drugs and hypoglycaemia
- medications—level of compliance with medications and any side effects experienced. A detailed drug history may be relevant in patients who may have been tried on different medications in the past; this may be a clue to the difficult-to-control epilepsy.

- whether the patient has ever been monitored in hospital with video-telemetry
- any previous episodes of self-harm due to fits.

Occupational issues are very important in the epileptic, so discuss operation of heavy machinery and driving. Discuss in detail any social issues and limitations that are important to the patient. Details about depression and/or the use of antidepressants are important, as all antidepressants (especially tricyclic agents) have a propensity to lower the seizure threshold. Never forget to ask about the reproductive plans of the female patient, as antiepileptic agents can be teratogenic. The oral contraceptive pill can be rendered ineffective by agents such as phenytoin.

Examination

Usually during non-ictal periods the examination is unremarkable in most epileptic patients. However, a thorough general neurological examination is indicated, particularly looking for evidence of focal neurologial signs. Cranial scars may testify to previous brain surgery or brain injury.

Investigations

1 If it is the first episode of fitting—serum calcium (hypocalcaemia), sodium (hyponatraemia) and magnesium (hypomagnesaemia) levels as well as serum glucose measurement, looking for hypoglycaemia. Screening for infection, hypoxia, drug effects and other metabolic derangements is also necessary.
2 Electroencephalograph (EEG)—to identify an underlying seizure focus if present. Recurrent fitting with normal EEG during the interictal period may warrant in-hospital video-telemetry to capture an event.
3 Cranial CT or MRI—looking for structural abnormality such as space-occupying mass, stroke or demyelination plaque.
4 Recurrence of fitting while on antiepileptic therapy warrants assessment of serum levels of the relevant agent.

Management

1 All symptomatic seizures with an underlying cause should be treated.
2 Treatment of idiopathic seizures (with normal EEG and MRI) should be initiated if the patient experiences more than two seizures. The most common cause of inadequate epilepsy control is poor drug compliance. Also be alert to the concurrent use of drugs that induce hepatic microsomal enzymes, which metabolise antiepileptic agents. Factors that would contribute to recurrent seizures include brain structural abnormalities, presence of focal neurological deficits and mental retardation.

Principles of antiepilepsy pharmacotherapy

Many factors need to be considered before deciding on the optimal drug or combination. These include seizure type, drug tolerability, drug interactions (and therefore comorbidities), and the patient's age and lifestyle. It is important to attempt monotherapy initially. Combination should be considered only after two sequential monotherapy attempts with two different agents have failed. Sodium valproate is considered a 'broad-spectrum' antiepileptic and can be used to treat most types of seizures. Generalised absence seizures (petit mal), which usually occur in children, are treated with ethosuximide. Generalised tonic–clonic seizures can be treated with carbamazepine and phenytoin.

Carbamazepine and sodium valproate should be avoided in severe liver failure. Phenytoin dose should also be reduced in such circumstances. Patients on carbamazepine should be monitored for development of rash, fever, bruising and leucopenia. Carbamazepine and phenytoin can cause interstitial nephritis. Because of its unique pharmacokinetics, a slight dose increase in phenytoin may result in major serum level elevation, especially in the elderly. Valproate can cause an increase in the hepatic transaminase levels as well as thrombocytopenia and platelet dysfunction leading to bleeding. Carbamazepine should not be used in generalised absence seizures. Carbamazepine and phenytoin cause induction of the hepatic cytochrome P-450 enzyme system, while valproate causes an inhibition of the same, and therefore it is important to make relevant dose adjustments to the concurrently administered other drugs that are metabolised by the liver. This is particularly important in female patients of childbearing age, because the efficacy of oral contraceptive agents will be compromised when administered concurrently with an agent that induces hepatic microsomal enzymes.

When these first-line agents are ineffective or are not tolerated, a second-line agent such as lamotrigine, topiramate, levetiracetam or gabapentin may be tried. Lamotrigine has a therapeutic profile similar to that of sodium valproate. It can be used as monotherapy or as add-on therapy in partial and generalised seizures. When given in combination, sodium valproate causes significant elevation of the lamotrigine level and the lamotrigine dose needs to be halved. The most significant side effect associated with this agent is severe rash, which can progress to Stevens-Johnson syndrome and is potentially life-threatening. Very slow titration is the key in lowering the rate of skin reaction. Topiramate is a novel agent that can be used in generalised as well as partial seizures. Some side effects of topiramate are somnolence, memory impairment, fatigue, anorexia and nausea. Levetiracetam is also a new agent effective in partial onset seizure control. Gabapentin is considered a safe drug, with no drug interactions and a minimal adverse-effect profile. The second-line agents overall have a lower side-effect profile and fewer concerns with drug interactions. These agents also do not require monitoring of serum levels.

All patients need counselling and help with occupational issues, the psychological impact of this chronic condition, and driving. Family and partner involvement in the management of patient, trigger factor control and drug compliance are important points to address in the discussion.

Summary of antiepileptic agents

- *Partial or generalised tonic–clonic seizures*—sodium valproate, carbamazepine, phenytoin
- *Absence seizures*—ethosuximide, sodium valproate
- *Myoclonic seizures*—sodium valproate, lamotrigine, topiramate
- *Second-line therapy for partial and generalised tonic–clonic seizures*—topiramate, gabapentin, lamotrigine, levetiracetam
- *Lennox-Gastaut syndrome*—felbamate (can cause fatal aplastic anaemia and severe liver toxicity)

MULTIPLE SCLEROSIS

The diagnosis of multiple sclerosis (MS) by definition requires evidence of central nervous system lesions separated in time and place.

Approach to the patient

History

Enquire about the onset, initial neurological deficit, any episodes of reversible visual loss or ocular pain, weakness, incoordination, lancinating pain, speech impairment, sphincter disturbances, sensory loss, seizures, vertigo and gait difficulty. Check for Lhermitte's phenomenon (electric shock-like pain radiating down the spine, triggered by neck flexion).

Try to determine the disease's pattern and the temporal profile. Most patients initially suffer from relapsing–remitting disease, with relapses of neurological symptoms followed by full or partial recovery. Many progress to develop secondary progressive disease with increasing disability. A minority of patients (10%) suffer from primary progressive multiple sclerosis, where there is progressive deterioration from the onset without any remissions.

Ask about complications associated with neurological deficit, such as aspiration pneumonia, urinary tract infection, mechanical injuries, limb contractures, pressure areas and painful muscle spasms.

It is important to assess the functional level of the patient, social and occupational difficulties, financial situation and the support available. Ask about activities of daily living and difficulties associated with sexual function.

Assess the mood of the patient, as this may vary from euphoria to severe depression at different times. Ask about the presence of severe fatigue, and also whether the patient has noticed exacerbation of symptoms with rises in body temperature.

Family history and the patient's place of birth may also reveal important information. Ask about pregnancy in the female patient, as there is a 20–30% increase in the relapse rate in the first month after delivery of the baby.

The patient should be questioned regarding different treatments given over the years and any adverse effects associated with them.

Examination

The history should be followed by a very detailed neurological examination. Look for disturbances of external ocular movements and other eye signs, such as internuclear ophthalmoplegia, optic atrophy and afferent pupillary defect. Examine for spinal cord signs such as spastic paraparesis (try to define the level), bulbar signs, cerebellar signs (especially cerebellar speech) and cerebral hemispheric signs. Perform a Mini-Mental State Examination to assess cognitive function, as multiple sclerosis can lead to cognitive impairment.

Investigations

1 MRI of the brain and spinal cord with gadolinium enhancement—looking for periventricular and callosal plaques in the brain and plaques in the brainstem and spinal cord.
2 Cerebrospinal fluid (CSF) examination—looking for oligoclonal immunoglobulin G bands (a serum sample checked at the same time should test negative for

oligoclonal bands) and mononuclear pleocytosis and also to exclude other infectious/inflammatory conditions.

3 CSF examination may be indicated in cases where there are no abnormalities detected in the MRI despite highly suggestive clinical features.

4 Visual, somatosensory and auditory evoked potentials, to demonstrate subclinical disease.

5 Exclusion of other metabolic/inflammatory conditions such as vitamin B_{12} deficiency (subacute combined degeneration), connective tissue disorders, sarcoidosis, Sjögren's disease, HIV etc.

Management

Mild attacks
Mild attacks of multiple sclerosis do not usually require treatment. Spontaneous improvement is the norm.

Acute attacks
More severe attacks with disabling or painful symptoms should be treated with high-dose parenteral pulsed methylprednisolone for 3–5 days. This therapy is known to accelerate remission but has no effect on the progression of the disease.

Long-term and secondary preventive therapy
Therapy with interferon beta-1a or 1b has been shown to retard the progression of relapsing–remitting disease. Interferon 1b has its use in secondary progressive disease too. Objectives of this therapy are to reduce the frequency and the severity of relapses. Some patients may develop neutralising antibodies to these agents, potentially rendering them ineffective. Interferon 1b is injected subcutaneously. Different formulations of interferon 1a can be injected subcutaneously or intramuscularly.

Patients may experience distressing flu-like symptoms with these therapies, and should be forewarned and at times premedicated with antipyretic agents.

A synthetic agent, glatiramer acetate, has been shown to be similarly helpful in the management of relapsing–remitting disease. This agent is useful for patients who do not tolerate interferon-beta. It has a slow onset of action (2–3 months) compared to the interferon preparations. A newly approved medication, natalizumab which is a monoclonal antibody to $alpha_4$-integrin, has been shown to be highly effective in relapsing–remitting MS but careful monitoring is required due to an association with an increased risk of progressive multifocal leucoencephalopathy (PML).

Management of complications
Painful muscle spasms can be managed with oral baclofen or diazepam. Botulinum toxin injections have also been used in severe cases. Distressing neurogenic pain can be managed with antiepileptic agents such as carbamazepine, phenytoin and gabapentin, or tricyclic antidepressants such as amytriptyline and nortriptyline. Urge incontinence is common and can be treated with anticholinergic agents, such as propantheline or oxybutynin. Those who suffer from urinary retention should be taught how to perform intermittent self-catheterisation. They may benefit from prophylactic antibiotics against the development of recurrent urinary tract infections.

Management of complications and symptomatic treatment should be approached in a multidisciplinary manner. Collaboration between the physiotherapist, the occupational therapist, the social worker and the psychologist is very important in formulating a comprehensive plan of management for the patient. Patient education and counselling should be given prominence. Patients who need assistance should be encouraged to join support groups such as the Multiple Sclerosis Society and other relevant local organisations.

MYASTHENIA GRAVIS

This disorder is characterised by a T-cell-dependent antibody-mediated autoimmune response to acetylcholine receptors in the neuromuscular junction.

Approach to the patient

History

Ask about:
- the onset
- the age at which the diagnosis was made
- duration
- details of exacerbations—frequency and trigger factors
- how the degree of weakness fluctuates in the different skeletal muscle groups. Involvement of ocular, bulbar, thoracic respiratory and limb musculature is a hallmark of this disorder.
- whether the patient has been treated with penicillamine in the past. Penicillamine therapy is a classic cause of drug-induced myasthenia gravis, and it almost always resolves once the medication is ceased.
- any history of thyroid disease (Graves' disease coexists in 2–5% of patients) or Addison's disease
- previous hospitalisations and any episodes where intubation and ventilation were necessary.

Patients suffer from diplopia, ptosis, dysphagia, dysarthria, weakness, lethargy and fatiguability of the muscles with repeated use. Complications of the condition include aspiration, respiratory failure and thromboembolism.

Ask about:
- therapy and therapy-related complications
- how the patient is coping with the condition
- support available in the community
- other known organ-specific autoimmune disorders that the patient may be suffering from
- drug-induced exacerbations of symptoms and the culprit agents—gentamicin is one such agent.

Examination

1 Look for cushingoid body habitus secondary to repeated therapy with corticosteroids, and for ptosis and drooling.
2 The patient may have a moist productive cough, dyspnoea and fever due to aspiration pneumonia.

3 Perform a thorough neurological examination, looking for weakness in the extraocular muscles, facial muscles, the bulbar area and the limbs. Note that the reflexes and the sensory function are preserved. In very chronic, 'burnt-out' myasthenia, wasting of the muscles can be a prominent feature.

4 Assess the patient's forced vital capacity.

Investigations

1 Radioimmunoassay—for anti-acetylcholine receptor antibody.

2 Tensilon (edrophonium chloride) test—an objective improvement of muscle strength after parenteral Tensilon® is diagnostic of myasthenia gravis. Remember that Tensilon®can cause severe, potentially lethal bradycardia, complete heart block and severe bronchospasm, so the patient must be monitored during this test. It is essential that atropine and a resuscitation trolley be available by the bedside during the study.

3 Ice pack test—can be performed in patients suffering from ptosis. Neuromuscular transmission is known to improve at lower temperatures. The test involves assessing for objective improvement of muscle power in the eyelids upon cooling. This test is a useful substitute for the Tensilon® test when the latter is contraindicated.

4 Neurophysiological tests—such as repetitive nerve stimulation test, looking for muscle fatiguability, and single-fibre electromyography, looking for features of block and jitter.

5 CT or MRI of the brain—to exclude other pathology.

6 Formal lung function studies, looking for a restrictive-type abnormality, and chest X-ray to exclude aspiration and atelectasis.

7 Thyroid function tests—to exclude thyroid ophthalmopathy.

8 ECG—looking for evidence of pulmonary hypertension associated with chronic hypoventilation and recurrent aspiration.

9 CT or MRI of the anterior mediastinum—looking for a thymic mass. If thymectomy has been performed, ask for the biopsy report during the discussion, to exclude thymoma.

Management

Management of myasthenia gravis should be individualised to each patient, based on the muscle groups involved and the level of their involvement.

1 Symptom management—achieved with anticholinesterase agents such as neostigmine and pyridostigmine. Note that overmedicating with anticholinesterase can also cause weakness together with other cholinergic side effects such as diarrhoea and abdominal cramps.

2 Immunosuppression—this is the mainstay of management and disease control. Immunosuppression with chronic systemic corticosteroid therapy is used for maintenance. Steroid-sparing therapy can also be achieved with the use of azathioprine, cyclosporine, mycophenolate mofetil or cyclophosphamide. Remember to raise the issue of complications associated with immunosuppression, such as opportunistic infections and secondary malignancies due to long-term cytotoxic use. Sometimes immunosuppressed myasthenia patients are treated with prophylactic sulfamethoxazole/trimethoprim against *Pneumocystis carinii*.

3   Thymectomy—should be performed in all patients with thymoma due to its propensity to spread locally. All patients with generalised myasthenia gravis under the age of 55 years may benefit from thymectomy even in the absence of thymic tumour. However, the value of thymectomy in myasthenia gravis is currently under investigation.

4   Plasmapheresis or IV immunoglobulins—for temporary and rapid control of symptoms in severe disease (such as myasthenia crisis) and prior to surgery.

5   Monitoring with regular spirometry—to diagnose respiratory exhaustion promptly.

Myasthenia crisis is a life-threatening exacerbation of the disease, with progressive inability to breathe due to severe muscle weakness. This must be differentiated from the *cholinergic crisis* due to excessive anticholinesterase therapy. This situation should be addressed in an intensive care setting, where facilities are available for intubation and ventilation.

The patient should be given adequate chest physiotherapy and meticulous nursing care to prevent complications and pressure sores. The patient may need prophylactic antibiotics to prevent sepsis, and parenteral or nasogastric feeding to ensure adequate nutrition. Caution should be exercised with the use of neuromuscular blocking agents in patients undergoing surgery under general anaesthesia, as these agents can cause prolonged paralysis.

Lambert-Eaton myasthenic syndrome (LEMS)

This disorder should be considered a differential diagnosis of a patient who presents with clinical signs of myasthenia gravis. Ask about the onset of early symptoms. Typically the patients initially experience proximal muscle weakness that manifests as difficulty in climbing stairs and getting out of a seat. This picture of weakness progresses to shoulder girdle weakness. Though ptosis may be seen, unlike myasthenia gravis the involvement of extraocular musculature and bulbar musculature is rare and the muscle weakness usually improves with exercise. In contrast to myasthenia, LEMS is commonly associated with autonomic dysfunction such as oromucosal dryness and impotence in men. LEMS could be a paraneoplastic phenomenon and therefore do not forget to ask about a diagnosis of a malignancy (such as small cell lung cancer). Investigations at the diagnosis of LEMS include repetitive nerve stimulation looking for an incremental response of the compound muscle action potential and antibodies to presynaptic voltage-dependent calcium channels.

DEPRESSION

Many a patient encountered as a long case will have a depressive component to their picture, simply due to their multiple and often chronic medical problems. It is important that the candidate be sensitive to the patient's mood and pick up clues that suggest possible depression.

Approach to the patient

History

Ask directly whether the patient has ever been depressed and, if so, whether he or she has been treated. If the patient denies depression, enquire about vegetative symptoms of depression, such as initial insomnia, anorexia, irritability and anhedonia.

Examination

Look for a depressive affect, paucity of direct eye contact and sometimes paucity of movement. It is very important to enquire about intention to self-harm and suicide in all patients with suspected depression. If the patient has been treated with antidepressants, ask about any adverse effects experienced and about the efficacy of therapy.

If you think a patient is depressed, remember to formulate a plan of action to manage the condition. If you recommend pharmaceutical therapy for depression, remember to warn the patient that most antidepressants take about 2 weeks to start acting. The most commonly used antidepressant agents are the tricyclic antidepressants and the selective serotinin reuptake inhibitors (SSRIs).

Management

Tricyclic antidepressants

These agents can also be used in chronic pain, migraine prophylaxis and obsessive-compulsive disorder in addition to depression. The best agent for use in pain is amitriptyline and the best for obsessive-compulsive disorder is clomipramine. Adverse effects of tricyclics include sedation, dry mouth, constipation, weight gain, orthostatic hypotension, urinary retention, excessive sweating and agitation. Prior to commencing therapy, remember to check for postural blood pressure; also counsel the patient about the more common side effects, such as blurred vision and dry mouth, and reassure the patient that these effects will subside within about 7 days. For the elderly, two suitable agents with minimal anticholinergic effects are nortriptyline and desipramine. These agents are also less likely to cause sedation.

Selective serotonin reuptake inhibitors

The side-effect profile of the SSRI agents includes nausea, agitation, insomnia, drowsiness, tremor, dry mouth, constipation and diarrhoea, and syndrome of inappropriate antidiuretic hormone secretion (SIADH). These agents are becoming popular due to their minimal anticholinergic effects. Some of the more commonly used SSRIs include citalopram, fluoxetine, paroxetine, sertraline and venlafaxine. The SSRI dose should be halved in renal failure.

All antidepressants are metabolised in the liver, so remember to halve the dose given to patients with liver failure.

ACUTE RENAL FAILURE

Acute renal failure is a comorbidity that can be encountered in the long case setting. It can also be incidentally encountered when an electrolyte profile with renal function indices is given to the candidate by an examiner during the discussion. In such situations it is important that the candidate correctly interpret the results and take charge of the discussion.

Case vignette

An 81-year-old man is admitted after an episode of syncope. On arrival in hospital his pulse rate is 30 bpm and blood pressure is 80/50 mmHg. He has a background history of paroxysmal atrial fibrillation, which has been managed with digoxin, and hypertension, managed with enalapril. He has been recently commenced on a non-steroidal antiinflammatory drug for painful arthritis of the knees. Investigations reveal his creatinine level to be 247 µmol/L and urea 26 mmol/L. His serum potassium level is 6.5 mmol/L. ECG reveals sinus bradycardia with tall tented T waves.

1 What is your approach to the management of this man's situation?
2 How would you explain his clinical picture?
3 Upon establishing haemodynamic stability, how would you address his renal function abnormality?

Approach to the patient

History

Ask about:
- the patient's family history suggestive of any hereditary renal disease
- a past history of renal conditions
- diabetes, vasculopathy, diseases such as gout or pseudogout (crystal-induced nephropathy) or vasculitic disorders

- whether the patient has taken any potentially renal-toxic drugs such as allopurinol, NSAIDs etc
- whether the patient has been recently commenced on or subjected to a dose increment of an agent such as a diuretic or an ACE inhibitor
- whether the patient has had recent vascular catheterisation procedures and/or radiocontrast exposure. Catheterisation can lead to cholesterol embolisation, which can cause acute renal damage. Radiocontrast material can be nephrotoxic.
- recent falls and prolonged immobilisation—these can lead to rhabdomyolysis, which in turn leads to acute renal failure due to myoglobin toxicity. It is important to rule this out in debilitated patients.

Remember: dehydration and hypovolaemia are the most common causes of acute renal failure, and assessment of the patient's state of hydration is of primary importance in this setting.

In order of frequency, the most common causes of acute renal failure are:

1 Acute tubular necrosis (ATN) due to ischaemia (hypovolaemia or hypotension) or nephrotoxins
2 Intrinsic renal disease
3 Obstructive disease.

Examination

1 Check the patient's fluid status by examining the oral mucosa and checking skin turgur.
2 Check blood pressure and pulse.
3 Assess the JVP, look for peripheral oedema, and auscultate the lung fields for creptations, looking for evidence of cardiac failure.
4 Look for rashes of vasculitis and evidence of connective tissue disease.
5 Examine the temperature chart for fevers, which would suggest sepsis.
6 Examine for wasting, hard mass lesions and lymphadenopathy, which would indicate malignancy.
7 Listen to the abdomen for a renal bruit, which may suggest renal artery stenosis.
8 In the anuric patient it is important to catheterise the bladder to exclude urethral obstruction and, if already catheterised, to flush the catheter to relieve any catheter obstruction.
9 Ask for the results of the urine analysis and the per rectum and per vagina examinations, looking for any pelvic mass lesions.
10 It is also important to request the results of microscopic examination of a fresh urine sample, looking for red cells, red cell casts and changes in the red cell morphology.

Causes of acute renal failure

- Impaired renal perfusion—shock, dehydration, severe left ventricular failure, renal artery obstruction
- Renal vein thrombosis
- Acute glomerular nephritis
- Acute vasculitis
- Acute interstitial nephritis—allergic, septic, infiltrative

- Acute tubular necrosis—ischaemic/toxic
- Exogenous renal toxins—drugs/ionic contrast agents
- Rhabdomyolysis
- Multiple myeloma
- Crystal-induced—e.g. urate, oxalate, pyrophosphate
- Haemolytic uraemic syndrome
- Thrombotic thrombocytopenic purpura
- Outflow tract obstruction—ureteric, bladder-related or urethral

Common causes of acute renal failure according to anatomy of location

1 *Prerenal causes*—severe congestive cardiac failure, hypovolaemia, dehydration, bilateral renal artery stenosis
2 *Intrinsic renal causes*—acute glomerulonephritis, tubulointerstitial nephritis, drug toxicity, fat embolism, cholesterol emboli, hepatorenal syndrome, haemolytic-uraemic syndrome, acute tubular necrosis.
3 *Postrenal causes*—renal outflow tract obstruction due to calculi, blood clots, trauma and retroperitoneal fibrosis.

Remember: both kidneys need to be affected to cause acute renal failure, unless only one kidney, anatomically or functionally, is present.

Investigations

In addition to serum biochemistry, the following investigations would be helpful:

1 Full blood count—looking for anaemia (may suggest chronicity), leucocytosis (may suggest sepsis or inflammation) and thrombocytopenia (possibly lupus nephritis).
2 Erythrocyte sedimentation rate—if elevated, can suggest multiple myeloma, connective tissue disease or vasculitis.
3 Urine analysis and midstream urine—for microscopy, culture and sensitivities. The presence of red cell casts and dysmorphic red cells in the phase-contrast microscopy would suggest glomerulonephritis; hyaline casts are non-specific; white blood cell casts suggest tubulointerstitial disease.
4 Urinary electrolytes and creatinine—the following findings, if present, would suggest a prerenal cause for the renal failure:
   - urinary osmolality > 500 mosm/L
   - urinary sodium < 20 mmol/L
   - fractional excretion of sodium < 1%.
5 Renal ultrasonography—looking for renal size, scarring and any evidence of urinary tract obstruction. If the ultrasound scan is inconclusive it should be followed up with spiral CT of the abdomen, looking for retroperitoneal fibrosis and renal cortical scarring.

6 Renal arterial Doppler study—looking for evidence of renal artery stenosis. The renal vascular resistive index should also be checked. This gives an assessment of the renal microvascular resistance and hence intrarenal vascular disease.

7 According to the clinical indication, the following tests can also be requested: serum electrophoresis, immunoelectrophoresis, antinuclear antibody test (ANA), extractable nuclear antibody tests (ENA), antineutrophil cytoplasmic antibody tests (ANCAs), serum complement levels, streptococcal serology (antistreptolysin-O test (ASOT) and anti-DNAseB), hepatitis B serology and hepatitis C RNA assay, HIV serology and blood cultures if the patient is febrile.

8 If the kidney size is normal and the diagnosis is still uncertain, a renal biopsy is indicated.

Management

Fundamental steps in management are as follows:

1 Stop all non-essential renal-toxic drugs (e.g. NSAIDs, ACE inhibitors, ARBs, gentamicin, amphotericin B, allopurinol) that would have potentially contributed to the current pathology. Decrease the dose of all renally excreted drugs.

2 Restore plasma volume and maintain a strict fluid balance, to avoid dehydration or volume overload. The daily fluid intake can be maintained at a volume equivalent to the previous day's losses + 500 mL. Correct electrolyte imbalances, particularly hyperkalaemia. Monitor the patient's body weight together with the fluid input and output on a daily basis.

3 Good nursing care is essential to prevent pressure sores and ensure hygiene.

4 Treat other acute medical conditions such as sepsis, vasculitis and thromboembolism.

5 Monitor renal function and electrolyte status regularly, to assess the need for renal replacement therapy.

CHRONIC KIDNEY DISEASE (CHRONIC RENAL FAILURE)

Case vignette

A 33-year-old woman presents with progressive lethargy, decreased appetite, insomnia, daytime somnolence and vomiting. She also complains of nocturia and amenorrhoea. She has been previously healthy and is not on any medication. Physical examination reveals conjunctival pallor, significantly elevated JVP, diffuse coarse pulmonary crepitations and peripheral oedema. Her blood pressure is 150/100 mmHg. Investigations reveal an Hb level of 8.7 g/dL, serum creatinine of 356 µmol/L and urea level of 31 mmol/L. Her serum potassium level is 5.1 mmol/L and serum albumin level 21 g/L.

1 How would you further work up this patient?

2 What are your differential diagnoses?

3 Renal biopsy reveals membranoproliferative glomerulonephritis with crescents. How does this additional information affect your plan of management?

4   Describe how you would plan renal replacement therapy for this
    woman.
5   What measures would you take to prevent other complications of renal
    failure?
6   Describe in detail your comprehensive plan of management for this
    woman.

Approach to the patient

History

Ask about:
- the precise cause of the kidney disease—if known (see box)
- uraemic symptoms such as fatigue, anorexia, polyuria, nocturia, sleep
  disturbance, decreased appetite, nausea and vomiting
- symptoms such as pleuritic chest pain of pericarditis and uraemic pruritus
- neurological symptoms of peripheral neuropathy, restless legs, pain, asterixis
  and seizures. Some patients may complain of bone pain.
- how and when the initial diagnosis was made, and what initial steps were taken
  for the management of the renal failure
- different renal replacement therapy the patient has received and how the patient
  has coped with the same
- any acute events associated with cardiac rhythm disturbances (severe bradycardia
  and syncope due to hyperkalaemia) and acute pulmonary oedema
- dialysis:
  - when the patient was commenced on dialysis
  - the different modalities of dialysis (peritoneal and machine)
  - complications of peritoneal dialysis, such as peritonitis etc
  - surgery for vascular access for dialysis and the complications thereof. Some
    patients may have had recurrent surgical procedures for fistula construction.
  - how the dialysis-dependent patient's lifestyle has been affected by the
    dialysis.

Patients with renal failure are at a higher risk of cardiac disease and it is important
to obtain details thereof. Ask about osteoporosis and fractures. Also ask about easy
bruising.

Patients who have had renal transplantation would be able to provide important
clinical information. Ask about the source of the grafted kidney, any previous
graft rejection and how it was managed. Check how the patient is tolerating
immunosuppression and chronic steroid therapy.

Obtain a detailed medication history, as patients with chronic renal failure are
managed with multiple medications. Enquire into the patient's diet and how they
maintain fluid balance. Ask about menstrual disturbance in the younger female
patient and erectile and sexual dysfunction in the male patient. Assess the patient's
psychological status and the social support available. Gain a good insight into the
patient's knowledge of this chronic disease condition.

Causes of chronic kidney disease

The causes of chronic kidney disease in our community in order of frequency are:

1 Diabetic nephropathy
2 Chronic glomerulonephritis
3 Artherosclerotic vascular disease (especially in the elderly)
4 Polycystic kidney disease
5 Reflux nephropathy
6 Hypertensive nephropathy,
7 Analgesic nephropathy
8 Chronic renal artery stenosis
9 Lupus nephritis
10 Vasculitides (particularly Wegener's granulomatosis, polyarteritis nodosa, microscopic polyarteritis)
11 Amyloidosis
12 Systemic sclerosis
13 Chronic urinary tract obstruction
14 Vasculopathy.

Examination

1 Look for a muddy brown complexion due to excess melanin deposition, and pallor due to anaemia. Confirm the pallor by looking at the mucosa. Examine the nails for brown discolouration. The patient may have generalised excoriations due to pruritus.

2 Perform a detailed cardiovascular examination, looking for evidence of fluid overload. Check the blood pressure and look for elevated JVP. Listen for cardiac murmurs (calcific stenosis of the aortic valve is not uncommon in this patient group) and pulmonary crepitations, and check for peripheral oedema.

3 Note abdominal scars of renal transplantation and palpate the transplanted kidney underneath.

4 If the patient is on haemodialysis, look for the form of vascular access. Note the vascular access device or the AV fistula (Fig 6.1). Check whether the fistula has a bruit. In patients on peritoneal dialysis, look for the Tenckhoff catheter (Fig 6.2) and for evidence of inflammation in the catheter site. These patients should be examined for any evidence of bacterial peritonitis (pus around the catheter entry point, tender or rigid abdomen, cloudy fluid in the bag).

5 Perform a detailed joint examination if the patient complains about arthritis (gouty arthritis can be associated with renal failure).

6 Perform a detailed neurological examination, as these patients can have a wide range of neurological signs.

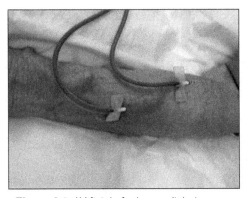

Figure 6.1 AV fistula for haemodialysis (courtesy of Brenton Shanahan and Paula McLeister)

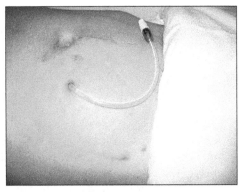

Figure 6.2 Peritoneal dialysis with Tenckhoff catheter (courtesy of Brenton Shanahan and Paula McLeister)

Investigations

1 Renal function indices and estimated glomerular filtration rate (eGFR)—persistent eGFR of less than 60 mL/min per 1.73 m² is defined as chronic kidney disease.
2 Kidney imaging studies (ultrasound/CT/MRI) and kidney biopsy.
3 Urine analysis—for osmolality and protein levels (albuminuria/microalbuminuria).
4 Electrolyte profile—especially Na, K, Ca and P levels and acid/base status.
5 Full blood count—looking for anaemia.
6 If the patient is anaemic it is important to check the serum iron studies (serum iron, total iron binding capacity, serum ferritin and transferring saturation), vitamin B_{12} and folate levels and examine the blood film for red cell morphology.
7 Most of the investigations discussed under 'acute renal failure' are also indicated in chronic renal failure.

Management

Management objectives in kidney disease are:
- to identify and remedy reversible causes
- to retard progression, and
- to prevent complications.

Early identification of the need for renal replacement, and institution of the same, is another important aspect of the management plan.

1 *Diet*—renal diet is an important aspect of the management of the renal failure patient, and the objective of the special diet is to retard the progression of the renal failure and minimise the complications of renal failure while maintaining adequate nutrition. Restriction of protein intake to 1 g/kg body weight has been shown to minimise the progression of renal failure in the diabetic as well as the non-diabetic patient with excessive proteinuria (> 3 g/day). Sodium and potassium intake should be restricted to 2 g per day to avoid salt loading and hyperkalaemia.
2 *Control blood pressure*—another remedy that has proven efficacy in retarding the progression of renal failure is the strict control of blood pressure, with a target blood pressure of 120/75 mmHg. This can be achieved with ACE inhibitor therapy, but alternative agents such as ARBs or calcium channel blockers can be used.

3   *Salt restriction and loop diuretics*—hypertension and volume overload can be managed with salt restriction and loop diuretics. Blood pressure control can be particularly difficult in these patients, and treatment with multiple antihypertensive agents may be necessary.

4   *Anaemia of chronic renal failure*—can be well managed with erythropoietin injections given subcutaneously once or twice a week. Darbepoetin alpha is a novel agent that can be used in this regard. Erythropoietin therapy should be commenced when the haematocrit falls below 30%. Common side effects of erythropoietin therapy are headache, encephalopathy and hypertension. Failure of haemoglobin to normalise despite adequate erythropoietin therapy would be due to haematinic deficiency (particularly iron, vitamin B_{12}, folate or vitamin C), hyperparathyroidism, sepsis, bleeding or malignancy. Iron deficiency is common among renal failure patients because their gastrointestinal iron absorption is usually impaired. Hence regular IV iron infusions should be carried out as guided by the serum iron indices. All renal failure patients should be supplemented with vitamin B complex (together with vitamin B_{12} and folate) and vitamin C daily.

5   *Renal osteodystrophy*—needs particular attention. Renal failure patients suffer from hyperphosphataemia and hypocalcaemia. To manage these electrolyte abnormalities, these patients should be placed on a low-phosphate diet and given phosphate binders such as calcium carbonate or calcium acetate to be taken with meals. They should also be given $1,25\text{-}(OH)_2D_3$ (calcitriol) supplements.

6   *Acidosis*—could become a difficult management problem, and the ideal treatment would be chronic oral sodium bicarbonate therapy. Patients can inadvertently be given a significant salt load with this therapy. Therefore, be alert to the development of pulmonary oedema and hypertension. Acidosis can manifest as hyperkalaemia, lethargy and dyspnoea.

7   *Cardiovascular status*—mortality of most patients with renal failure is due to a cardiovascular event. Therefore it is extremely important to investigate the cardiovascular status and the risk profile of the patient. Check the cholesterol level, fasting blood sugar level and Hb A_{1c} level. Perform an echocardiogram to study left ventricular wall anatomy, myocardial function and valvular anatomy and function. Perform a stress test or a perfusion study if the patient complains of ischaemic symptoms such as exertional angina.

8   *Team approach*—management of the patient with chronic renal failure should be done with the full participation of a qualified and experienced multidisciplinary team, including the physician (nephrologist), clinical nurse consultant or educator, dietitian, social worker, occupational therapist and a psychologist.

Renal osteodystrophy

Renal osteodystrophy is a specific condition about which some knowledge would be very useful. There are five broad types of abnormalities in bone metabolism associated with chronic renal failure that come to play in this situation:

*   hyperparathyroid bone disease, leading to excessive bone resorption and cyst formation
*   osteoporosis, with decreased bone mineral density
*   osteomalacia
*   osteosclerosis
*   adynamic bone disease, where bone formation as well as bone resorption is impaired.

Other complications of chronic renal failure

1 *Platelet dysfunction*—can cause a coagulopathy leading to bruising and epistaxis

2 *Dermatological problems*—such as pigmentation and pruritus. Pruritus is due to a combination of hypercalcaemia, hyperphosphataemia, hyperparathyroidism and iron deficiency.

3 *Gastrointestinal complications*—such as anorexia, nausea, vomiting, diarrhoea, peptic ulcer disease, acute pancreatitis and constipation

4 *Endocrinological problems*—such as amenorrhoea, erectile dysfunction and infertility

5 *Neurological complications*—such as peripheral neuropathy, carpal tunnel syndrome, confusion, coma and seizures

6 *Cardiovascular disorders*—such as pericarditis, hypertension, peripheral vascular disease, congestive cardiac failure and myocardial fibrosis

7 *Urinary symptoms*—such as nocturia and polyuria

8 *Gouty arthritis*—due to hyperuricaemia

9 *Hypercholesterolaemia, hypertriglyceridaemia* and *insulin resistance*

10 *Pancreatitis*

11 *Renal osteodystrophy*

To help remember these problems, they can be rearranged by forming the mnemonic: A B C D E P, which stands for:

A—anaemia, arthritis, acidosis, anorexia

B—blood pressure, bleeding, bone disease

C—cholesterol elevation, cardiac failure, constipation

D—planning dialysis

E—endocrine problems, entrapment neuropathy

P—pruritus, peripheral neuropathy, pancreatitis, peptic ulcer disease, platelet dysfunction.

Hyperparathyroidism of renal failure is a compensatory response to alterations in calcium and phosphate metabolism in chronic renal failure, and generally can be attributed to decreased absorption of calcium due to decreased production of $1,25(OH)D_3$ by the failing kidney, phosphate retention with diminishing GFR, and alteration in free calcium levels by the shifts in the calcium phosphate product. This results in decreased calcium levels and high phosphate levels, and both stimulate parathyroid hormone production—Ca by the calcium receptor and PO_4 by a direct effect on gene induction.

Secondary hyperparathyroidism causes osteitis fibrosis cystica due to the increased activity of the osteoclasts. This manifests as digital subperiosteal erosions and a 'pepper pot' appearance of the skull in X-ray images (Figs 6.3, 6.4). Hyperparathyroidism also causes osteosclerosis. Long-standing secondary hyperparathyroidism evolves into tertiary hyperparathyroidism, leading to semi-autonomous hypersecretion of parathyroid hormone that is related to the volume of the gland. Osteomalacia is now rarely seen, because of the reduced use of aluminium-based phosphate binder. Adynamic bone disease is now increasing and, while the cause is yet to be fully determined, it seems that overtreatment of hyperparathyroidism may be a factor (i.e. some degree of hyperparathyroidism seems to give protection from adynamic bone disease).

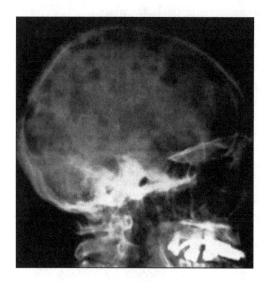

Figure 6.3 X-ray of pepper pot skull (reprinted from Kumar V, Abbas A K, Fausto N 2005 *Robbins and Cotran Pathologic Basis of Disease*, 7th edn. Elsevier, p 679, fig 14.15)

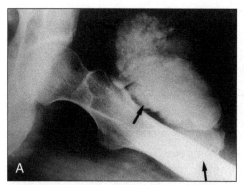
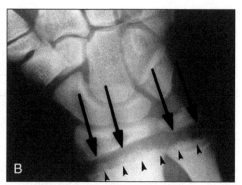

Figure 6.4 X-ray of renal osteodystrophy (A) Calcified 'tumoral' paraarticular masses (arrows) (B) Rickets-like changes in renal osteodystrophy. Widening of the physes (arrows) and cupping, widening, disorganisation and demineralisation of the metaphyses (arrowheads) (reprinted from Jevtic V 2003 Imaging of renal osteodystrophy. *European Journal of Radiology* 46:11)

Dialysis planning

Renal replacement is usually begun when the GFR falls below 10 mL/min. This can be timed and projected by plotting 1/(serum creatinine in mmol/L) against time in months. When the level falls below 1.3 mL/min, dialysis is usually commenced. A multidisciplinary team approach (as described above) is important in dialysis planning.

Principles of renal replacement are:

- daily weighing
- regular evaluation of the serum electrolyte profile and the blood pH
- restriction of fluid intake
- monitoring of dialysis adequacy by urea reduction methods.

Be ready to discuss issues related to placing the patient on the transplant list and issues of immunosuppression (further discussed in Long case 4).

Indications for renal replacement therapy

The absolute and acute indications for renal replacement therapy are:

- Hyperkalaemia with $K^+ > 6.5$ (or rapidly rising K^+ levels) not responding to medical measures
- Uraemic pericarditis
- Uraemic pleurisy
- Uraemic encephalopathy of any form and acute uraemic neuropathy
- Bleeding diathesis secondary to severe uraemia—this is also described as an urgent and absolute indication
- Drug overdose—if the agent is amenable to dialysis
- Fluid overload resistant to diuretics
- Metabolic disturbances—including metabolic acidosis with pH < 7.1 not responding to other medical measures (others include hypercalcaemia, hypocalcaemia and hyperphosphataemia)
- Blood urea > 40.0 mmol/L tends to automatically trigger dialysis in an ICU setting, but not on the ward
- Persistent and intractable nausea and vomiting

Nephrotic syndrome

- Severe proteinuria
- Hypoalbuminaemia
- Peripheral oedema
- Hyperlipidaemia
- Thromboembolic propensity

07
Oncology

COMMON MALIGNANCIES

A good grasp of the basic principles of cancer management is expected of all candidates. Identification of common malignancies, staging protocols, evaluation of prognosis and issues of therapy are the major areas of interest.

Approach to the patient

History

Ask about:

- initial presenting symptoms
- diagnostic investigations that have been carried out
- treatment received so far
- the patient's risk factor profile
- exposure to carcinogens (quantification of the exposure may be necessary)
- past medical history (ulcerative colitis in patients with colonic carcinoma and cirrhosis in hepatic carcinoma)
- previous history of malignancy
- relevant family history
- relevant social habits (smoking, alcohol consumption, sexual promiscuity, sun exposure, asbestos exposure etc).

Treatment-related cancer is becoming common. Ask about immunosuppressive therapy, hormonal agents, past exposure to chemotherapeutic agents and exposure to radiation.

Enquire about chemotherapy, radiotherapy and surgery for the current diagnosis of cancer. Relevant information about chemotherapy includes the agents that have been used (if known), number of cycles the patient has had and is yet to have, any side effects experienced and the response to therapy. Ask about early side effects such as hypersensitivity, nausea, vomiting and oral mucositis, and how these side effects were managed. Other side effects such as hair loss, sepsis due to immunosuppression, debility, fatigue as well as organ-specific toxicity (pulmonary toxicity, hepatotoxicity, cardiotoxicity and bladder toxicity) should be enquired into.

Ask about sperm or ova harvesting in the young patient who has been treated with agents having gonadal toxicity. Ask about adverse effects associated with other therapeutic modalities, such as radiotherapy and surgery. Enquire about the patient's insight into his or her condition and what expectations they have for the future.

Ask about pain and how it is managed. Ask whether the patient is depressed. Try to gain an insight into their social support network. Check how the patient is coping and whether any professional psychological help has been received.

Examination

1 Look for cachexia, alopecia, cushingoid body habitus, flat affect and any vascular access devices (e.g. Hickman catheter).
2 Look for radiation dermatitis, radiation burns, radiation tattoos (markings of the radiotherapy field) and surgical scars.
3 Look for organomegaly, particularly in the abdomen, lymphadenopathy and bone tenderness.
4 Define all mass lesions by quoting the exact measurements. With mass lesions, describe the consistency, fixation, mobility of skin above the lesion, temperature and shape.
5 Perform a detailed neurological examination to exclude deficit due to cord compression, cerebral metastases, paraneoplastic phenomena and neurotoxic chemotherapy.
6 Look for evidence of pneumonitis or pulmonary fibrosis in those who have received pulmonary toxic agents, such as cyclophosphamide or busulphan, as well as those who have received thoracic radiotherapy.
7 Check for evidence of cardiac failure in those who have been treated with cardiotoxic agents, such as the anthracyclines.

Investigations

Investigations should be tailored according to the clinical presentation, location of the malignancy, type of malignancy and the spread. Radiological imaging (X-ray, CT or MRI scan), basic blood tests (full blood count, electrolyte profile), invasive tests (e.g. endoscopy), organ-specific functional tests and tumour markers are other investigations of relevance.

Imaging tests help define the tumour and the staging process. Biopsy and anatomical pathology is important for defining the diagnosis and grading the cancer.

The candidate should be able to discuss the different investigations that need to be performed in the initial diagnostic work-up as well as in the staging process of different cancers.

Curative and palliative management

In discussing therapeutic options, the candidate should demonstrate a good working knowledge of chemotherapy, radiotherapy and surgical management. The candidate should be thoroughly familiar with the different means of monitoring for chemotherapy toxicity and the preventive and remedial steps that have to be taken.

Assess the patient's performance status, as this has significant influence on the choice of therapy. Performance status is usually described according to the Eastern Cooperative Oncology Group (ECOG) classification system (see box overleaf) or Karnofsky Performance Scale. Patients who score poorly on these scales have poor tolerance to chemotherapy, and consideration should be given to the palliative options. It is important to possess some knowledge of the principles of palliative care, pain management and care of the terminally ill. Suitable patients should be referred to a palliative care service early in the management. Patients with terminal cancer should be referred to a community outreach palliative care service, which would work in liaison with a hospice facility. Hospice care is indicated for patients living in the community or discharged to the community but who require ongoing nursing care and have a life expectancy of less than 6 months. Following is a discussion on the different cancer types likely to be encountered in the long case setting.

ECOG (Eastern Cooperative Oncology Group) Performance Scale

0 Active with no restriction of performance.

1 Ambulatory and able to attend to light work activity. Unable to carry out strenuous physical activity.

2 Can manage self-care but unable to attend to any form of work activity. Ambulatory for more than 50% of the time while awake.

3 Can manage only limited amount of self-care. Bed-bound for more than 50% of the time while awake.

4 Disabled, with complete inability to attend to self-care. Completely bed bound.

(Adapted from Oken M M, Creech R H, Tormey D C et al 1982 Toxicity and response criteria of the Eastern Cooperative Oncology Group. *American Journal of Clinical Oncology* 5(6):649–655)

BREAST CANCER

Case vignette

A 35-year-old woman presents with a painless, hard and immobile lump in her left breast. She has a family history of breast cancer, with her mother having been treated with mastectomy at the age of 56. Since the initial presentation she has had multiple tests and doctors have planned curative treatment. After definitive primary surgery she has had one cycle of chemotherapy so far. She has experienced distressing side effects and is currently feeling very debilitated and depressed. She has taken 3 months off from her job as a computer analyst and she has a 3-year-old daughter who is cared for by her partner.

1 What is the best approach to the management of this case?
2 What investigations are critical to decide on the appropriate plan of management?
3 How is she coping currently?
4 What further information is required to assess her prognosis?

The current screening recommendation for breast cancer surveillance is for all women between the ages of 50 and 70 to have a mammogram every 2 years. A discovery of a suspicious lump on palpation should be followed up with mammography, to further assess its anatomy and pattern of calcification, and ultrasonography, to define its consistency (cystic or solid). This should be followed up with fine-needle aspiration biopsy or core biopsy to obtain a tissue diagnosis. A thorough physical examination should be carried out to exclude any additional lumps in either breast, axillary lymphadenopathy, lymphadenopathy elsewhere, hepatomegaly and bone tenderness. If the lesion is confined to the breast alone, no staging is necessary, or minimal staging is carried out with chest X-ray and liver function tests (especially looking for an elevation of the alkaline phosphatase level) for apparent early disease. If there is evidence of significant nodal involvement at surgery, further staging investigations should be carried out. These include a bone scan and an ultrasound or CT scan of the liver, in addition to chest X-ray and liver function tests.

Management

Management of localised breast cancer is dependent upon the patient's age, menopausal status, tumour size, axillary lymph node status, hormone receptor status and expression of protein HER2. Localised breast cancer with positive expression of protein HER2 benefits from treatment with humanised monoclonal antibody trastuzumab (Herceptin®). Patients with axillary-node-positive breast cancer should receive adjuvant systemic therapy upon complete local resection of the primary tumour. Premenopausal women have low rates of hormone receptor/protein-positive tumour, and therefore have better response to adjuvant chemotherapy. Older/postmenopausal patients are more likely to express hormone receptors and therefore be more responsive to hormonal therapy; however, they are also less likely to respond to chemotherapy.

Early-stage disease

Locally confined disease can be managed with breast-conserving surgery and radiotherapy, or modified radical mastectomy. Adjuvant therapy in early-stage disease may be either systemic chemotherapy or hormonal therapy. Treatment with adjuvant chemotherapy is dependent on the lymph node status, tumour size, histology of the tumour, hormone receptor status, and age and menopausal status of the patient.

Premenopausal patient
- *Hormone-receptor-negative tumour* is treated with adjuvant chemotherapy. The agents of preference include taxanes and anthracyclines. Trastuzumab can be given together with cytotoxics in node-positive tumours; however, when combined with anthracyclines, significant cardiotoxicity should be watched for.
- *Hormone-receptor-positive tumour* is treated with chemotherapy together with ovarian ablation or tamoxifen for a period of 5 years. With tamoxifen therapy it is important to be vigilant for ocular and endometrial side effects.

Postmenopausal patient
- *Hormone-receptor-negative tumour* is treated with adjuvant chemotherapy or radiotherapy.
- *Hormone-receptor-positive tumour* is treated with aromatase inhibitors or tamoxifen with or without cytotoxic chemotherapy. Follow-up after curative therapy for early-stage disease includes regular physical examination together with yearly mammography.
- *HER2-positive disease* is treated with trastuzumab.

Advanced-stage disease

Advanced-stage cancer could be locally advanced large tumours, those with significant nodal or cutaneous spread, recurrent cancer or metastatic disease. A decision to treat aggressively in a patient with good performance status who has locally advanced tumour would require multimodality combination therapy. This would include induction chemotherapy followed by loco-regional therapy in the form of surgery and/or radiotherapy. Inflammatory breast cancer is another form of locally advanced breast cancer that requires aggressive systemic and loco-regional therapy. High-dose chemotherapy with autologous stem cell transplantation has not shown any significant benefit over conventional therapy, and should therefore be considered only in the setting of a clinical trial. Younger patients with oestrogen-receptor-positive disease may benefit from oophorectomy or chemical castration with luteinising hormone receptor agonists. Other options of therapy in metastatic disease include tamoxifen, palliative chemotherapy or combination therapy.

For the older patient with receptor-positive metastatic disease, the management options include tamoxifen, aromatase inhibitor therapy or single-agent palliative chemotherapy with an agent such as mitozantrone. The postmenopausal patient with receptor-negative metastatic disease may benefit from palliative chemotherapy. Radiotherapy is indicated in this setting for pain management.

Screening of relatives

Screening of other first-degree female relatives of a young patient with breast cancer is a contentious issue and may be a subject of discussion at the examination. The implications of such screening should be discussed with the family members and the choice should be offered, if appropriate.

The cosmetic effects of mastectomy may be distressing, and options available to address such situations (e.g. breast reconstruction surgery) should be offered to the patient.

CARCINOMA OF UNKNOWN PRIMARY

Case vignette

A 58-year-old man has been hospitalised with fevers, rigors and severe mucositis. He has presented initially with a newly discovered lump above his left clavicle, which has grown in size rapidly. Upon biopsy, a diagnosis of cancer has been made and he has had multiple further tests. He has been told that the primary site of his cancer remains unknown, despite extensive investigation. He has had two cycles of chemotherapy so far, and has just completed the second cycle 4 days ago. He has recently retired from his job and has been planning to move back to Europe, where the rest of his family live.

1 Discuss how you would plan his diagnostic work-up as per his initial presentation.

2 Discuss the possible primary sites that could be associated with his presentation.

3 Discuss your approach to the clinical picture associated with his current presentation.

4 What impact has his condition had on his life? Describe how you could help him.

An occult primary malignancy can manifest as metastases discovered incidentally for the first time in the lymph nodes, bone, liver or lung. Diagnosis is made by biopsy of the lesion. Further investigations to ascertain the origin of the tumour are directed at excluding potentially curable disease and deciding on appropriate treatment for symptomatic disease. Using the relatively novel techniques of immunohistochemistry, molecular genetics and electron microscopy, more precise characterisation of the origin of the tumour may be possible. Some immunoperoxidase tumour markers that help define the possible primary site of the cancer include vimentin for mesenchymal sarcoma, desmin for rhabdomyosarcoma, oestrogen or progesterone receptor status for breast cancer, prostate-specific antigen (PSA) for prostate cancer, S-100 or HMB-45 for malignant melanoma, and cytokeratin for squamous cell carcinoma.

The level of tumour differentiation has significant diagnostic and management implications. Elevated levels of tumour markers in the blood may give further clues to the origin of the tumour. Some such markers are CA125 for ovarian cancer, CA19-9 for cholangiocarcinoma, alpha-fetoprotein (AFP) for testicular carcinoma and hepatoma, and human chorionic gonadotrophin (hCG) for testicular carcinoma and choriocarcinoma. But the usefulness of these markers in the initial diagnostic process is questionable. They are more useful for the monitoring of tumour response to treatment.

Adenocarcinoma at different levels of differentiation is the most common pathological diagnosis in patients presenting with carcinoma of unknown primary site. Commonly, the origin will be in the lungs or the gastrointestinal tract, but an exhaustive search for the primary site is often not useful.

In the assessment process, in addition to a thorough history, physical examination and basic haematological and biochemical tests, PSA level should be checked in the male patient and a mammography should be performed in the female patient. All patients should have urine analysis and a chest X-ray performed. Other investigations should be performed as guided by the patient's symptoms and signs. Most patients with this condition have a very poor prognosis, with life expectancy limited to a few months. However, some patients may respond favourably to chemotherapy, so this option should be given serious consideration.

Poorly differentiated carcinoma is the next most common pathology identified in patients presenting with carcinoma of unknown primary site. The patient may be relatively young and present with rapid progression of the disease. In addition to routine haematological and biochemical investigations, the patient should have a chest X-ray as well as CT of the thorax and abdomen, looking for mediastinal and retroperitoneal disease. Serum levels of hCG and AFP should be assessed to exclude germ cell tumour in the young male patient. These patients always warrant a trial of chemotherapy, as some (mostly those treated with platinum-based or taxane-based combined chemotherapy regimens) may show significant disease response and improvement of the clinical status.

CARCINOMA OF THE PROSTATE

Case vignette

A 61-year-old man has been admitted to the hospital with dyspnoea. He has a background history of acute myocardial infarction and significant heart failure. He was also diagnosed with prostate carcinoma 1 year ago and has been treated with radiotherapy. He has experienced multiple local complications from this. He has been told that he had localised disease and has been cured of his malignancy. Examination reveals stony dullness all over his left hemithorax posteriorly. Chest X-ray shows a complete white-out of the left lung.

1 Discuss his prognosis, taking into account the current clinical findings, his cardiac condition and the possible differential diagnoses.
2 How would you monitor for recurrent disease in prostate cancer. In cases of recurrence, what management is optimal?
3 What complications could he have had with radiotherapy?
4 What is the role of androgen blockade in prostate cancer management?

Approach to the patient

History

An older patient with multiple medical problems may also have a diagnosis of prostate cancer. In such a situation it is important to identify the relative importance of the prostate cancer in the patient's clinical context. Ask about the initial diagnosis and the presenting symptoms. Some patients may present with prostatic symptoms such as frequency, urgency, hesitancy, urinary retention, or with urinary tract infection.

Enquire about the biopsy process and complications such as haematuria. Enquire about the different treatment protocols the patient has had, including prostatectomy. Ask about side effects such as incontinence, impotency and the management of them. Patients may complain about refractory bone pain. Check the patient's mood and also the support structure that is in place. Ask how the patient is monitored for recurrence with regular assessment of serum PSA level.

Examination

Initial diagnosis is made by digital per rectum examination or measurement of serum PSA levels (case finding). In the physical examination look for surgical scars and radiotherapy tattoos. Do not forget to look for gynaecomastia and bone tenderness.

At the first presentation on clinical diagnosis, a transrectal biopsy is performed for histological diagnosis; however, this has limited sensitivity and therefore a series of core biopsies from multiple sites is preferred. Serum PSA level should be assessed in all patients, as its level correlates well with the extent of the disease. Other investigations in this setting include renal function indices, looking for any obstructive nephropathy, and IV pyelography, looking for irregularity of the prostatic urethra and dilatation of the renal pelvi-caliceal system. Staging investigations include, in addition to serum

PSA level, pelvic CT scan, looking for local spread, and a three-phase radioisotope bone scan, looking for occult bony metastases. Staging is done according to the TNM (*t*umour, lymph *n*odes, *m*etastases) classification system.

Investigations

1 Full blood count, electrolyte profile and renal function indices
2 Serum PSA level
3 Transrectal ultrasound
4 Intravenous pyelogram
5 Abdominal and pelvic CT (for staging)/MRI
6 Chest X-ray
7 Radioisotope bone scan
8 Core biopsy and staging biopsy
9 Most prostatic tumours are adenocarcinomas. Histological grading of the tumour has significant prognostic implications. Grading is interpreted according to the Gleason score (see box).

Gleason histological grade of prostate carcinoma

Grade 1—Well-differentiated tumour with a uniform glandular pattern
Grade 2—Well-differentiated tumour with glandular tissue of varying shape and type
Grade 3—Moderately differentiated tumour
Grade 4—Poorly differentiated tumour
Grade 5—Very poorly differentiated tumour with minimal or no glandular tissue formation

---

Management
Early disease

Clinical as well as pathological staging will determine the appropriate therapeutic approach. Other factors that influence the management approach include the patient's functional capacity, age, other comorbidities and patient expectations.

Management of carcinoma of the prostate is complicated because opinions vary widely among the experts. The treatment options include radical prostatectomy, radical radiation therapy or active surveillance. However, most believe that localised disease should be treated aggressively with a curative intent. Radical radiotherapy, radical surgery or a combination is indicated for patients with disease confined to the prostate within the capsule with no lymph node metastases. Radiotherapy could be administered as external beam or brachytherapy. Complications associated with radiotherapy include bladder irritation, proctitis, impotence, diarrhoea, dysuria and severe perineal cutaneous reaction and, in the long term, urethral stricture formation. Complications of radical surgery include permanent impotence (in 90% of patients), urinary incontinence and, very rarely, rectovesical fistula formation. There is an operative mortality of less than 5%.

Active surveillance is preferred in elderly patients with multiple other medical problems. This process involves digital rectal examination and serum PSA assessment at regular intervals (usually every 3 months initially) and occasional re-biopsy. Detection of an abnormality indicating progression of disease would warrant active treatment.

Advanced disease

Locally advanced disease and recurrent disease together with metastatic disease have a worse prognosis. Palliative management of widespread disease is with androgen deprivation therapy and radiotherapy for painful bony metastases. Androgen deprivation also helps reduce bone pain and also effect some primary and secondary tumour regression. Even hormone-responsive tumours may become hormone refractory after a period of time (usually within 2 years). Attempts at managing hormone-resistant disease can be made with palliative radiotherapy, IV strontium-89 and chemotherapy with mitozantrone.

Hormonal therapy is the option for those not suitable for radical therapy and those with metastatic disease. This involves surgical or pharmacological castration together with antiandrogen therapy. The objective of this form of therapy is total androgen blockade (to block gonadal as well as adrenal androgen production). Pharmacological castration is achieved by the administration of luteinising hormone-releasing hormone agonist agents such as luprelide or goserelin. Concurrent administration of a non-steroidal antiandrogen drug such as flutamide (also bicalutamide/nilutamide) helps prevent the exacerbation of bone pain associated with the commencement of the luteinising hormone agonist. Cyproterone acetate is a steroidal antiandrogen that has also shown to be beneficial in this regard. With this form of palliative therapy, the patient's survival could be expected to be around 3 years.

Hormonal therapy has side effects that need to be discussed with the patient. Many patients suffer from sexual dysfunction, gynaecomastia and hot flushes. Counselling the patient as well as the partner and offering support is important. Another significant side effect is osteoporosis and pathological fracture, which needs preventive therapy with vitamin D, calcium supplements and bisphosphonates.

Patients with hormone-therapy-refractory advanced prostate cancer may benefit from antiandrogen withdrawal, antifungal agent ketoconazole, corticosteroids or chemotherapy with docetaxel-based regimens.

CARCINOMA OF THE LUNG

Case vignette

A 69-year-old man presents with fevers, rigors and a productive cough. He reports significant weight loss over the preceding 3 months. He also complains of dry mouth, erectile dysfunction and progressive severe proximal muscle weakness. He has a history of chronic airways limitation and intermittent claudication. He has a significant smoking history. He also consumes 2–4 standard drinks of alcohol each day. On examination he has bronchial breath sounds in the left upper zone and a fixed inspiratory and expiratory wheeze. His sputum mug shows purulent sputum with large amounts of fresh blood.

1   **What is the most likely diagnosis?**
2   **What investigations would be helpful in the confirmation of the diagnosis?**
3   **What are this man's main problems currently, and how would you propose to address those?**
4   **What is the significance of his neuromuscular complaints?**

A long case patient with a significant smoking history may present with chronic airways limitation, ischaemic heart disease and peripheral vascular disease, together with a recent diagnosis of lung cancer. As with prostate cancer, an important basic knowledge of the management of lung cancer will help you identify the stage of disease and decide on the relevant management plan.

Investigations

For the purpose of diagnosis of lung cancer, the following tests should be performed:
1   Chest X-ray
2   Flexible fibreoptic bronchoscopy and biopsy of the lesion
3   Fine-needle aspiration biopsy of the lesion if it is not accessible by bronchoscopy
4   Thoracoscopic or open biopsy of the lesion, if the above methods are not feasible
5   Sputum cytology may be useful, but usually its sensitivity is very low.

The following additional investigations should be carried out for the purpose of staging the disease:
1   CT of the chest, abdomen and head
2   Three-phase nuclear medicine bone scan
3   Positron emission tomography (PET), where available—this has proved a very useful tool in the staging process.

Management

Non-small-cell lung cancer

For non-small-cell cancer of stages I and II, where the disease is confined to the lung or has spread only to ipsilateral peribronchial or hilar lymph nodes, surgical intervention in the form of lobectomy or pneumonectomy is indicated as a curative measure. Upon curative therapy, patients need surveillance every 3 months, with clinical assessment and a chest X-ray if indicated, for 2 years, and thereafter every 6 months for up to 5 years. Screening should continue annually thereafter.

In stage IIIA disease, where there is involvement of the mediastinal or subcarinal lymph nodes or there is spread to the chest wall, pleura or pericardium, management involves a combination of surgery, radiotherapy and chemotherapy. Locally advanced disease (IIIB) is usually treated with radiotherapy and chemotherapy.

For stage IV disease with systemic metastases, treatment objectives are best supportive care, palliation and prolongation of life. The patient's performance status is crucial in the choice of best palliative modality. Double- or single-agent palliative chemotherapy is indicated, based on performance status. Patients with better performance status benefit from doublet chemotherapy (cisplatin with another agent). With this therapy, life expectancy can be marginally improved, with some preservation of quality of life.

Chemotherapeutic agents that can be used in this situation include cisplatin, taxanes, gemcitabine, vinorelbine or camphothecin.

Small-cell lung cancer

Small-cell lung cancer behaves in a very aggressive manner—it has a rapid doubling time and a propensity to spread widely within a very short period of time. Small-cell lung cancer is staged as either *limited disease*, where the disease can be encompassed in a single radiation field, or *extensive disease*, where there is metastatic disease or the involvement of the contralateral supraclavicular nodes, pleural effusion or pericardial effusion. This tumour is highly responsive to chemotherapy as well as radiotherapy. However, terminal and therapy-refractory recurrence happens within the first 2 years. Limited-stage disease is usually treated with a platinum-based agent and etoposide, where the life expectancy is expected to increase to about 18 months. The untreated patient has an average life expectancy of 9–12 months. In addition, the patient should be offered mediastinal radiotherapy and prophylactic cranial irradiation. Metastatic disease, too, can be treated with palliative gentle chemotherapy, but the prognosis is usually grave. Many patients may also manifest paraneoplastic syndromes with neurological features (e.g. Lambert-Eaton myasthenic syndrome), SIADH or Cushing's syndrome.

CANCER OF THE COLON

Case vignette

A 74-year-old female presents with progressive exertional dyspnoea, weight loss and prolonged constipation followed by watery diarrhoea over a period of 2 months. She has also noted blood in her bowel motions. She has been well until the development of the current symptoms. She is not on any regular medications and denies any allergies or significant past medical history. She is the main carer of her husband, who has progressive Alzheimer's disease.

1 What are the possible differential diagnoses in this case?
2 What investigations would be indicated initially?
3 What social issues are of significance in this case, and what is your proposed plan of action to address these?

Approach to the patient

History

Colon cancer is a common malignancy and a leading cause of death. Ask about the initial presentation. Most patients present with abdominal discomfort of varying degree, altered bowel habits (chronic constipation followed by spurious diarrhoea), melaena and per rectal bleeding. The patient may also have constitutional symptoms of malignancy, such as weight loss, weakness and lethargy, and features secondary to anaemia. Significantly advanced disease can present with bowel obstruction, bowel perforation or neurological symptoms due to the spread to the pelvic nerves. Advanced cancer can also present with regional lymphadenopathy or hepatic metastasis. Check for any family history of colon or other cancer. Familial adenomatous polyposis and hereditary non-polyposis colon cancer are genetic risk factors for colon cancer with an onset at a younger age. A history of ulcerative colitis is a definite risk factor for colonic cancer. Other risk factors include high alcohol consumption, obesity and diabetes. Ask about staging investigations and treatment so far. Ask how the patient manages the colostomy if relevant.

Examination
Look for evidence of generalised wasting, cachexia and features of anaemia. Perform a thorough abdominal examination and clearly define any mass lesions by location, magnitude, mobility and consistency. Exclude hepatomegaly and ascites. Look for lymphadenopathy by drainage zone. Look for obvious or occult blood in the rectal examination. Look for pigmented lesions in the buccal mucosa that may suggest Peutz-Jeghers syndrome, which is a risk factor for colon cancer. Look in the colostomy site for evidence of inflammation or infection.

Investigations
1 Full blood count, electrolyte profile, liver function tests (especially alkaline phosphatase (ALP) level), iron studies
2 Colonoscopy and biopsy/double contrast barium enema/sigmoidoscopy
3 Transrectal ultrasound—for evaluation of the degree of local invasion and local lymph node spread
4 Fine-needle aspiration biopsy—for detection of lymph node spread
5 CT scan of abdomen and pelvis
6 MRI or PET scans—may help in more occult disease
7 Chest X-ray—looking for metastasis
8 Serum carcinoembryonic antigen (CEA) and CA19-9 levels—particularly useful in prognostication of new diagnoses and monitoring of recurrence
9 Supine and erect abdominal X-rays in case of perforation/obstruction
10 Intraoperative evaluation for metastasis

Management
Management depends on the tumour stage (see box). Locally confined disease can be treated with surgery (hemicolectomy) with a curative intent. Isolated liver or pulmonary metastasis too may be amenable to curative surgery. Node-positive disease benefits from adjuvant chemotherapy with 5-fluorouracil (5-FU) or a combination of 5-FU with leucovorin and oxaliplatin. Neoadjuvant chemotherapy (with 5-FU) and radiotherapy has a potential role in rectal carcinoma prior to curative resection. Metastatic and advanced cancer may benefit from palliative surgery and/or chemotherapy.

Dukes' staging classification

Stage A Localised to mucosa or submucosa
Stage B Spread to muscularis but no lymph node spread
Stage C Lymph node spread
Stage D Distant metastasis

CANCER OF THE HEAD AND NECK

Cancers of the head and neck are common among heavy smokers and those who abuse alcohol. They are staged according to the TNM staging system.

Early-stage disease (stage 1 and stage 2) can be treated with radiotherapy or surgery. Decision on the therapeutic modality is influenced by the performance status of the patient and the anatomical site. Where preservation of the architecture and organ function is required, radiotherapy may be preferred over surgery.

Advanced-stage disease (stage 3 or stage 4) should be treated with concurrent chemotherapy, radiotherapy and/or surgery in combination. Chemotherapy agents commonly used in the treatment of cancer of the head and neck are cisplatin and 5-FU.

All patients with cancer of the head and neck should have panendoscopy performed, to look for other primary lesions in the vicinity.

ANAEMIA

Case vignette

An 81-year-old female is admitted to the coronary care unit with crescendo angina. She also complains of early satiety, nocturia and pedal oedema. She reports a 10 kg weight loss over 3 months. She has a background history of rheumatoid arthritis. She is currently managed on a non-steroidal antiinflammatory agent and aspirin. On examination she is hypertensive with a pulse rate of 100 bpm. She has significant conjunctival and palmar crease pallor. The ECG shows evidence of left ventricular hypertrophy and diffuse ST segment depression, together with T wave inversion in the inferior leads. Her blood tests reveal an Hb level of 7 g/dL.

1 **What are the possible precipitating factors of her coronary ischaemia?**
2 **What is your diagnostic work-up?**
3 **What may be the causative factors behind her anaemia?**
4 **How would you plan this patient's management—short term and long term?**

Approach to the patient

An Hb level of < 13 g/dL in men and < 12 g/dL in women is considered anaemic in common practice.

History

Ask about:

- the symptoms at presentation—patients may present with constitutional symptoms such as lethargy, malaise, exertional dyspnoea, fatigue or gastrointestinal blood loss in the form of haematemesis or melaena
- how long the patient has had anaemia—if they have had it since childhood, the likely diagnosis of a haemoglobinopathy should be considered

- easy bruising, uncontrolled blood loss, large joint arthropathy and excessive bleeding post-surgery—features suggesting a coagulation disorder/bleeding diathesis
- other symptoms that would help identify the aetiology, such as change in bowel habits or weight loss suggesting colonic cancer, abdominal discomfort, bloating, anorexia and weight loss of gastric carcinoma, abdominal pain suggesting peptic ulcer disease, night sweats, weight loss and fevers suggesting lymphoma.

Take a detailed medication history, looking for evidence of therapy with non-steroidal antiinflammatory agents, sulfur-containing medications (haemolysis) and myelosuppressive agents. Enquire about alcoholism and general nutrition. Check whether the patient has had any transfusions and whether there have been any adverse transfusion reactions or transmission of blood-borne infections such as hepatitis C and HIV. It is also useful to know the patient's blood group.

Examination

Look for features of anaemia such as palmar crease pallor, conjunctival pallor, tachypnoea, tachycardia and evidence of high-output cardiac failure. Look for signs that suggest the likely aetiology (see box): characteristic copper-hue pigmentation (the combined effect of melanin deposition, icterus and pallor) of the thalassaemia patient with malar hyperplasia and often stunted growth, pigmented lesions in the mouth (Peutz-Jeghers syndrome), scleral icterus (haemolysis), epigastric tenderness (peptic ulcer disease), abdominal distension or mass lesions, splenomegaly, hepatomegaly, bony tenderness (malignancy), lymphadenopathy (lymphoma), impaired cognition, peripheral neuropathy and dorsal column signs (vitamin B_{12} deficiency), arthropathy (anaemia of chronic disease or gastro-intestinal blood loss secondary to NSAID use), slate-grey pigmentation, peripheral arterio-venous fistula, vascular access device or abdominal Tenckhoff catheter (renal anaemia).

Causes of anaemia

1 Bleeding (acute/chronic)
2 Haematinic deficiency (iron, vitamin B_{12}, folate, vitamin C)
3 Haemolysis (immune/mechanical/toxic/paroxysmal nocturnal haemoglobinuria)
4 Chronic inflammation
5 Chronic renal failure
6 Bone marrow infiltration
7 Bone marrow suppression (e.g. cytotoxics, carbimazole, gold, irradiation)
8 Sepsis (e.g. malaria, *Clostridium welchii*)
9 Marrow aplasia
10 Myelodysplasia
11 Myelofibrosis
12 Haemoglobinopathies (sickle cell disease, thalassaemia)
13 Sideroblastic anaemia

Anaemia in the long case patient is often multifactorial. The diagnostic work-up should include a comprehensive battery of tests as guided by the clinical setting. Iron deficiency secondary to chronic blood loss, commonly from the gastrointestinal tract, is the most common cause of anaemia in this group of patients. Other differential diagnoses encountered commonly include anaemia of chronic disease, vitamin B_{12} and folate deficiency, myelodysplasia, aplastic anaemia, sideroblastic anaemia, myelosuppression, chronic renal failure, myelofibrosis and chronic alcoholism (due to a combination of bone marrow toxicity of alcohol, iron and folate deficiency and gastrointestinal bleeding).

Investigations

Investigation of anaemia should be guided by the clinical picture. The more common conditions should be excluded first. Relevant investigations in the anaemic patient include:

1 Full blood count, mean cell volume, reticulocyte count/haematocrit and blood film—to assess the severity of the anaemia and to ascertain the red cell morphology. Also look at the white cell count and the platelet count.

Blood picture: Patients with anaemia of chronic disease usually have normocytic, normochromic anaemia. Those with iron deficiency, thallasaemia or sideroblastic anaemia have microcytic, hypochromic anaemia. Microcytic, hypochromic anaemia is also seen in myelodysplastic syndrome.

2 Coagulation profile—international normalised ratio (INR), activated partial thromboplastin time (APTT), bleeding time and clotting time, to exclude a bleeding diathesis
3 Haematinics—iron studies in the form of serum ferritin, serum iron and transferrin saturation, to exclude iron deficiency
4 Serum vitamin B_{12} and serum and red cell folate levels
5 Haemolytic screen—including blood film, serum haptoglobin level, serum lactate dehydrogenase (LDH) level, serum bilirubin level, the direct Coombs' test, haemoglobin electrophoresis, Heinz body preparation and, if indicated, the cold agglutinin test
6 Erythrocyte sedimentation rate (ESR)—looking for evidence of chronic inflammation and paraproteinaemia
7 Electrolyte profile and the renal function indices—to exclude renal failure as a cause
8 Erythropoietin levels
9 Thyroid function tests—to exclude hypothyroidism, which can cause a macrocytic anaemia
10 Chest X-ray—to exclude chronic pulmonary disease and pulmonary malignances
11 Serum protein electrophoresis and immunoelectrophoresis—to exclude any paraproteinaemia
12 If all non-invasive and minimally invasive tests do not help in the correct diagnosis, the next investigation is a bone marrow biopsy with both aspiration and trephine.

Management

Management depends on severity (level of Hb) and the patient's cardiopulmonary status. Initial steps include identification and correction of reversible, causative factors and replacement of blood with packed cell transfusions and/or the supplementation of haematinics as indicated.

As a general rule, blood transfusion is indicated if Hb is < 7 g/dL. If Hb remains > 10 g/dL, transfusion should be considered only if there is a compelling clinical indication such as precipitation of coronary ischaemia or heart failure.

Gastrointestinal bleeding warrants endoscopy (colonoscopy or gastroscopy) to identify the exact location of the bleeding and for possible therapy or biopsy of suspicious lesions. If gastroscopy and colonoscopy fail to identify the source of bleeding, capsule endoscopy may be warranted, to look for a small intestinal focus.

Patients with chronic renal failure need iron supplementation and at times may need IV iron infusion. Patients with kidney disease may benefit from therapy with erythropoietin or darbapoietin.

It is recommended that patients with chronic kidney disease be maintained at an Hb level of 11 g/dL or more.

Patients with anaemia of chronic disease improve when the underlying disease is well treated. Haematinic replacement and therapy with erythropoietin or darbapoietin is also indicated in this group.

Management of anaemia due to cytotoxic chemotherapy in patients with non-myeloid malignancies is similar to the management of anaemia of chronic disease.

HAEMATOLOGICAL MALIGNANCIES

Haematological malignances are commonly encountered in the long case. History taking should enquire into the events surrounding the diagnosis, such as presenting symptoms of fatigue, lethargy, weight loss, fever, night sweats, bone pain, how the diagnosis was made, the various investigations that have been carried out, including bone marrow biopsy and/or excision biopsy of lymph nodes, and the treatment given so far, including blood transfusions, chemotherapy and bone marrow or stem cell transplantation. Ask about the side effects of chemotherapy and any episodes of febrile neutropenia, life-threatening sepsis etc. Ask how the patient is coping with the disease, what knowledge they have about the prognosis of the condition, what expectations they have for the future, and the level of social support available.

Following is a discussion of the salient points relevant to the commonly encountered haematological malignancies. The candidate is expected to have an up-to-date knowledge of each disease and to be able to handle wisely the complicated clinical issues associated with the management of these conditions.

MULTIPLE MYELOMA

Case vignette

A 56-year-old man presents with significant lethargy, severe back pain, loss of sensation in the lower extremities and dizziness. He also complains of bleeding gums and frequent blurring of vision. Physical examination reveals mucosal and conjunctival pallor and bony tenderness of the lower back. There are signs of peripheral neuropathy. His blood tests reveal anaemia, renal impairment and hypercalcaemia.

1 What further tests would you carry out to confirm your diagnosis?
2 How would you assess this man's prognosis?
3 Discuss the management at hand and long-term therapeutic options.

Approach to the patient

Multiple myeloma is a common malignant condition encountered in the long case setting, because patients with multiple myeloma can have many secondary medical complications. Multiple myeloma is due to disordered proliferation of a clone of plasma cells secreting monoclonal immunoglobulins. The clinical presentation of multiple myeloma is variable.

History

Ask about pain, bony fractures, lethargy, fatigue, dyspnoea, mucosal bleeding, fevers and rigors. Enquire about loss of sensation, limb weakness, visual problems and dizziness.

Some common presentations are intractable bone pain, pathological fracture, symptomatic anaemia, pancytopenia, sepsis, renal failure or acute symptomatic hypercalcaemia. Some may present with the hyperviscosity syndrome, with associated neuropathy and coagulopathy (oral and nasal bleeding, blurred vision, headache and vertigo) or amyloidosis. Hyperviscosity syndrome is more common in Waldenström's macroglobulinaemia, where the paraprotein is IgM. The most common presenting symptom, however, is bone pain, particularly in the vertebral column. Multiple myeloma should be suspected in any patient over the age of 40 years presenting with bone pain, pathological fracture, osteoporosis, lethargy, anaemia and recurrent infections. Incidental discovery of proteinuria, hypercalcaemia, acute renal failure, high ESR or rouleaux formation should alert the clinician to look for multiple myeloma.

Examination

Look for evidence of anaemia and sepsis. Do not forget to look at the temperature chart. Check the mucosa for bleeding. Perform a thorough neurological examination. Look for bony fractures and assess for bone tenderness.

Investigations

1 Full blood count—looking for anaemia or pancytopenia
2 Blood film—looking for a normocytic normochromic picture and rouleaux formation
4 Serum electrolyte profile
5 Renal function indices—looking for renal failure due to light-chain toxicity, sepsis, amyloidosis and hypercalcaemia
6 Serum calcium level and serum albumin level—looking for hypercalcaemia and hypoalbuminaemia
8 Serum uric acid level—can be elevated
9 Serum and urine protein electrophoresis and immunoelectrophoresis—looking for a paraprotein band
10 Skeletal survey—looking for lytic bone lesions
11 Bone marrow biopsy (both aspirate and trephine)—looking for plasma cell

infiltration. Bone marrow immunoperoxidase staining will identify kappa or lambda light chains in the plasma cells, confirming its monoclonal nature.

12 Cytogenetic analysis by interphase fluorescence in situ hybridisation (FISH)

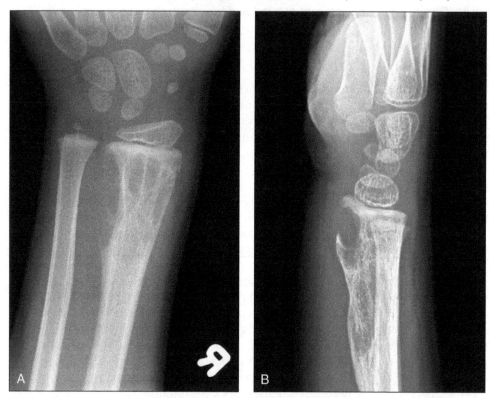

Figure 8.1 Lytic bone lesions: anteroposterior (A) and lateral (B) radiographs of the distal forearm demonstrate an expansile destructive lytic lesion with its epicentre in the diametaphysis of the distal radius which abuts the epiphyseal plate (reprinted from Kai B, Ryan A, Munk P L et al 2006 Gorham disease of bone: three cases and review of radiological features. *Clinical Radiology* 61:7).

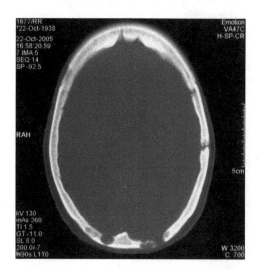

Figure 8.2 Axial CT image of the head in bone window, revealing irregular lytic lesions of the cranial vault in the occipital and left temporal regions (reprinted from Dinkar A D, Spadigam A, Sahai S 2007 Oral radiographic and clinico-pathologic presentation of Erdheim-Chester disease: a case report. *Oral Surgery, Oral Medicine, Oral Pathology, Oral Radiology, and Endodontology* 103:5)

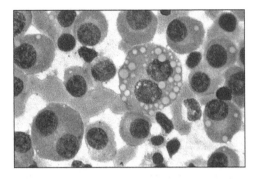

Figure 8.3 Bone marrow film of a myeloma patient (reprinted from Kumar V, Abbas A K, Fausto N 2005 *Robbins and Cotran Pathologic Basis of Disease*, 7th edn. Elsevier, Philadelphia, p 679, fig 14.16)

Diagnostic criteria for multiple myeloma

For the diagnosis of multiple myeloma there should be one major criterion together with one minor criterion or three minor criteria present—these should be clinically manifest.

Major criteria

1   > 30% plasma cells in the bone marrow (a smaller proportion of patients may have a lesser percentage).
2   M-band in serum protein electrophoresis (> 3.5 g/dL IgG or > 2 g/dL IgA)
3   More than 1 g/24 hr Bence-Jones protein in urine
4   Plasmacytoma confirmed on biopsy

Minor criteria

1   10–30% plasma cells in the bone marrow
2   M-band in serum electrophoresis and Bence-Jones protein in urine at a lesser level than above
3   Lytic bone lesions on skeletal survey
4   Low immunoglobulin levels (< 50% normal)

(Adapted from Grogan T M 2001 Plasma cell neoplasms. In: Jaffe E S, Harris N L, Stein H et al (eds) *World Health Organization classification of tumours. Pathology and genetics of tumours of haematopoietic and lymphoid tissues*. IARC Press, Lyon, p 142)

International staging system for multiple myeloma

Stage:

I   Serum beta 2 microglobulin (B2M) < 3.5 mg/L and serum albumin ≥ 35 g/L
     Median survival 62 months
II   Not belonging to stage I or stage III
     Median survival 44 months
III Serum B2M equal to or more than 5.5 mg/L
     Median survival 29 months

(From Greipp P R, San Miguel J, Durie B J et al 2005 International staging system for multiple myeloma. *Journal of Clinical Oncology* 23(15):3412–3420)

Management

Emergent management of acute complications:

1   Hypercalcaemia—hydration, bisphosphonates, high-dose steroids
2   Renal failure—renal replacement therapy/dialysis
3   Spinal cord compression—radiotherapy

General management strategy:

1   If the patient is suitable for autologous bone marrow transplantation (patients aged less than 70 years and with good prognostic features)—initial cytoreduction with combination chemotherapy such as VAD (vincristine, doxorubicin, dexamethasone)/stem cell collection at maximal response/high-dose melphalan followed by stem cell rescue.
2   A second autologous bone marrow transplantation may be indicated if there is less than very good partial response (VGPR; a response less than 90%).
3   Maintenance therapy with thalidomide with or without steroids if in remission.
4   If the patient is not suitable for autologous bone marrow transplantation—thalidomide-based therapy with melphalan and prednisone or dexamethasone.

If the disease relapses or is progressive:

1   Thalidomide-based therapy—for those who have not been treated with thalidomide previously.
2   Bortezomib—for those who have been treated with thalidomide before.
3   Lenalidomide (a thalidomide analogue).
4   Non-ablative allograft bone marrow transplantation from a human leucocyte antigen (HLA)-matched sibling (especially for those aged < 65 years)—this is associated with significant toxicity and therapy-related mortality (e.g. graft-versus-host disease).
5   If the disease is still not responding, consider new and experimental biological therapies or unrelated donor allograft bone marrow transplantation (if the patient is aged < 50 years and in the absence of bad prognostic cytogenetics).

Supportive care:

1   Bisphosphonates—to reduce the risk of pathological bone fracture
2   Transfusion—if significantly anaemic/pancytopenic
3   IV normal immunoglobulin—if IgG is very low and there is recurrent serious sepsis
4   Radiotherapy—for painful osteolytic lesions

Differential diagnoses for paraproteinaemias

1   Monoclonal gammopathy of unknown significance (MGUS)—in this condition the patient is asymptomatic, the M component in the serum is < 30 g/L, the plasma cell component in the bone marrow is < 10%, there is no M protein in the urine, there are no bony lytic lesions, there is no anaemia or hypercalcaemia, and the renal function is not impaired.

Risk of progression to multiple myeloma depends on:

  • height of the M band on protein electrophoresis
  • predominance of isotype IgA against IgG
  • presence of an abnormal free light chain ratio.

2   Smouldering myeloma—in this condition the M protein level in the serum is elevated enough to suggest a diagnosis of multiple myeloma. There are > 10% myeloma cells in the bone marrow, but there is no anaemia, renal failure or skeletal lesions.

3   Solitary plasmacytoma—this disease presents with a single bony lesion. Serum M protein component is not seen. This can be treated with a curative intent using local radiotherapy. Average survival with this condition is 10 years.

4   Waldenström's macroglobulinaemia—patients with this condition present with fatigue, weight loss, anaemia and the syndrome of hyperviscosity. The patient may also have retinal bleeds, lymphadenopathy, hepatosplenomegaly, an elevated ESR and very high serum IgM levels. Therapeutic options include plasma exchange for hyperviscosity syndrome and/or management of lymphoma with fludarabine or chlorambucil and rituximab.

5   Primary or light chain (AL) amyloidosis

6   Lymphoma

7   Chronic lymphocytic leukaemia (CLL)

Signs of poor prognosis in multiple myeloma

1   Cytogenetic abnormalities—(cytogenetic abnormalities associated with poor prognosis are: del 13q, t(4:14), del 17p)

2   Significant anaemia with a haemoglobin level of < 8.5

3   Hypercalcaemia

4   High M protein production rate

5   Acute or chronic renal failure

6   Low serum albumin level (30 g/L)

7   Elevated beta 2 microglobulin level (5.5 mg/L)

8   Elevated LDH levels

9   Age over 70 years

10   Poor performance status

CHRONIC MYELOGENOUS LEUKAEMIA

Case vignette

A 45-year-old man with massive hepatosplenomegaly was diagnosed with chronic myeloid leukaemia when he saw his GP to discuss his recent significant weight loss. He has a young family and he remains the sole breadwinner.

1   **What is the best therapeutic option you can offer him?**

2   **What are the prognostic markers of his condition?**

Approach to the patient

Chronic myelogenous leukaemia (CML) is a clonal myeloid stem cell disorder charac-terised by three discrete phases:

1 Chronic phase
2 Accelerated phase
3 Blast phase.

Without therapeutic intervention, the disease eventually and inevitably progresses to blast phase.

Individuals of all age groups can be affected by this condition, but it is particularly common among those over the age of 55 years.

History

Ask about the diagnosis and the initial symptoms. Ask about fatigue, weight loss, spontaneous bleeding and abdominal fullness. Patients present with the symptoms of fatigue, anorexia and weight loss. However, about 40% of patients are diagnosed incidentally.

Examination

Examine for abdominal organomegaly. On presentation the patient may have massive splenomegaly or hepatosplenomegaly.

Investigations

1 Full blood count and differential—looking for elevation of the white blood cell (WBC) count (with a left shift showing myeloid precursor cells) and the platelet count and sometimes the haemoglobin level. There is basophilia and eosinophilia in the differential WBC count.
2 Bone marrow biopsy—usually shows a hypercellular picture with myeloid hyperplasia.
3 Diagnosis of CML depends on the detection of the BCR-ABL (break point cluster region) transcript (translocation of c-ABL proto-oncogene from chromosome 9 to 22). This is the product of the t (9:22) Philadelphia chromosome.
4 Leucocyte alkaline phosphatase activity is low or normal—this test is only rarely done.

Management

Initial therapy:

1 While awaiting the results of the cytogenetic and molecular tests, the patient's blood counts can be stabilised with hydroxyurea. Prophylactic therapy with allopurinol against gout due to hyperuricaemia associated with cytoreduction is also important at this stage.
2 Standard therapy during the chronic phase: imatinib (400–600 mg/day)—this agent is a tyrosine kinase inhibitor that has revolutionised the treatment of CML in the chronic phase.

The therapeutic response is monitored by:

- full blood count
- bone marrow examination and cytogenetics
- quantitative assessment of BCR-ABL transcript by polymerase chain reaction (PCR).

3   Good response to the above therapy with maintenance of remission is an indication to continue therapy with regular monitoring (3-monthly bone marrow examinations for 1 year). If the response is maintained, therapy is continued further with annual bone marrow examinations. Dose increases can be considered for suboptimal responses.

4   Allograft bone marrow transplantation is considered for suitable patients in accelerated or blast phase or for those not responding to imatinib therapy. Suitability for allografting depends on patient's age, performance status and the availability of HLA-matched related or unrelated donors.

5   Second-line tyrosine kinase inhibitors (dasatinib/nilotinib) should be considered for those who do not respond to imatinib therapy even at a higher dose and are not suitable for allografting.

Other therapy:

- In the past, CML was treated with interferon and busulfan. However, these have fallen out of favour.

ACUTE MYELOID LEUKAEMIA

Case vignette

A 63-year-old female presents with left-sided hemiparesis and visual impairment. She also complains of excessive fatigue preceding the neurological event, together with recent onset of back pain. She has a background history of Hodgkin's lymphoma, treated curatively 5 years ago. Examination reveals, in addition to the neurological deficit, retinal ischaemia, evidence of anaemia, mucosal bleeding and gum hypertrophy. Blood tests reveal leucocytosis with myeloblasts.

1   How would you put this clinical picture together?

2   What is the most likely diagnosis?

3   Discuss the prognosis of this patient.

Approach to the patient

The incidence of this condition increases with age, peaking at around age 65 years.

History

Ask about:

- presenting symptoms—patients usually present with fatigue, pallor, dyspnoea, fever, bone pain, gum hypertrophy and spontaneous bleeding
- any visual problems
- monarthritis
- previous malignancies, such as lymphoma, and therapy thereof—secondary acute myeloid leukaemia (AML) due to prior chemotherapy or radiotherapy has a grave prognosis.

Examination

Look for evidence of anaemia, mucosal bleeding, bone tenderness, lymphadenopathy and organomegaly. Lymphadenopathy, hepatomegaly and splenomegaly are less common manifestations. Increased leucocyte count can lead to leucostasis, causing visual impairment due to retinal ischaemia, stroke, bleeding diathesis and acute respiratory distress syndrome. Collectively this is called 'hyperleucocytosis syndrome'.

Some patients may present with hyperuricaemia, manifesting as gouty arthritis and ureteric colic, or with symptomatic hypercalcaemia. Check the temperature chart for fevers.

Investigations

1   Full blood count—may show circulating myeloblasts with or without a leucocytosis and associated anaemia and thrombocytopenia
2   Electrolyte profile, renal function indices, liver function indices
3   Bone marrow biopsy—this is diagnostic and shows > 20% blast cells
4   Immunophenotyping, cytogenetics and molecular studies—looking for abnormalities such as PML-RARA transcript, CBF leukaemia. These are very important in the diagnostic work-up.
5   Coagulation profile, D-dimers
6   Echocardiogram

Management

Management options differ depending on the patient's age, performance status and cytogenetic risk category. Patients of good performance state and aged < 70 years are either recruited into a novel chemotherapy trial or treated with induction chemotherapy (e.g. ICE—idarubicin, cytarabine, etoposide or FLAG—fludarabine, cytarabine, combinations) followed by consolidation therapy.

This is followed by further therapy depending on the patient's cytogenetic risk group (see box):

*   *Poor risk*—allografting from a related or unrelated donor, or non-ablative conditioning
*   *Intermediate risk*—consider ablative sibling allografting after first complete remission if the patient is < 60 years old
*   *Good risk*—observe after first complete remission.

Patients with acute promyelocytic leukaemia (APML) should be investigated for evidence of disseminated intravascular coagulation.

Cytogenetic associations of AML

Based on the cytogenetic analysis, patients are divided into good risk, standard risk and poor risk categories:

*   Good risk—t(15:17), t(8:12), inv 16
*   Poor risk—del 7, complex karyotypes

There are an evolving number of molecular variants of AML which, hopefully, will further stratify these cytogenetic subtypes.

Factors indicating poor prognosis

1   Secondary leukaemia (upon treatment of previous myelodysplastic or myeloproliferative disorders)
2   Poor performance status
3   Age over 60 years
4   Adverse cytogenetics—most important prognostic indicator

These patients can be treated with all-*trans*retinoic acid (ATRA) and idarubicin. Maintenance therapy consists of a combination of ATRA, methotrexate and 6-mercaptopurine.

At relapse, treatment is with arsenic trioxide (As_2O_3) and ATRA.

ACUTE LYMPHOBLASTIC LEUKAEMIA

Acute lymphoblastic leukaemia (ALL) is less common, and in the adult patient the prognosis is relatively guarded. The prognosis depends on the cytogenetic analysis. Poor prognostic cytogenetic markers include t (4:11) and t (9:22). Patients are enrolled in a therapeutic clinical trial if eligible. The therapeutic regimen usually consists of multiple courses of high-dose prednisolone, combination chemotherapy and central nervous system prophylaxis (intrathecal methotrexate and cranial irradiation).

Consider allograft transplantation after first remission if the patient is less than 60 years old.

CHRONIC LYMPHOCYTIC LEUKAEMIA

Due to the chronicity and the relative stability of the patient in the early stages, it is more likely for a candidate to encounter a patient with chronic lympohocytic leukaemia (CLL) in the examination setting. Patients usually present with lymphadenopathy, anaemia, infections and hepatosplenomegaly. Sometimes the diagnosis is made on incidental observation of an elevated WBC count. Disease stage and severity is classified according to the Rai or the Binet classification. The Binet classification is easy to remember, and goes as follows:

Stage A—disease involving two or fewer lymph node regions
Stage B—disease involving more than two lymph node regions
Stage C—presence of anaemia or thrombocytopenia.

Staging has therapeutic as well as prognostic implications. Stages A and B disease warrant only watchful waiting in the older patient.

Therapy is indicated in advanced disease. Other indications for therapeutic intervention include bulky disease, B symptoms, autoimmune phenomena (autoimmune haemolytic anaemia), rapid doubling time (< 6 months), young age (< 40 years) and poor risk features (see box).

It is ideal to enrol the patient in a therapeutic clinical trial if suitable.

Those less than 70 years of age with good prognostic signs are treated with chemotherapy (fludarabine/cyclophosphamide) and rituximab. Relapses may be treated with alemtuzumab-based therapy. However, if the patient is less than 50 years of age, non-ablative sibling allografting should be considered.

Those aged over 70 or with poor prognostic signs may be treated with fludarabine or chlorambucil together with rituximab.

Poor risk features of CLL
- CD 38 positivity
- Adverse cytogenetics (trisomy 12, 11q, del 17p etc)
- Unmutated IgH status
- ZAP 70 positivity
- Rapid lymphocyte doubling time ($<$ 6 months)
- Bone marrow failure
- Advanced stage

HODGKIN'S DISEASE

Case vignette
A 35-year-old male presents to the emergency department with fevers, rigors and a productive cough. Examination reveals bronchial breath sounds in the right lower zone on his chest. Sputum mug contains rusty purulent sputum. Chest X-ray shows evidence of consolidation in the right lower zone. In addition, the chest X-ray displays a mass lesion in the mediastinum.
1 What are the management objectives in this patient?
2 What are the differential diagnoses of the mediastinal mass?
3 What investigations would you plan to further investigate his clinical picture?

Approach to the patient
History
Ask about the initial diagnosis. Note the patient's age. Hodgkin's disease has a bimodal age-related prevalence with an initial peak in the third to fourth decade and a second peak in the sixth decade. The most common presentation is with singular or localised lymphadenopathy without any other symptoms. Some get diagnosed upon the incidental finding of a mediastinal mass on chest X-ray. However, upon enquiry, the patient may describe retrosternal chest discomfort, dyspnoea or cough. Ask about fevers, night sweats and recent weight loss. Some patients may complain of intractable pruritis and rash. Alcohol-induced pain is another late feature of this condition. Ask about any previous history of malignancies and family history of Hodgkin's disease.

Examination

Identify the distribution of lymphadenopathy and establish its classic rubbery consistency. Examination of the neck region should be very thorough. Listen to the chest for evidence of tracheal or bronchial obstruction due to mediastinal mass. Examine the abdomen for splenomegaly and, less commonly, hepatomegaly. Study the temperature chart to establish the pattern of the fever, which classically is intermittent and often nocturnal (Pel-Ebstein fever). Look for a mediastinal mass in the chest X-ray.

Investigations

1 Histology by excision lymph node biopsy
2 Staging (see box), with the following investigations: CT scan of chest, abdomen and pelvis, bone marrow aspiration biopsy, PET scan
Other investigations of prognostic significance:
1 Full blood count
2 Serum albumin level
3 ESR

Staging classification of Hodgkin's disease

The Ann Arbor staging classification of Hodgkin's disease is as follows:

Stage 1—disease involving a single lymph node region

Stage 2—disease involving two or more lymph node regions located on the same side of the diaphragm

Stage 3—disease involving lymph node regions on both sides of the diaphragm

Stage 4—disseminated disease.

B symptoms—night sweats, fevers and weight loss of > 10% of the body weight within 6 months.

Management

The disease is classified into *early-stage* disease (stage I, IB, IIA, non-bulky disease) and *advanced-stage* disease (bulky disease, stage IIB, III or IV) from a therapeutic perspective. Response to treatment is monitored with CT imaging and PET scanning.

Early-stage Hodgkin's lymphoma

1 If the patient has more favourable prognostic markers (see box), consider combination chemotherapy (doxorubicin, bleomycin, vinblastine, dacarbazine: ABVD) for 4 months followed by radiotherapy to the sites that were involved at diagnosis.
2 In the absence of good prognostic markers, combination chemotherapy is given for a longer period (6 months).
3 Patients with impaired cardiopulmonary function or of poor performance status or advanced age may not tolerate the ABVD combination. If the patient has demonstrated reduction of the DLCO50 due to bleomycin toxicity, continuation of the combination of AVD (with bleomycin omission) can be considered. Mechlorethamine, vincristine, prednisone and procarbazine (MOPP) is also an alternative combination in this setting.

Favourable risk features in early-stage Hodgkin's lymphoma

- Involvement of three or fewer nodal sites
- Age 40 or less
- ESR of 70 or less
- Absence of large mediastinal mass

Advanced-stage Hodgkin's lymphoma

1 Patients with better prognostic signs with an international prognostic score (IPS) less than four (see box) are treated with combination chemotherapy (ABVD) for 6 months followed by radiotherapy to the sites of bulky disease at the diagnosis and those sites that failed to achieve complete remission after chemotherapy.

2 If the prognostic signs are poor (IPS > 4), consider intensified combination chemotherapy (bleomycin, etoposide, doxorubicin, cyclophophamide, vincristine, prednisolone, procarbazine: BEACOP) provided the patient is younger than 60 years and of good performance status. Otherwise consider longer-term ABVD for 8 months. Combination chemotherapy may be followed by radiotherapy as described above.

3 Some centres enrol patients in novel therapeutic trials and this should be considered if suitable.

4 Long-term adverse effects of combination therapy include acute myeloid leukaemia, non-Hodgkin's lymphoma (after 10 years), and solid tumours (after 15 years). Resistant disease can be treated with autologous bone marrow transplantation.

International Prognostic Score (IPS)

Each adverse factor scores 1 point:

- Serum albumin < 40
- Hb < 10.5
- Male sex
- Age > 45 years
- Stage IV
- WCC > 15
- Lymphocytes < 0.6

(From Hasenclever D, Diehl V 1998 A prognostic score for advanced Hodgkin's disease. International Prognostic Factors Project on Advanced Hodgkin's Disease. *New England Journal of Medicine* 339(21):1506–1514)

NON-HODGKIN'S LYMPHOMA

Approach to the patient

History

Ask about:

- the circumstances of diagnosis
- symptoms at presentation
- any evidence of precipitating conditions such as previous malignancies, Sjögren's syndrome, radiation exposure, immunosuppression, immunodeficiency and infections with HIV or hepatitis C
- any family history of lymphoma or other malignancy.

Patients with gastrointestinal lymphoma may have a history of coeliac disease. Ask about B symptoms of fevers, night sweats and weight loss.

Examination

Perform a thorough lymph node assessment for lymphadenopathy. Check for abdominal organomegaly. Don't forget to look at the temperature chart.

Investigations

CT scan, PET scan and bone marrow biopsy are used in the staging process.

1 Excisional biopsy of a lymph node
2 Full blood count—looking for anaemia, pancytopenia or lymphocytosis
3 Serum electrolyte profile and renal function indices
4 Liver function tests—looking for abnormalities due to hepatic involvement
5 Serum uric acid level—looking for an elevation
6 Serum calcium level—looking for hypercalcaemia
7 Serum lactate dehydrogenase level—looking for an elevation
8 Serum protein electrophoresis and immunoelectrophoresis
9 Serum beta 2 microglobulin level—looking for an elevation
10 Chest X-ray
11 CT of chest, abdomen and pelvis
12 Bone marrow biopsy
13 PET scan
14 Serology for HIV and tests for hepatitis C infection

Management

The histological subtype of the disease is important in deciding on the management option. Disease is often categorised into *aggressive* disease or *indolent* disease, based on the histology.

The stage of the disease and the prognostic score, calculated according to the systems described in the boxes (for aggressive disease and indolent disease respectively), are important factors that influence the therapeutic plan. The scoring system also includes the patient's age and the functional status, which have a major bearing on the management strategies.

Aggressive lymphomas include diffuse large B-cell lymphoma, mantle cell lymphoma, T-cell lymphoma, Burkitt's lymphoma and lymphoblastic lymphoma. Indolent lymphomas include follicular lymphoma.

Prognostic grading of intermediate grade/aggressive non-Hodgkin's lymphoma

Prognosis in non-Hodgkin's lymphoma is described according to the International Prognostic Index (IPI). The disease is graded according to a scoring system, as follows:

1   Age over 60 years—1 point
2   Stage III or IV—1 point
3   LDH level above 10 mmol/L—1 point
4   Extranodal spread— > 1 point
5   Poor performance score (ECOG 2–4) — 1 point

Risk scores:
- Low risk = 0,1
- Intermediate risk = 2
- Intermediate/high risk = 3
- High risk = 4, 5

(After Shipp M A, Harrington D P, Anderson J R et al 1993 A predictive model for aggressive non-Hodgkin's lymphoma. The International Non-Hodgkin's Lymphoma Prognostic Factors Project. *New England Journal of Medicine* 329(14):987–994)

Follicular Lymphoma International Prognostic Index (FLIPI)

1   Age > 60 years—1 point
2   Stage III–IV—1 point
3   Hb <12 g/dL—1 point
4   Elevated LDH—1 point
5   Number of nodal sites > 4—1 point

(After Solal-Céligny P, Roy P, Colombat P et al 2004 Follicular Lymphoma International Prognostic Index. *Blood* 104:1258–1265)

Intermediate grade/aggressive lymphoma (excluding Burkitt's lymphoma and lymphoblastic lymphoma)

Diffuse large B-cell lymphoma

This disease has a higher therapeutic response. Aggressive therapy is indicated if the patient's cardiopulmonary performance status is adequate. Standard therapy is combination chemotherapy with cyclophosphamide, doxorubicin hydrochloride, vincristine and prednisolone (R-CHOP) and radiotherapy. Treatment intensification is considered for younger patients with poor prognostic indicators.

Consider intrathecal methotrexate if there is a high risk of central nervous system relapse. Features that suggest this possibility include high or high/intermediate IPI score, testicular or sinus involvement or stage IV disease.

Relapse of the disease is treated with second-line chemotherapy (fludarabine) followed by autologous stem cell transplants for those responsive to chemotherapy. If this strategy fails, further therapy with hypomethylating agents (epigenetic strategies), new monoclonal antibodies and non-ablative allograft transplantation should be considered.

Mantle cell lymphoma
Though this was considered a 'low-grade' lymphoma according to the working formulation, it is treated where feasible as an 'aggressive lymphoma' due to its poor prognosis.
* Combination chemotherapy such as R-Hyper CVAD (MDACC), R-CHOP or FCR (fludarabine, cyclophosphamide, rituximab)
* Consideration may be given to upfront autografting.

T-cell lymphoma
There is no standard therapy for aggressive T-cell lymphomas. Generally CHOP with (or without) upfront autografting is considered.
* Alternative hyperCVAD can also be considered.
* Enrolling patients in promising randomised control treatment trials is encouraged.

Burkitt's lymphoma and lymphoblastic lymphoma
These are managed according to the protocols used for the management of ALL (see p 121).

Indolent lymphoma
Indolent lymphomas such as follicular lymphoma are managed with watchful waiting, and active therapy when required (chemotherapy or radiation to localised disease)—similar to the indications for treatment in CLL (see p 121). Generally these diseases are considered incurable, though novel strategies (e.g. rituximab in combination) are starting to show survival benefits.

MYELODYSPLASIC SYNDROME
Myelodysplasic syndrome should be considered a possible diagnosis in the elderly patient who has a combination of macrocytic anaemia, neutropenia and thrombocytopenia. The condition could be idiopathic, or secondary to previous exposure to cytotoxic chemotherapy or radiotherapy. Diagnosis is made by bone marrow biopsy.

Management
Supportive therapy:
1 The patient needs supportive care with regular transfusions of packed cells and platelets if bleeding.
2 Antibiotics against sepsis
3 Fe chelation
4 Erythropoietin
Specific:
1 Chemotherapy
2 Epigenetic approaches such as hypomethylating agents

3   Some patients with myelodysplasic syndrome may progress to develop AML. If the blast cell count is high, therapy should be as for AML (see p 120). In the younger patient, consideration should be given to allogenic bone marrow transplantation.

POLYCYTHAEMIA VERA

Case vignette

A 45-year-old female presents with progressive abdominal enlargement and bilateral pain in the upper abdominal quadrant. She denies smoking, alcohol excess or recent overseas travel, and her medication history is negative for potentially hepatotoxic agents. She denies ingestion of any herbal medications. On examination she is jaundiced. She has ascites, caput medusae and hepatosplenomegaly. She is particularly tender in the left upper quadrant with guarding. Liver function tests are grossly abnormal and ultrasonography reveals paucity of venous architecture. Full blood count shows erythrocytosis with low plasma erythropoietin levels. Hepatitis and HIV screen comes negative.

1   **Explain the clinical picture in light of the available information.**
2   **What further information is required to arrive at a definitive diagnosis?**
3   **Formulate a plan of management for the short term and the long term.**

Approach to the patient

Polycythaemia vera is a myeloid stem cell disorder characterised by trilineage (erythrocytes, granulocytes and platelets) hyperplasia, high blood counts and splenomegaly. Polycythaemia rubra vera is characterised by predominant erythrocyte hyperplasia. Prior to the diagnosis of polycythaemia vera in any patient with erythrocytosis it is essential to exclude spurious polycythaemia and secondary polycythaemia.

History

Polycythaemia vera is common among middle-aged and older patients. Often it is an incidental diagnosis in a patient with a high haemoglobin level in the full blood count done for some other reason. Ask about constitutional symptoms of lethargy, malaise and weight loss. Check for neurological symptoms, such as headache, vertigo, tinnitus and visual disturbances. Thrombotic stroke is a possible complication. Some complain of pruritus, of which the precise aetiology is not clear. Ask about diaphoresis, which is due to hyperviscosity associated with erythrocytosis. Patients who present with erythema, warmness and pain in the distal extremities may be suffering from the condition called erythromelalgia, an association of polycythaemia vera. Enquire about bleeding in the form of epistaxis or gastrointestinal haemorrhage, which is a common presentation of this disease. Ask about acute joint pain due to gout.

Examination

Physical examination may reveal plethoric facies, easy bruising, hypertension, neurological deficit and splenomegaly. Perform a thorough neurological assessment. Some may manifest evidence of portal hypertension, because these patients are susceptible to Budd-Chiari syndrome and portal vein thrombosis. Left upper quadrant tenderness mimicking acute abdomen may be due to splenic infarction. Check for abdominal organomegaly. Although rare, do not forget to look for digital infarcts due to erythromelalgia. Some patients may have excoriations due to severe pruritis and gouty tophi (with or without acute joint tenderness). Look in the fundus for venous engorgement.

Investigations

1 Full blood count—looking for raised haematocrit, leucocytosis and thrombocytosis. Ask for red cell mass to exclude relative or spurious polycythaemia due to decreased plasma volume (decreased plasma volume can cause erythrocytosis, and this is called stress erythrocytosis or Gaisböck's syndrome). Sometimes the red cell mass may still be elevated in secondary polycythaemia due to excess erythropoietin secretion.
2 Serum erythropoietin level (which is elevated in secondary polycythaemia but in polycythaemia vera is usually < 4 munits/mL)
3 Oxygen saturation—to exclude hypoxia as a possible cause
4 Overnight pulse oximetry—to exclude sleep apnoea causing hypoxia
5 Depleted iron reserves, elevated uric acid and elevated serum vitamin B_{12} levels— would further support the diagnosis of polycythaemia vera
6 Abdominal ultrasound—to exclude erythropoietin-secreting mass lesions
7 Bone marrow biopsy—looking for myeloid cell hyperplasia and typical megakaryocyte morphology
8 Cytogenetic studies
9 Molecular testing for the JAK 2 gene mutation—this has a 95% sensitivity for the diagnosis of polycythaemia vera.

Management

Broad management objectives include: 1) prevent complications of raised haematocrit, such as thrombosis and hyperviscosity; 2) control organomegaly; and 3) manage the symptoms.
1 Raised haematocrit is controlled by venesection.
2 Low-dose aspirin is indicated for the prevention of thrombosis.
3 Chemotherapy with busulfan or P32 is indicated in resistant cases. However, this could increase the risk of secondary leukaemia.
4 Erythromelalgia is managed successfully with salicylate therapy.
5 Hyperuricaemia is managed with allopurinol.
6 Massive splenomegaly may warrant splenectomy.

DIABETES MELLITUS

Case vignette

A 58-year-old female presents with nausea and vomiting in the background of progressive exertional dyspnoea.

She is a smoker with a 10-pack per year history. She was diagnosed with diabetes 2 years ago and has been managed on metformin 500 mg twice daily.

On examination she has coarse crepitations in the lung bases bilaterally. She has an S3 gallop in the precordium. She is obese and has moderate bipedal pitting oedema. Blood pressure is 140/90 mmHg.

On the ECG, ST segment depression is observed in the lateral leads. Her fasting blood sugar levels are 11.2 mmo/L with an Hb A_{1c} of 8.2%. Serum troponin level is not elevated.

1   Discuss the risk of a coronary event in this woman.
2   What is your immediate management?
3   How would you optimise her glycaemic control?
4   Discuss your plan to optimise her cardiovascular risk profile.
5   Prepare a comprehensive diabetes care plan for this woman.

Approach to the patient

Diabetes is a very commonly encountered condition in the long case setting. Most diabetic patients have multiple associated medical conditions, and this makes them favourite long case material. A candidate is expected to be able to address diabetic cases thoroughly and extensively. Ascertain whether the patient has the metabolic syndrome (see box) that is associated with high cardiovascular risk. The following is a discussion of the integral issues that should never be missed in any diabetic case.

Metabolic syndrome

- Central obesity
- Raised TG levels (> 1.7 mmol/L)
- Reduced HDL cholesterol level (males < 1.03 mmol/L, females < 1.29 mmol/L)
- Hypertension (> 130/85 mmHg)
- Elevated fasting plasma glucose levels (> 5.6 mmol/L) or previous diagnosis of type 2 diabetes

(Adapted from International Diabetes Federation 2006 Consensus worldwide definition of metabolic syndrome. Online. Available: http://www.idf.org/webdata/docs/MetS_def_update2006.pdf)

History

Ask about:
- when and how the diagnosis was made, and symptoms at presentation, such as loss of weight, polyuria, polydypsia, and other associated presenting features such as diabetic ketoacidosis, hyperosmolar coma and infection
- initial treatment, subsequent treatment and the current medical regimen
- age at disease onset
- the type of diabetes the patient has—this has implications for the risk of diabetic ketoacidosis and for the therapeutic regimens
- the insulin treatment, such as previous and/or current regimens, types of insulin, dose and frequency of administration, who injects the insulin, the method of delivery (pen or syringe) and adverse effects associated with insulin treatment
- medication history, in detail—note the different classes of drugs that have been used to treat the diabetes, and also other medications that would interfere with adequate glycaemic control
- the patient's knowledge of and compliance with the diabetic diet, and knowledge of the concept of the glycaemic index of various carbohydrate-containing foods
- who monitors the blood sugar levels and how often this is done—ask for the most recent readings
- episodes of ketoacidosis, hyperosmolar coma and other acute events that have necessitated hospitalisation
- whether the patient suffers from hypoglycaemic episodes and how he or she recognises early warning signs, and what remedial measures the patient takes in such situations
- other vascular risk factors, such as smoking, hyperlipidaemia and hypertension
- diabetic complications:
  - macrovascular complications—ischaemic heart disease, heart failure, intermittent claudication and stroke (remember that diabetic cardiomyopathy may dominate the picture, leading to silent ischaemic episodes)
  - microvascular complications:
    - *ocular complications*—such as diabetic retinopathy. Ask how often the patient visits the ophthalmologist and the current level of vision and any

visual symptoms. Ask about any laser therapy for diabetic retinopathy. While discussing the eye, ask about cataracts.

◻ *neurological complications*—ask about peripheral paraesthesias, painful peripheries, burns, neuropathic ulcers and Charcot's joints. Ask whether the patient has ever had nerve conduction studies done. Enquire about symptoms of autonomic neuropathy, such as persistent postural dizziness, bloating, nocturnal diarrhoea, impotence and incontinence.

◻ *nephropathy*—ask whether the patient has any urinary symptoms, such as frequency, polyuria and nocturia. Has the patient observed peripheral oedema that would suggest early-stage renal failure? Enquire about any previous investigations, such as 24-hour urinary collection for proteinuria, and whether the patient is aware of their level of renal function.

- other complications:
  - *infections/sepsis*—ask about previous or current oral or vaginal candidiasis, impetigo, ulcers, abscesses, carbuncles, furuncles and recurrent urinary tract infections
  - *diabetic foot*—the presence of painful callosities, corns or ulcers. Any anatomical foot deformities that predispose to foot injury should be enquired into. Ask whether the patient sees a podiatrist and, if so, how often.

The social and occupational impact of diabetes on the patient should be discussed in detail. Talk about impotence, if relevant to the patient. Social and marital issues associated with this condition should be dealt with in detail. Check for a family history of diabetes mellitus and obtain details thereof.

Exclude possible secondary causes for the diabetes, such as chronic pancreatitis, cystic fibrosis, Cushing's syndrome, acromegaly, polycystic ovary syndrome and consumption of drugs such as corticosteroids, thiazides and the oral contraceptive pill (see box).

Causes of secondary diabetes mellitus

1 Medications—glucocorticoids, diazoxide, thiazides, oral contraceptive pill
2 Cushing's disease
3 Acromegaly
4 Polycystic ovary syndrome
5 Pancreatic insufficiency (e.g. chronic pancreatitis, cystic fibrosis)
6 Obesity
7 Gestation
8 Haemochromatosis
9 Ataxia telangiectasia
10 Glucagonoma/vipoma

Examination

1 Body habitus—particularly looking for obesity, endocrinopathic appearance suggesting Cushing's syndrome (see box), polycystic ovary syndrome or acromegaly (see box), and evidence of recent weight loss or weight gain. Measure

the waist circumference and calculate the body mass index (BMI). Patients who have had type 1 diabetes from an early age may have stunted growth.

2 Postural blood pressure and postural pulse (postural response is absent in autonomic neuropathy)

3 State of hydration, injection marks, amputations, impetigo, acanthosis nigricans

4 Eye examination—looking for cataract, visual acuity, diabetic retinopathy and oculomotor nerve palsy with pupillary sparing

5 Oral cavity—for hygiene, periodontal disease and candidiasis

6 Abdomen—for hepatomegaly associated with diabetic fatty liver

7 Peripheral neuropathy (motor and sensory) and diabetic amyotrophy (in the quadriceps femoris musculature)—the 10 g Semmes-Weinstein monofilament test, looking for peripheral neuropathy (assesses the foot at risk)

8 Cutaneous stigmata—such as diabetic dermopathy, necrobiosis lipoidica diabeticorum and lipodystrophy associated with frequent injections (particularly in patients with poor technique)

9 Presence or absence of all peripheral pulses

10 A detailed diabetic foot examination.

Clinical features of Cushing's syndrome

- Weight gain leading to central obesity
- Moon facies
- Excessive sweating
- Telangiectasia, straie, increased skin fragility (easy bruising)
- Hyperpigmentation
- Proximal myopathy
- Hirsutism
- Buffalo hump
- Decreased libido, impotence, amenorrhoea
- Mood disturbances (euphoria, depression and delirium)
- Hypertension
- Diabetes

Clinical features of acromegaly

- Enlargement of the hands and feet
- Protrusion of eyebrows and jaw
- Arthritis, carpal tunnel syndrome
- Increased spacing between the teeth
- Macroglossia
- Cardiac failure

- Compression of the optic chiasma leading to bitemporal hemianopia
- Diabetes mellitus
- Hypertension
- Increased palmar sweating and seborrhea of the face

Investigations

Investigations that should be performed in the diabetic patient include:

1 Blood sugar level (capillary or venous)
2 Glycosylated haemoglobin (Hb A_{1c}) level
3 Serum fructosamine level (not a very reliable test)
4 Full blood count
5 Fasting serum lipid profile
6 Electrolyte profile and the renal function indices—looking for evidence of renal impairment
7 Spot urine specimen—for proteinuria and for albumin-to-creatinine ratio (a ratio of > 2.5 is considered significant). If urine is positive for protein, a 24-hour urine collection should be carried out, looking for microalbuminuria. An albumin excretion of 30–300 mg over 24 hours is defined as microalbuminuria and is predictive of early diabetic nephropathy. The positive tests should be repeated within 3 months, and if there is persistent microalbuminuria on two occasions the patient should be commenced on an ACE inhibitor.
8 ECG—for evidence of ischaemic heart disease

Management

Discussion of therapeutic options revolves around the diabetic diet, regular physical exercise, oral hypoglycaemic agents and their side effects, and insulin therapy. Objectives of diabetes management include: 1) adequate control of the blood sugar level (fasting levels to be maintained below 6.1 mmol/L and postprandial levels below 7.8 mmol/L) and the glycosylated haemoglobin level (should be maintained below 7% in most cases, based on the patient's clinical status); 2) prevention of end-organ complications; and 3) control of other vascular risk factors.

1 *Hypoglycaemic agents*—If the diabetic diet and physical exercise fail to provide adequate glycaemic control in the patient with type 2 diabetes, consider commencing an oral hypoglycaemic agent. Commonly used agents are:
   - *biguanides*—metformin is the most common and the first line of pharmacotherapy in type 2 diabetes. Act to enhance peripheral insulin sensitivity. Side effects of this class of drugs include diarrhoea, nausea, impaired vitamin B_{12} absorption and lactic acidosis, particularly in patients with hepatic or renal failure.
   - *sulfonylureas*—act via stimulation of pancreatic insulin secretion. Side effects of this class of drugs include hypoglycaemia, weight gain, rash and, very rarely, bone marrow suppression and cholestasis. Sulfonylureas have been associated with an increased mortality rate in post myocardial infarction patients.
   - *thiazolidinediones*—rosiglitazone and pioglitazone are the thiazolidinediones currently available. These agents act mainly by improving insulin sensitivity

and preserving pancreatic beta cell function. These agents have beneficial effects on cardiovascular health and have been observed to be able to prevent in-stent restenosis. According to the guidelines these agents are considered third-line therapy in difficult-to-control diabetes and should be added to the regimen when glycaemic control is suboptimal on biguanides and sulfonylureas. First-generation agent troglitazone was associated with hepatotoxicity, but other agents of this class (e.g. rosiglitazone) are believed to be safe. Thiazolidinediones give good blood sugar control when used in combination with insulin, metformin or sulfonylureas, but have a tendency to cause weight gain. In heart failure patients these agents may contribute to an exacerbation of the condition and they also have a negative impact on bone density, contributing to osteoporosis. It is very important to avoid this agent in patients with heart failure. Peripheral oedema is another commonly observed side effect. Rosiglitazone can elevate LDL as well as HDL levels, while pioglitazone has a neutral effect on LDL levels and a beneficial effect on HDL levels.
- *meglitinides*—repaglinide is a short-acting agent that acts by stimulating pancreatic insulin secretion, but can cause weight gain and hypoglycaemia. This agent can be given in combination with metformin.
- alpha-glucosidase inhibitor agents such as acarbose act to inhibit the activity of intestinal glucosidase enzymes. Their side effect profile includes bloating, abdominal discomfort, diarrhoea and flatulence.

2   *Insulin therapy*—Type 2 diabetic patients whose glycaemic control is suboptimal on oral agents alone need therapy with insulin, as do all type 1 diabetics. Insulin therapy can be commenced as an outpatient at a dose of 0.25 units per kg (in an inpatient it can be commenced at up to 1 unit per kg) and the dose increased according to the blood sugar control achieved. Different centres have different protocols for insulin therapy, so it is best to know thoroughly the one used at your centre. A combination short- and long-acting insulin 30/70 units twice daily divided into a ratio of 2:1, before lunch and before dinner, is a good starting regimen for the patient with type 2 diabetes. Premixed rapid-acting insulin 25 units is another attractive option for the mature-onset diabetes patient. This is composed of 25% insulin lispro (rapid-acting) with 75% insulin lispro-protamine (intermediate-acting), and should be administered preprandially twice daily. Because of its very rapid onset of action, it can be given immediately before meals, thus ensuring convenience of use and better compliance. Insulin regimens for the patient with type 1 diabetes are different from those for the patient with type 2 diabetes and are usually a four-times-a-day regimen.
Once-daily, long-acting insulin analogues such as glargine can be given to patients with type 2 diabetes on oral agents requiring insulin therapy.

3   *Education*—This is often overlooked in the management of diabetes. Patient education should be discussed in detail and should take the following format:
- Educate the patient on the need to control blood sugar levels adequately, to prevent end-organ damage, and warn about the severe adverse consequences of poor control. Teach them how to monitor blood sugar levels, giving instructions on the methods and frequency. Initially it is wise to monitor the blood sugar level several times daily at regular intervals. This can be done immediately before each meal and 2 hours postprandially. Once stable levels

are achieved, twice-daily monitoring is adequate—this should be done at different times on different days, so that a good estimate of the overall control can be gained. A satisfactory level at which to maintain blood sugar is 4–8 mmol/L.

- Advise on the optimal diabetic diet and the benefits of regular, light physical exercise. Diet should comprise at least 50% carbohydrate, made up of food with a low glycaemic index and containing complex carbohydrates. Food should contain minimum amounts of saturated fat. A high fibre content and mono- or polyunsaturated fats are highly desirable. The patient should take smaller portions at regular intervals (three main meals and one snack between each meal) to maintain blood sugar levels at a uniform range and avoid rapid fluctuations.

4 *Prevention of end-organ damage*—When a patient tests positive for microalbuminuria it is important to ensure strict blood pressure control to prevent progression to diabetic nephropathy. Ideally the blood pressure in the diabetic patient will be below 130/85 mmHg. All nephrotoxic drugs should be stopped and care should be exercised when administering ionic radiocontrast material to the patient. To prevent atherosclerotic vascular disease, the patient should be strongly advised against smoking, and strict control of serum cholesterol levels should be ensured (aim at LDL < 2.0 mmol/L). Global risk factor modification also involves strict control of blood pressure too.

5 *Weight reduction*—Should be promoted if the patient is overweight or obese. Losing 5–10 kg is of significant benefit. This can be achieved by joule restriction and regular exercise. A suitable form of exercise is brisk walking for at least 30 minutes a day, 4 days a week. Resistant cases may benefit from agents such as orlistat, which is an inhibitor of gastrointestinal lipase. Warn the patient about the side effects of greasy stool, frequency of defecation and bulky stool.

6 *Family education and support*—Do not forget to stress the importance of providing education and support to the patient's family. Diabetes is best managed in a multidisciplinary setting with the participation of the physician, general practitioner, nurse educator, podiatrist, nutritionist and social worker.

7 In some jurisdictions the local department in charge of roads and traffic may require notification of a person's diagnosis with diabetes.

Cholesterol target guidelines

- LDL cholesterol < 2.0 mmol/L
- Total cholesterol < 4.0 mmol/L
- HDL cholesterol > 1.0 mmol/L
- Triglycerides < 1.5 mmol/L

Cholesterol-lowering drug therapy is indicated for any patient with a diagnosis of coronary artery disease, peripheral vascular disease, diabetes with either age > 60 years or microalbuminuria or Aboriginal ethnicity or a significant family history of coronary heart disease at a younger age. These patients do not need a lipid level done prior to commencement of therapy.

OBESITY

Case vignette

A 45-year-old obese female is admitted after a suicide attempt with ingestion of and overdose of tricyclic antidepressant. She has recovered from the acute episode but complains of early morning headache of long-standing duration, exertional dyspnoea, bilateral knee pain on walking, lower back pain, cold intolerance and easy bruising. She has known diabetes mellitus managed on metformin and rosiglitazone. On examination she is obese with a BMI of 35. She is tachycardic at 100 bpm and hypertensive at 140/95 mmHg and there is a loud P_2 in the precordium. There is evidence of hirsutism, acanthosis nigricans and bipedal oedema.

1   What other clinical information is required to consider the most likely differential diagnosis?
2   What are the possible contributing factors to her obesity?
3   What investigations would you request?
4   What are the psychosocial issues related to her obesity and how do you propose to manage these?
5   Suggest a treatment plan for this patient.

Approach to the patient

Obesity may be central to many a medical problem that a long case patient presents with. It may be an incidental observation, but obesity needs addressing if present. Obesity is associated with an increased all-cause mortality and in particular cardiovascular mortality. A BMI of > 30 is defined as obesity according to the US National Institute of Health criteria. A BMI of 19–25 is considered healthy and desirable.

$$\text{Body mass index (BMI)} = \text{weight (kg)/height squared (m}^2)$$

History

Ask about:
- family history of obesity
- age of onset of obesity
- any recent weight gain
- vascular risk factors such as diabetes mellitus, hypertension, hyperlipidaemia and smoking
- symptoms such as excessive sweating, headache, visual disturbance (bitemporal hemianopia), easy bruising and cold intolerance—may suggest endocrinological disorders known to cause obesity, such as Cushing's syndrome, myxoedema or pituitary tumour
- medications that contribute to weight gain, such as corticosteroids, insulin and rosiglitazone
- snoring (bed partner's report)
- daytime somnolence
- early-morning headache

- early-morning diuresis and waking in the morning not feeling fresh—may suggest obstructive sleep apnoea (common in the obese)
- medications that would cause weight gain, such as sulfonylureas and thiazolidinediones
- detailed dietary history—this is very important, with information about the types of food consumed and the frequency of meals. Ask whether the patient is on a particular diet (in particular enquire about popular diets) and if so, ask about the benefits and side effects experienced.
- details of the occupational and social problems associated with obesity
- previous attempts at weight loss and reasons for failure.
Estimate the level of insight the patient has into his or her condition.

Examination

Calculate the BMI and the waist-to-hip ratio. Check the exact distribution of fat. Check blood pressure. Look for features of any associated endocrinological disorder, such as cushingoid body habitus, easy bruising and buffalo hump (suggestive of Cushing's syndrome), peach complexion, goitre and bradycardia (suggestive of myxoedema), and virilisation in a female patient (suggestive of polycystic ovary syndrome).

Investigations

1 Random or fasting blood sugar level—looking for hyperglycaemia
2 Fasting lipid profile—looking for hyperlipidaemia
3 Liver function tests—looking for abnormalities that may be due to non-alcoholic steatohepatitis
4 Thyroid function tests—looking for hypothyroidism
5 24-hour urinary cortisol excretion—to screen for Cushing's syndrome.

The major predictor of health risks associated with primary obesity is body fat distribution. Android distribution or central obesity (adiposity preferentially located in the abdomen) is associated with a variety of metabolic derangements, including dyslipidaemia, hypertension and glucose intolerance. Obesity is also associated with type 2 diabetes, ischaemic heart disease, stroke, gallbladder disease, liver function abnormalities due to non-alcoholic steatohepatitis (NASH), and osteoarthritis of the weight-bearing joints (see box).

Morbidities associated with obesity

- Coronary artery disease
- Atrial fibrillation
- Congestive cardiac failure/right heart failure (cor pulmonale)
- Stroke
- Deep venous thrombosis
- Hypertension
- Hyperinsulinaemia
- Diabetes mellitus
- Hypercholesterolaemia

- Obstructive sleep apnoea
- Restrictive lung disease
- Hypoventilation
- Reflux
- Hirsutism
- Acanthosis nigricans
- Gout
- Osteoarthritis
- Cancer
- Depression

Management

1 Educate the patient about the ills of obesity and the need for significant weight loss.
2 Formulate a practical weight-loss program with definite goals and a timetable.
3 Prescribe a low-joule/high-fibre diet in consultation with a dietitian. Educate the patient about joule counting and fat counting. Encourage the patient to eat only small portions of food.
4 Encourage regular physical exercise. Light exercise to the level of slight breathlessness for 20–30 minutes, four times a week, would be adequate. This may take the form of fast walking, jogging or swimming.
5 For refractory patients, prescription of anti-obesity medications such as orlistat may be beneficial. But when prescribing a lipase inhibitor such as orlistat, warn the patient about the side effects of faecal urgency, greasy stool, increased frequency of defecation and, at times, faecal incontinence.
6 Other pharmacotherapeutic agents include phentermine and sibutramine (Reductil®).
7 Bariatric surgery should be considered for morbidly obese patients who respond poorly to non-surgical measures.
8 Rimonabant is a new cannabinoid receptor antagonist that has shown promise as an antiobesity and smoking cessation agent. However, it should not be used in the setting of depression.

CORTICOSTEROID USE

Case vignette

A 74-year-old woman presents with recent weight gain, occasional blurred vision and polyuria. She has been commenced on prednisolone 25 mg daily for a recent diagnosis of giant cell arteritis. On examination she has cutaneous striae and evidence of easy bruising together with abdominal obesity and a moon facies.

1 What further investigations would you order?
2 How would you plan her management?

Approach to the patient

History

When assessing patients commenced or maintained on long-term corticosteroid therapy, it is important to find out whether the patient is aware of the multiple adverse effects associated with such therapy and the precautionary measures that need to be taken to minimise such effects. If the patient has been on steroids for a considerable period of time, ask about weight gain, easy bruising, insomnia, polyphagia, ankle oedema, irritability and the psychological symptoms of depression or psychosis. Ask whether the patient has ever been tested for diabetes and, if so, how often and using which test. Also ask whether the patient's blood pressure is monitored closely. Ask whether the patient has had cataracts diagnosed or experienced any visual impairment. Some patients may develop glaucoma associated with steroid use.

Corticosteroids at a dose higher than the replacement dose (equivalent of 7.5 mg per day of prednisolone) for more than 6 months can predispose the patient to osteoporosis, and it is important to enquire whether the patient has ever been diagnosed with osteoporosis and, if so, what treatment he or she has received. If not, ask whether they have ever had bone densitometry done. Ask about any fractures on minimum impact, and bone pain, and whether a radioisotope bone scan has been performed. Patients on corticosteroids benefit from calcium and vitamin D supplementation (steroids can impair vitamin D absorption in the gut) in addition to bisphosphonates and hormone replacement therapy in the setting of established osteoporosis. Ask about hip pain on movement, a feature that may suggest aseptic necrosis of the femoral head. Ask about infections, particularly atypical infections such as *Pneumocystis carinii*, cytomegalovirus infections, tuberculosis, *Cryptococcus neoformans* and recurrent oral and genital candidiasis.

Examination

Look for moon-shaped facies, cushingoid body habitus, multiple cutaneous ecchymoses, evidence of skin fragility, cataract, oral candidiasis, buffalo hump, proximal muscle loss and weakness, tenderness in the hip joints and tenderness in the vertebral column (see box).

Adverse effects of chronic corticosteroid therapy

- Obesity
- Cushingoid body habitus
- Hypertension
- Diabetes mellitus
- Hirsutism
- Cutaneous fragility/striae
- Acne
- Immunosuppression/opportunistic infection
- Oral/vaginal candidiasis
- Cataract
- Glaucoma

- Osteoporosis
- Proximal myopathy
- Avascular necrosis of bone (especially head of femur)
- Mood disorders/psychosis
- Peptic ulcer disease
- Pancreatitis
- Hypokalaemia
- Peripheral oedema
- Suppression of hypothalamic–pituitary axis

It is highly recommended that these patients be regularly vaccinated with pneumococcal vaccine every 5 years and influenza vaccine every year.

Ask about any steroid-sparing agents that have been tried, and their effects.

OSTEOPOROSIS

Approach to the patient

History

Ask about back pain, any falls or fractures and the treatment received. Check whether the patient is on any therapeutic agents that would contribute to osteoporosis. Ask about family history of osteoporosis and enquire into the menopausal status. Post-menopausal osteoporosis is common, but do not forget other contributing factors relevant to the patient's circumstances, such as chronic corticosteroid use, chronic renal failure, vitamin D deficiency, hyperthyroidism, hyperparathyroidism, multiple myeloma and Cushing's syndrome.

Examination

Look for bone tenderness, vertebral column abnormalities and exclude physical signs of endocrine disorders such as Cushing's syndrome.

Osteoporosis is common and the cause can be multifactorial. If clinical assessment suggests the existence of osteoporosis in the patient, ask the examiner for the report of the dual-energy X-ray densitometry (DEXA) study to establish a definite diagnosis. Candidates should be able to quickly and accurately interpret the Z and T scores in the bone densitometry report (Fig 9.1). A bone mineral density value lower than 1 standard deviation below the mean bone densitometry value of the young normal (T score < 1) should be considered an indication for the initiation of preventive measures. A T score of −2.5 or below is considered diagnostic of osteoporosis and an indication for treatment. A significantly abnormal Z score should alert the candidate to secondary causes of osteoporosis. Remember, most pathological fractures due to osteoporosis occur in the mid- and lower thoracic and upper lumbar regions of the vertebral column. Pathological fractures elsewhere in the vertebral column should arouse suspicion of other causes, such as malignancy.

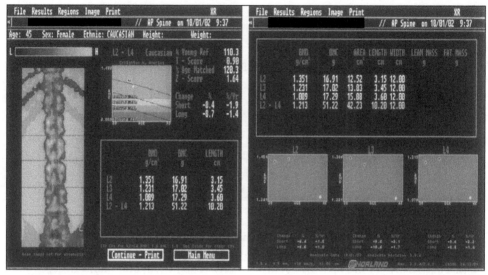

Figure 9.1 DEXA bone scan depicting near-normal bone density (note the T score of 0.90 and Z score of 1.64). A T score of < 1 warrants initiation of preventive measures against osteoporosis.

Investigations

1   Bone densitometry
2   Serum testosterone levels in male patients, to exclude hypogonadism
3   Thyroid function tests
4   Serum 25-hydroxyvitamin D level and serum calcium and phosphate levels
5   Renal function indices—to exclude chronic renal failure
6   Serum electrophoresis and immunoelectrophoresis—to exclude multiple myeloma
7   24-hour urinary cortisol levels—to exclude Cushing's syndrome

Management

1   *Correct the underlying cause*, if there is one—this is the first step in the management of osteoporosis.
2   *Education*—educate and encourage the patient to adopt lifestyle measures that will prevent the progression of osteoporosis, such as ingestion of food with high calcium content, calcium supplements, adequate amounts of vitamin D, regular low-impact and weight-bearing physical exercise, cessation of smoking and reduction of alcohol intake. Postmenopausal women should aim at ingesting 1.5 g of calcium daily.
3   *Pharmacology*—pharmacological treatment of osteoporosis is a judicious decision that needs to be taken on further consideration of the patient's clinical condition. If the bone mineral density is significantly low, or the patient is older, or if there is an established pathological fracture, the need for pharmacological intervention is significantly high, and hence can be justified:
    • Hormone replacement therapy (HRT) is an initial treatment option and this can be commenced in any postmenopausal woman with no contraindication. HRT has also been found useful as prophylactic therapy.

- Bisphosphonate therapy is of proven benefit in osteoporosis. The oral agents alendronate, etidronate and risedronate are useful in the prevention and treatment of osteoporosis. They have been shown to decrease the rate of new fractures occurring in the vertebrae and hips. These agents, however, can cause severe oesophagitis. To prevent this adverse effect, the patient should be advised to take the drug first thing in the morning with a glass of water, at least 30 minutes before breakfast. The patient should also avoid lying down for at least 30 minutes after the ingestion of the drug. For patients intolerant of oral forms, once-a-month IV pamidronate infusion is a suitable alternative.
- Other agents that should be considered include raloxifene, the selective oestrogen receptor modulator (SERM) and calcitriol (vitamin D). Calcium supplements should be recommended for all osteoporosis patients. Venous thromboembolism is a serious side effect of raloxifene.

Intermittent dosing of recombinant human parathyroid hormone (teriparatide) has been shown to benefit postmenopausal women and men with osteoporosis. Anabolic steroids too have been shown to be beneficial in this group of patients.

Strontium ranelate is approved for the treatment of postmenopausal osteoporosis and has been shown to reduce vertebral and hip fractures.

Often a combination of different agents based on the clinical scenario is necessary to optimise the management of osteoporosis.

PAGET'S DISEASE

Approach to the patient

Paget's disease is encountered in the long case patient, but often as an inactive disease condition. Usually the active disease presents with bone pain, deformity and pathological fracture.

History

Ask when and how the diagnosis was made and what treatment has been received so far. Ask about any change in hat size (though not many people wear hats these days!) or the size of spectacle frames, bone deformity, joint pain and symptoms of cardiac failure. By now you may have noticed whether the patient has any hearing impairment, which may be due to Paget's disease of the ear ossicles or compression of the acoustic nerve. Check whether the patient suffers from ureteric colic.

Examination

Observe skull enlargement (skull diameter > 55 cm is abnormal), back deformity and limb deformity. Note lateral bowing of the femur and anterior bowing of the tibia. A bony mass lesion in the lower limb should alert the candidate to osteosarcoma. Auscultate for bruits in the skull and other bones. Look for osteoarthritis, particularly in the knees. Perform a detailed cardiovascular examination, looking for evidence of high-output cardiac failure. Conduct a detailed neurological examination, looking for deficit due to compression of cranial nerves at the cranial foramina and of brainstem due to platybasia. Look in the fundi for angioid streaks and optic atrophy.

Investigations

If there is an index of suspicion or a clinical indication, ask for confirmatory tests for Paget's disease, which include:

1 Serum alkaline phosphatase levels— > 600 mmol/L is considered highly suggestive
2 Urinary deoxypyridinoline and *N*-telopeptide levels—levels of these markers also reflect disease activity
3 Skeletal X-rays of the relevant regions—when sclerotic bony lesions are seen, differential diagnoses that should also be considered are carcinoma of the prostate in the male and carcinoma of breast in the female
4 Three-phase bone scan—to exclude fractures and the complication of osteosarcoma.

Management

Symptomatic treatment is with analgesics, paracetamol or non-steroidal anti-inflammatory drugs (NSAIDs).

Disease-specific pharmacological treatment is indicated only if there is pain or active disease near a major joint or in a long bone.

The mainstay of treatment is oral bisphosphonates in the form of alendronate, tiludronate, risedronate or IV pamidronate. Calcitonin is used only rarely these days. Treatment should be continued until disease activity ceases, as indicated by symptoms and biochemical markers.

HYPERTHYROIDISM

Case vignette

A 61-year-old man presents with acute dyspnoea, delirium and high fevers after a CT coronary angiogram. He is agitated and has diarrhoea. On examination his blood pressure is 130/85 mmHg and pulse is 120 bpm and irregularly regular. He has diffuse crepitations in the lower zones of both lungs and pitting bipedal oedema. In the background history it is revealed that he has been investigated by his general practitioner for paroxysmal atrial fibrillation, heat intolerance and recent weight loss.

1 What are the possible differential diagnoses in this case and what investigations would you request?
2 He has a palpable nodule in the thyroid region and the thyroid function tests reveal elevated T3 levels and significantly suppressed thyroid-stimulating hormone (TSH) levels. What is the most likely reason for his clinical picture?
3 What is your acute management plan?
4 Develop a comprehensive long-term and definitive plan of management for this man upon his recovery from the acute crisis.

Approach to the patient

The patient's age may give some clues to the aetiology. Younger patients are more likely to get hyperthyroidism from Graves' disease and older patients from toxic adenomata or toxic nodular goitres.

History

Ask about:

- visual impairment and headache—may be clues to a pituitary adenoma secreting TSH, although this is very rare
- recent fevers (viral illness) and tenderness over the thyroid gland—suggestive of acute or subacute thyroiditis as a possible differential diagnosis
- whether the patient has had recent iodine-containing contrast dose (coronary angiography etc)—would suggest the possibility of iodine-induced hyperthyroidism
- symptoms such as anxiety, excessive sweating, tearfulness and palpitations
- how the patient handles heat—heat intolerance is a salient feature
- significant weight loss in spite of an increased appetite
- sexual function—loss of libido and impotence in the male can be associated with hyperthyroidism
- menstrual period in females—menstrual abnormalities are common with this condition
- weakness—elderly patients with clinical hyperthyroidism may manifest only weakness and this phenomenon is called apathetic thyrotoxicosis
- whether the patient has ever been treated with amiodarone and whether they have had radiation exposure, particularly to the neck area—remember that the most common cause of hyperthyroidism is Graves' disease.

Examination

Look for warm, clammy skin and evidence of wasting/weight loss. Check the pulse for AF or tachycardia. Perform an eye examination, looking for lid retraction and lid lag. Patients with cardiac involvement may show evidence of heart failure. Perform a detailed neck examination, looking for a goitre and also lymphadenopathy. If a goitre is found, define the features in detail, including the size, consistency, tenderness and nodularity. Check the limbs for muscle weakness due to thyroid myopathy. Neurological examination shows brisk reflexes and a fine tremor of the upper extremities. Male patients may have gynaecomastia. Look in the extremities for clubbing-like thyroid acropachy and the nail bed for onycholysis. Patients with Graves' disease may have the eye signs of exophthalmos, conjunctival oedema and periorbital oedema. They may also have skin infiltration manifesting as pretibial myxoedema.

Investigations

1 Serum TSH and free T4/T3 levels—usually TSH is suppressed due to T4/T3 elevation in primary hyperthyroidism. Elevated levels of TSH and T4 are seen with amiodarone therapy. Elevated TSH may indicate secondary (pituitary) hyperthyroidism, which is extremely rare.
2 Thyroid-stimulating immunoglobulins of Graves' disease or Hashimoto's thyroiditis.

3   Radioactive iodine uptake thyroid scan—increased activity is indicative of Graves' disease, toxic adenoma or toxic nodular goitre, whereas decreased uptake is suggestive of inflammation (thyroiditis).
4   If clinical features suggest and serum TSH is normal or elevated, a cranial CT or MRI—to exclude pituitary tumour.
5   ECG looking for AF, and echocardiogram to assess left ventricular function.

Management

1   Symptomatic treatment with a beta-blocker
2   Carbimazole or propylthiouracil—to achieve euthyroid state. Iodine therapy alone at high doses or in combination with carbimazole can also help achieve euthyroid state.
3   Radioactive iodine—for ablation of the hyperactive thyroid gland
4   Surgery—if relevant for large goitres

HORMONE REPLACEMENT THERAPY

Many patients in the long case examination may be on hormone replacement therapy (HRT). The question of continuation of this therapy may be a subject of interest in the discussion. HRT has proven benefits in the prevention and management of senile osteoporosis. There is observational evidence to support the usefulness of HRT in lowering LDL and lipoprotein-a and in elevating HDL levels, and therefore would seem to have a cardiovascular benefit. However, recently completed controlled trials have failed to demonstrate any objective benefits of HRT in improving the clinical end-points of cardiovascular disease. It has further demonstrated that HRT can increase the incidence of DVT and thromboembolism in some treated patients. Anecdotal risks of malignancies, too, should be acknowledged.

Raloxifene is a selective oestrogen receptor modulator that has shown promise as an alternative to conventional HRT. It acts as an oestrogen receptor agonist in the skeletal tissue and the cardiovascular system, and as an oestrogen receptor antagonist in the breast and the uterus. It is not very useful in the management of perimenopausal symptoms. The incidence of DVT with its use is similar to that of conventional hormonal therapy. The other distressing side effect of this agent is persistent cramps in the legs. Its main indication is for the prevention and treatment of senile osteoporosis. There are observational data supporting its beneficial effect on the serum lipid profile, but end-point data are still awaited. It has also been shown to be helpful in decreasing the incidence of breast cancer. The above information should help the clinician in making a decision regarding the continuation of HRT and deciding on an alternative if indicated.

PYREXIA OF UNKNOWN ORIGIN

Case vignette

A 66-year-old man of Greek descent has been investigated in hospital for a period of 1 week for a swinging fever of 1 month's duration and associated headache, weight loss, arthralgia, myalgia and lethargy. He complains of drenching night sweats and rigors. The patient denies any localising symptoms. He has a background history of myocardial infarction treated with angioplasty and stent 1 year ago. He is currently on metoprolol 25 mg twice daily and aspirin 150 mg daily. He denies any allergies or family history of significant illness. He has recently travelled to the west coast of the United States for a family reunion. On examination his pulse rate is 100 bpm and his temperature is 38°C. His temperature chart shows a regular pattern of temperature spikes up to 39°C. No other significant signs are evident.

1 List the possible differential diagnoses in this man.

2 What investigations may help in arriving at a more definitive diagnosis?

On further enquiry the patient reveals that he noticed an expanding erythematous maculopapular rash, which disappeared spontaneously. The lesion was painless. According to the detailed description, the lesion had a clear central core and a well-defined border.

3 How would this information help you to narrow your list of diagnoses?

4 Discuss a suitable plan of management for this patient's condition.

Approach to the patient

Pyrexia of unknown origin is defined as intermittent or continuous fever for more than 3 weeks in a patient in whom the cause of the fever has not been identified in spite of repeated investigations for more than a week.

History

Ask about:

- the onset and duration of the illness
- any treatment received so far
- other associated symptoms that may give some clues to the likely aetiology of the fever—such as weight loss, cough, rashes
- symptoms that may help in the localisation of the focus
- the temporal pattern of the febrile episodes
- past medical history—focusing on infectious conditions, connective tissue diseases, vasculitic conditions and malignancies
- detailed medication history—looking particularly for drugs that may cause fever
- history of alcohol intake and recreational drug use
- pets, farm animals, hobbies, sexual activity
- travel—be familiar with region-specific rare infections such as kala-azar, Lassa fever, Q fever, Lyme disease
- specific features of rather rare diseases such as erythema migrans of Lyme disease (as was the case in the above case vignette) when there is a suspicion
- detailed family history—important in excluding diseases such as familial Mediterranean fever.

Examination

The condition could be due to multiple causes, both infective and non-infective (see box). A detailed physical examination should be carried out, looking first for a focus of sepsis. Look for areas of inflammation in the skin and check for lymphadenopathy and/or hepatosplenomegaly. Look for rashes, inflamed joints, painless mass lesions etc. Study the temperature chart. Perform the examination with a particular focus on the most likely body system to be involved, based on the overall clinical picture.

Some of the commonly encountered causes of undiagnosed persistent fever are occult abscesses in the abdomen, tuberculosis, cytomegalovirus (CMV) infection, HIV infection, haematological malignancy, solid cancer, pulmonary embolism, Wegener's granulomatosis, undiagnosed vasculitis (especially polymyalgia rheumatica and giant cell arteritis), granulomatous conditions such as sarcoidosis, Still's disease and drugs. The remainder of the physical examination should be focused on looking for features of non-infective causes of fever.

Causes of pyrexia of unknown origin

- Bacterial sepsis—e.g. bacterial endocarditis, subphrenic abscess, typhoid fever, brucellosis
- Viral sepsis—e.g. HIV, Epstein-Barr virus, parvovirus, Ross River virus, Barmah Forest virus
- Fungal sepsis
- Rickettsial sepsis—e.g. Q fever
- Mycobacterial sepsis—tuberculosis/atypical varieties
- Connective tissue disease—e.g. systemic lupus erythematosus (SLE), mixed connective disease, rheumatoid arthritis

---

- Systemic vasculitis—e.g. Wegener's granulomatosis, polyarteritis nodosa, Behçet's disease
- Granulomatous conditions—e.g. sarcoidosis, Crohn's disease
- Neoplasms—e.g. sarcoma, renal carcinoma, Hodgkin's disease
- Drug fever—sulfa drugs, vancomycin, hydralazine, methyldopa
- Pulmonary embolism
- Haematoma
- Gout
- Dressler's syndrome
- Alcoholic hepatitis
- Hypothalamic lesions—impaired thermoregulation
- Factitious fever

Investigations

Initial investigations should be aimed at excluding infection, and a standard septic work-up may already have been done. If the results are inconclusive, it is most appropriate to repeat the septic work-up. The standard septic work-up includes:

1 Full blood count and differential white cell count, to exclude leucocytosis or leucopenia
2 ESR and C-reactive protein (CRP), looking for persisting inflammation
3 At least three sets of blood cultures from different sites of the body at different intervals
4 Alerting the microbiology lab to the need for prolonged cultures for fungi and fastidious organisms
5 Chest X-ray
6 Urine analysis and midstream urine for microscopy and culture
7 Sputum microscopy and culture
8 Stool culture, for *Salmonella*
9 Lumbar puncture if neurological features are present.

If these investigations are non-diagnostic and the patient is still febrile, further investigations should be ordered, looking for specific diagnostic clues. These include:

1 CT of the thorax, abdomen and pelvis—looking for abscesses and unsuspected lymph node enlargement
2 Transoesophageal echocardiography—looking for valvular vegetations, to exclude subacute infective endocarditis
3 Gallium scan, looking for areas of active inflammation or lymphoma
4 Indium-labelled white cell scan, looking for foci of sepsis
5 Three-phase bone scan (or bone first gallium record)—looking for osteomyelitis or other bony lesions (inflammation or metastatic deposits)
6 Swabs as clinically indicated (e.g. cannula site)
7 Serology for CMV and HIV
8 Autoimmune serology
9 Serology for rheumatic fever—antistreptolysin-O titre, a reading of > 200 units/mL is abnormal

10 Temporal artery biopsy if there is clinical suggestion of temporal arteritis

11 Liver biopsy

Management

Very ill patients should be treated as for septicaemia, with broad-spectrum, potent parenteral antibiotic combinations. Otherwise, therapy should be guided by the clinical circumstances and the above investigational results.

THE IMMUNOCOMPROMISED HOST

Approach to the patient

There is a high likelihood that a patient presented as a long case will have some form of immunodeficiency, either as the primary presentation or as a comorbidity. Immunodeficiency could be granulocytopenia, cellular immunodeficiency (see box) or humoral immunodeficiency (see box).

Causes of cellular immunodeficiency

- Lymphoma
- Chronic lymphocytic leukaemia
- High-dose corticosteroid therapy
- Cytotoxic therapy
- HIV/AIDS
- Immunosuppression associated with solid organ or bone marrow transplantation. (Viral infections due to agents such as herpes simplex, varicella zoster and cytomegalovirus are common in this group of patients. In the setting of solid organ transplantation, the most common causative organism of opportunistic sepsis is cytomegalovirus—with the exception of heart transplantation, where it is toxoplasmosis. Other opportunistic infections of importance are *Pneumocystis carinii* pneumonia and reactivation of tuberculosis.)

Causes of humoral immunodeficiency

- Multiple myeloma
- Lymphoma
- Splenectomy
- Complement deficiency
- X-linked agammaglobulinaemia
- Common variable immunodeficiency

Therapy for humoral immunodeficiency may include IV infusion of immunoglobulins at regular intervals. Encapsulated bacteria such as *Streptococcus pneumoniae* and *Haemophilus influenzae* usually cause sepsis in this setting. In terminal component complement and properdin deficiency, *Neisseria meningitidis* is the organism that causes the most sepsis.

History

Ask about:

- the current symptoms the patient presents with, to ascertain the focus of sepsis
- recurrent infections and, if known, investigations performed so far
- other medical conditions—diabetes mellitus, renal failure, HIV, haematological malignancy
- details of any relevant family history
- medications consumed—immunosuppressive agents
- alcohol abuse, recreational drug use
- sexual behaviour.

Examination

Search for the focus of sepsis. You should carry out a detailed examination of the systems involved. Check the temperature chart to ascertain the temporal pattern of the fevers. Look for clues to the predisposing condition, such as stigmata of liver disease or chronic renal failure, venepuncture marks of injecting drug use, lymphadenopathy, hepatosplenomegaly, splenectomy scar and central venous catheters.

Sepsis in injecting drug use (causative organisms)

- *Staphylococcus aureus*
- Gram-negative coccobacilli
- *Candida* sp.
- Hepatitis B and C
- HIV

Sepsis in chronic liver disease and cirrhosis (causative organisms)

- *Streptococcus pneumoniae*
- *Listeria monocytogenes*
- *Vibrio vulnificus*
- *Pasteurella*
- *Yersinia*

The following is an outline of some of the different forms of immunodeficiency that can be expected in the long case setting and some information that may be useful in approaching the management of such patients.

Granulocytopenia

A patient is absolutely granulocytopenic by the classic definition when the neutrophil count goes below 0.5×10^9/L. The risk of sepsis is increased in this setting.

If a granulocytopenic patient is febrile, possible foci of sepsis are: oropharynx, lung, distal oesophagus, colon, perianal skin, intravenous cannula site and the urinary tract.

Investigations

Standard septic work-up, including:

1 Chest X-ray
2 Multiple blood cultures for both aerobic and anaerobic organisms
3 Multiple bacteriological swabs from relevant sites
4 Urine analysis followed by microscopy, culture and sensitivities.

Management

Empiric therapy should generally be commenced with a beta-lactamase inhibitor agent with anti-pseudomonal activity together with an aminoglycoside. If the patient fails to respond to the Gram-negative regimen or there is suspected peripheral or central-line sepsis, or if there are Gram-positive organisms identified in the blood microscopy, add vancomycin to the antibiotic combination. If the patient does not defervesce after 3–7 days of antibiotic therapy, consider commencing empiric antifungal therapy with an agent such as IV amphotericin-B or fluconazole. Remember to ask the microbiology lab to perform prolonged cultures to identify fungal organisms. Administration of granulo-cyte colony-stimulating factor or granulocyte-macrophage colony-stimulating factor would help shorten the duration of neutropenia, but its use in the setting of sepsis has not been proved to be of any benefit.

Sepsis in hyperalimentation (causative organisms)

• Coagulase-negative staphylococci
• *Staphylococcus aureus*
• Fungal organisms such as *Candida*

Metabolic acidosis

This is seen in conditions such as diabetes mellitus, acute myeloid leukaemia and renal failure. Acidosis impairs the optimal functioning of the granulocytes and the complement system. The causative organisms of infections include *Pseudomonas aeruginosa* and fungi.

Fungal infections

In a septic patient, if the following risk factors are present, consider the possibility of candidaemia:

• Neutropenia
• Multiple antibiotic use

- Prolonged broad-spectrum antibiotic use
- Corticosteroid use
- Indwelling urinary catheter
- Central venous catheters
- Renal failure
- Sarcoidosis.

Investigations
1 Microscopy of biological specimens using fungal stains
2 Prolonged fungal cultures

Management
1 Fungal prophylaxis for susceptible patients
2 Antifungal therapy
3 Exclusion of resistant fungal organisms (e.g. *Candida krusei*, resistant to fluconazole)

Febrile neutropenia

This condition is common among patients treated with cytotoxic chemotherapy as well as those suffering from aggressive haematological malignancies. There is a high likelihood that the discussion of a long case with the above pathology will also involve the management of febrile neutropenia. Examiners expect the candidate to be confident with the management of such life-threatening conditions.

Febrile neutropenia is defined as a body temperature of more than 38°C, in a patient whose white cell count is less than 1×10^9/L. The causative organism is more often a Gram-positive than a Gram-negative bacterium; however, if the agent is *Pseudomonas aeruginosa*, mortality is expected to be extremely high, so the empiric antibiotic regimen should include agents that would be active also against *Pseudomonas* sp.

Management

The therapeutic regimen is usually determined according to the data on causative organisms of sepsis in patients at that particular institution. A standard regimen in febrile neutropenia is gentamicin 5 mg/kg together with ceftazadime 1 g three times a day, or ticarcillin and clavulanic acid 3 g four times a day. Addition of vancomycin should be strongly considered if the patient is known to be colonised with methicillin-resistant *Staphylococcus aureus*, if the patient is in septic shock, or if the fever continues despite the above antibiotic therapy.

BACTERIAL ENDOCARDITIS

Case vignette

A 41-year-old man presents with severe dyspnoea, orthopnoea with fevers and chills progressive with associated arthralgia over a period of 2 weeks. He reports feeling extremely lethargic prior to the onset of fevers. He also reports significant weight loss over a period of about 1 month. He has been healthy otherwise. He denies any intravenous drug use, smoking or alcohol excess. He reports allergy to penicillin. On examination the patient is saturating at 95% on 100% oxygen via the non-rebreather mask. He is febrile at 39°C. He has splinter haemorrhages in the upper extremities. His JVP is significantly elevated with a prominent V wave. There is a harsh pansystolic murmur audible across the precordium. There are coarse crepitations in all lung fields bilaterally.

1 **What investigations would you perform to work up this patient further?**
2 **Discuss your plan of management, focusing on the immediate and long-term objectives.**
3 **Discuss the possible predisposing factors in this man for endocarditis.**
4 **What are the possible causative organisms in this case and what are your therapeutic options?**

Approach to the patient

History

Ask about the presenting symptoms and their duration. Ask about previous cardiac surgery, valvular repair or replacement, and any past history of a known cardiac murmur. Check what investigations have been performed so far (transoesophageal echocardiogram should not escape a patient's memory!). Ask about the treatment received and any side effects. Enquire about predisposing conditions, such as previous valvular heart disease, rheumatic fever during childhood, injecting drug use, and recent dental work or invasive procedures. Ask about other medical conditions such as gastrointestinal malignancy etc. *Streptococcus bovis* infection may be associated with colonic malignancy.

Examination

Check the temperature chart and look for peripheral stigmata (petechiae, finger clubbing, splinter haemorrhages, Osler's nodes (tender nodules in the finger pads) and Janeway lesions (non-tender macular lesions on the palms and soles)). Look in the fundus for Roth spots. Perform a detailed cardiovascular examination, looking for signs of valve pathology and congestive cardiac failure. A sternotomy scar would testify to previous cardiac surgery. Check for neurological deficit and palpate the abdomen for splenomegaly. Don't forget to look for ports or percutaneous indwelling central venous catheter (PICC) lines meant for chronic parenteral antibiotic therapy. Inflammation or cellulitis around such foreign bodies is of major concern.

Investigations

Investigation of suspected subacute bacterial endocarditis should include:
1 Three sets of blood cultures taken from different sites of the body at different intervals (of > 1 hour apart) within the first 24 hours of presentation. Negative cultures should be maintained for 3–4 weeks to facilitate the detection of fastidious and slow-growing HACEK (*Haemophilus, Actinobacillus* sp., *Cardiobacterium hominis, Eikenella, Kingella*) organisms. Unusual organisms that should be considered in this setting include *Coxiella burnetii, Chlamydia* sp., *Legionella* sp., *Bartonella* sp. and fungi.
2 Full blood count—looking for anaemia and leucocytosis
3 ESR and CRP

4 Urine analysis—looking for haematuria

5 Transthoracic echocardiogram—looking for valvular regurgitation, ventricular septal defect (VSD), large vegetations and cardiac failure. Transoesophageal echocardiography—looking for valvular vegetations and/or cardiac abscess.

6 Chest X-ray—looking for features of cardiac failure.

Remember Duke's criteria for the diagnosis of bacterial endocarditis:

- *Major criteria*—vegetations on echocardiography, bacteraemia and a new regurgitant murmur
- *Minor criteria*—predisposing cardiac lesions, injecting drug abuse, fever of >38°C and vasculitic phenomena on physical examination.

For a conclusive diagnosis of endocarditis, one should have a combination of two major criteria or one major criterion with three minor criteria.

Management of infective endocarditis

1 Sensitive streptococcal endocarditis (minimal inhibitory concentration (MIC) < 0.1) may be treated with 2 weeks of IV penicillin and gentamicin. Also high-dose ceftriaxone (2 g daily) can be used intravenously for 4 weeks. Patients with penicillin allergy can be treated with vancomycin for 4 weeks.
   If the disease is complicated or the symptoms have been present for more than 3 months, the antibiotic regimen should be changed to 4 weeks of IV penicillin together with 2 weeks of IV gentamicin.

2 Enterococcal endocarditis can be treated with penicillin/gentamicin combination for 4–6 weeks or ampicillin/gentamicin combination for 4–6 weeks. Penicillin-allergic patients may be treated with vancomycin.

3 Staphylococcal endocarditis can be treated with flucloxacillin or nafcillin for 4–6 weeks. If the organism is methycillin resistant or if the patient is penicillin intolerant, vancomycin should be given for 6 weeks.

4 Treatment for prosthetic valve endocarditis caused by *Staphylococcus aureus*, *S. epidermidis* or diphtheroids will be guided by sensitivity testing. Methicillin-resistant *S. aureus* is treated with vancomycin combined with gentamicin for a total of 2 months.
   Clinical progress is monitored with the observation of the temperature pattern, follow-up blood cultures, ESR and CRP, as well as urine analysis looking for resolution of haematuria.

5 Patients with significant haemodynamic instability, heart failure, significant valve damage, septic emboli or cardiac abscess need surgical intervention.

6 Patients with a previous history of endocarditis, known valve disease, mitral valve prolapse with regurgitation, prosthetic valves and intracardiac shunts need antibiotic prophylaxis (see box) prior to invasive procedures that can cause bacteraemia such as dental work, large bowel surgery or genitourinary surgery.

Antibiotic prophylaxis regimens

1 For oral, upper respiratory tract and oesophageal procedures:
   - Amoxycillin 2 g orally 1 hour before the procedure, or ampicillin 2 g intravenously or intramuscularly 30 minutes before the procedure if the patient is fasted

---

- For penicillin-allergic patients, clindamycin 600 mg orally 1 hour before the procedure.
2   For genitourinary and lower gastrointestinal procedures:
- Amoxycillin 2 g orally 1 hour before the procedure for low-risk patients
- Ampicillin 2 g intravenously or intramuscularly, together with gentamicin 1.5 mg/kg intravenously or intramuscularly within 30 minutes followed by ampicillin 1 g intravenously or intramuscularly 6 hours after the procedure (for high-risk patients)
- For penicillin-allergic patients vancomycin can be substituted.

(Adapted from Dajanis A S, Taubert K A, Wison W et al 1997 Prevention of bacterial endocarditis. Recommendations by the American Heart Association. *Circulation* 96(1): 358–366)

THE HIV PATIENT

Human immunodeficiency virus (HIV) infection with its multiple opportunistic infections, drug interactions and adverse drug effects, together with numerous sociocultural and economic problems, is ideal for a long case at the examination. Although it is a complex disorder, there are certain basic HIV/AIDS concepts with which the candidate must be familiar.

Case vignette

A 35-year-old female is admitted with acute confusion. She has a history of haemophilia and multiple blood transfusions. She has also had transfusion-acquired HIV for the past 14 years. She was managed on lamivudine, zidovudine and the combination of ritonavir and lopinavir. Due to a recent rise in the viral load, her HAART regimen has been changed with the addition of efavirenz. She has not experienced any AIDS-defining illness in the recent past. She works as a shop assistant and has had a steady male partner for the past 3 months who is not known to have HIV. She is sexually active. On examination the patient is confused to place and time but not to person. Her vital signs are stable. There is evidence of treatment-related lipodystrophy and generalised lymphadenopathy. She has no overt signs of opportunistic infections or wasting.

1   What are the possible differential diagnoses for her confusion?
2   What additional information, including investigations, would you require to work this patient up?
3   What is your initial approach to the management of this patient?
4   Her urine beta-hCG is positive. What concerns do you have and how would her management be affected by this finding?
5   How would you monitor the response to therapy?
6   What options are available to manage treatment-resistant HIV-1?

Approach to the patient

History

Enquire about how and when the diagnosis was made, whether the patient experienced any seroconversion illness, the initial viral load and the initial CD4 cell count. Ask about all risk-prone behaviour, partner infection, and any deaths among previous or current partners due to AIDS. Ask about opportunistic infections and other infections, particularly candidiasis, varicella zoster, *Mycobacterium avium* complex (MAC), tuberculosis, and hepatitis A, B and C. Enquire about the symptoms, such as fever, weight loss, diarrhoea, night sweats, dyspnoea, cough, anorexia, depression and symptoms of neurological impairment. Other important aspects of the history are psychosocial problems, travel history, living circumstances, relationships, financial problems, employment and details of available community resources. It is important to learn about the various drugs that have been used to treat the patient and the complications encountered. The candidate has to gain a very good understanding of the patient's insight into this serious disease condition and the associated prognosis.

Examination

Physical examination of the HIV patient needs to be extensive.

1 Check the oral cavity—looking at the general hygiene and for candidiasis, oral hairy leucoplakia, Kaposi's sarcoma and herpes simplex infection.
2 Perform fundoscopy—looking for retinitis, generally due to HIV or CMV.
3 Check for lymphadenopathy.
4 Thoroughly examine the respiratory system, abdomen and pelvis—looking for evidence of opportunistic infection and malignancy.
5 Perform a Mini-Mental State Examination—looking for cognitive impairment.
6 Perform a neurological examination—looking especially for peripheral neuropathy.

Investigations

Diagnosis

Early detection, prior to seroconversion, can be made by serum assays of p24 antigen level or detection of HIV RNA in the patient's blood by polymerase chain reaction (PCR) assay. Remember that there is a possibility of false-positive results with radioimmunoassays. Seroconversion takes place usually 1–3 weeks after infection and the serological test can be performed for the purpose of diagnosis thereafter. However, sometimes the antibody test will not yield a positive result for as long as 3 months. The standard enzyme-linked immunosorbent assay (ELISA) test is highly sensitive. A repeat ELISA test and/or a Western blot test may be carried out for confirmation. A positive Western blot result includes the standard determination of the number of viral components. Indeterminate results (positive ELISA test and indeterminate Western blot test) occur in about 4 in 1000 tests and are reviewed by repeat testing to see if progression to a positive Western blot has occurred. Rapid serological tests for HIV are now available. These tests are convenient to use. However, these test results need to be validated with a standard enzyme immunoassay (EIA) or by Western blot test. For the newly diagnosed HIV patient it is necessary to organise pre-test and post-test counselling, with partner notification and contact tracing.

On diagnosis of HIV, the viral load together with the CD4 lymphocyte subset count should be checked. Viral load and CD4 count should be checked three to four times a year unless the clinical course is very stable.

After diagnosis
Upon diagnosis, the basic investigational battery includes:
1 Full blood count—looking for anaemia, leucopenia and thrombocytopenia.
2 CD4 lymphocyte count (per mL) and the viral load (copies per mL), genotype testing for drug resistance. (The CD4 subset lymphocyte count in the blood gives an impression of the short-term prognosis of the patient and the viral load gives an idea of the patient's long-term prognosis.)
3 Electrolyte profile and renal function indices
4 Liver function indices and amylase level
5 Serum cholesterol levels (preferably fasting)
6 Serology for syphilis, toxoplasmosis, CMV, hepatitis B and hepatitis C
7 Tuberculin skin test (Mantoux)—a positive test proves that the patient has had previous exposure or the BCG vaccination; however, false-negative tests are seen due to immunosuppression in AIDS
8 Pap smear—important in the female patient
9 Chest X-ray—as a baseline test
10 Testing for therapeutic drug resistance in patients who have a higher viral load (> 1000 copies/mL)

Management
1 All patients should be immunised against hepatitis A, hepatitis B, and annually against the influenza virus. A tuberculin reaction of 5 mm or more is an indication for isoniazid prophylaxis for 12 months.
2 An HIV-specific flowchart of clinical events should be commenced on every new case.
3 HIV infection is divided into stages depending on the patient's CD4 count, and these divisions indicate what opportunistic infections the patient is prone to and what prophylactic therapy is indicated.
4 Objectives of therapy include suppression of HIV viral load, maintenance of immunocompetence and maintenance of quality of life.
5 A detailed review of the patient's socioeconomic circumstances is vital in the planning of the management strategy. Extensive counselling is important, particularly about sexual activity and protection, drug compliance, surveillance for opportunistic infections and drug toxicity/interactions in those who are commenced on HAART regimens.

Stages of HIV
HIV is divided into several clinical stages from a management and prognostic point of view.

Early stage
CD4 count of 500 or above. The clinical findings may be confined to persisting lymphadenopathy alone. Other possible presentations at this stage include aseptic meningitis and idiopathic thrombocytopenic purpura.

Intermediate stage

CD4 count of 200–500. The clinical associations include oral hairy leucoplakia, oral candidiasis, herpes simplex virus (HSV) infection, herpes zoster infection, seborrhoeic dermatitis, tuberculosis, Kaposi's sarcoma (human herpesvirus 8), bacterial sinusitis, bronchitis and pneumonia.

Late stage

CD4 count of 50–200. Opportunistic infections with *Pneumocystis carinii* and chronic diarrhoea due to *Cryptosporidium* are likely, and prophylaxis with oral co-trimoxazole against *P. carinii* should be commenced.

Advanced stage

CD4 count of less than 50. The patient is susceptible to numerous opportunistic infections, such as MAC, *Bartonella*, histoplasmosis, aspergillosis, CMV infection, cryptococcal infection, toxoplasmosis, microsporidiosis, extrapulmonary tuberculosis, Epstein-Barr virus infection, disseminated *Mycobacterium avium* complex infection, disseminated herpes simplex or disseminated herpes zoster, and progressive multifocal leucoencephalopathy. At this stage the patient is also susceptible to primary central nervous system lymphoma as well as wasting and dementia due to HIV.

Terminal stage

Therapeutic decisions should be made with the aim of best palliation and psychological comfort. The change of classification to terminal stage from the advanced stage should be based on the patient's overall clinical status, the patient's perspective on his or her condition and expectations. A decision should be made regarding the continuation of active therapy. Strong consideration should be given to stopping active treatment if signs and symptoms of the disease are not controlled with available therapy or if therapy is not tolerated. At this stage the focus of management should shift to comfort care, with psychological support, family support and pain management.

Drug therapy in HIV

The current management approach to the HIV patient is to commence HAART early so as to prolong life expectancy and maintain good quality of life. There is still some debate as to exactly when the treatment should commence. It is important to be cognisant of other factors that would influence the decision whether to treat or not. These include the patient's expectations, resistance, and tolerance to side effects, drug interactions, affordability and psychosocial factors that would affect compliance.

Recommendations: Current consensus is to commence antiretroviral therapy when the CD4 count is < 200 or the viral load is > 30000 copies per mL. Symptomatic HIV and/or AIDS-defining illnesses are additional indications for therapy with antiretroviral agents. A CD4 count of 200–350 is a grey area where patients may or may not benefit from HAART therapy. In this regard an individualised decision should be made based on the clinical merits. Pregnant women require therapy to mitigate vertical transmission.

Compliance is the critical issue in treatment. The therapeutic objective is to achieve an undetectable viral load. The candidate is expected to possess a good knowledge of the commonly used antiretroviral drugs and the compatible combinations. It is important to be able to identify adverse reactions associated with these therapeutic agents.

The four classes of drugs in common usage are: nucleoside/nucleotide reverse transcriptase inhibitors, non-nucleoside reverse transcriptase inhibitors, protease inhibitors and fusion inhibitors. These are discussed below.

Protease inhibitors

These are: indinavir, ritonavir, saquinavir (available in two forms: hard-gel and soft-gel formulation), nelfinavir, atazanavir, fosamprenavir and amprenavir.

Indinavir has the propensity to cause nephrolithiasis, so adequate hydration of the patient should be ensured. Ritonavir has significant side effects, including nausea, diarrhoea, circumoral paraesthesias and hepatitis. It is important to establish the baseline liver function prior to commencement of therapy and to follow up with regular liver function tests. Ritonavir can augment the activity of other protease inhibitors by blocking hepatic drug metabolism, and therefore it can be used in combination at low dose to boost the activity of another agent of the same class, which is an accepted practice.

The hard-gel formulation of sequinavir is well tolerated but has compromised efficacy due to poor gastrointestinal absorption; the soft-gel formulation has better absorption. Nelfinavir has the gastrointestinal side effects of nausea, vomiting and diarrhoea. Amprenavir causes rash and gastrointestinal discomfort.

Protease inhibitors cause a lipodystrophy in treated patients, with significant cosmetic implications. Redistribution of peripheral adiposity to the trunk, particularly to the dorsum of the neck and the abdominal region, is observed. There is potential for the acceleration of atherosclerosis; therefore, close supervision of the serum lipid profile is important.

Protease inhibitors have many serious interactions with other therapeutic agents, so it is important to be vigilant about polypharmacy in these patients. Rifampicin, astemizole, midazolam and cisapride should not be administered to patients who are being treated with protease inhibitors.

Nucleoside analogue reverse transcriptase inhibitors

These include: entecavir, emtricitabine, zidovudine, zalcitabine, stavudine, didanosine, lamivudine, tenofovir and abacavir.

Zidovudine can cause the side effects of headache, nausea, myelosuppression, myopathy and neuropathy. Zalcitabine is known to cause peripheral neuropathy. Stavudine, too, can cause peripheral neuropathy, in addition to fatty liver and lactic acidosis. Didanosine is another agent that causes peripheral neuropathy, and it can also cause pancreatitis.

Lamivudine is a relatively safe drug that has a minimal side-effect profile.

Abacavir is reported to cause serious hypersensitivity reactions, so the patient should be warned of early signs of hypersensitivity and the necessary steps to be taken in such an event.

Non-nucleoside reverse transcriptase inhibitors

These are nevirapine, delavirdine and efavirenz. These drugs cause a transient rash. They also have significant interactions with the hepatic cytochrome P-450 enzyme system.

Nevirapine has the highest incidence of Stevens-Johnson syndrome of any licensed drug and can also cause a severe (often fatal) hepatitis. Efavirenz can cause neurocognitive side effects. It is also teratogenic. Nevirapine is preferred in pregnancy.

Viral resistance testing should guide change of therapy if viral load rebound occurs. But it is important to check the level of compliance prior to attributing viral load rebound to drug resistance.

Fusion inhibitors

The approved agent is enfuvirtide, an amino acid synthetic peptide. This agent blocks the fusion of HIV with CD4 cells. It is indicated in HIV-1 treatment-experienced patients who have ongoing viral replication despite therapy with other agents. It is also indicated in treatment-experienced patients who are becoming intolerant to previous antiretroviral agents. No data are available on treatment-naive patients. Injection site reaction and pneumonia are known side effects.

Commonly used combinations

Two nucleoside reverse transcriptase inhibitors in combination with a protease inhibitor or with a non-nucleoside reverse transcriptase inhibitor are commonly used.

It should be noted that zidovudine and stavudine should not be used in combination because they antagonise each other's effect; and it is contraindicated to give didanosine and zalcitabine in combination due to enhanced neurotoxicity.

Upon commencement of antiretroviral therapy, treatment response can be monitored by checking the CD4 count and viral load at regular intervals. Initial response can be checked at 4 weeks. Then monitoring should continue at increasing intervals to every 3 months until viral load is recorded as undetectable. Thereafter, monitoring every 3–4 months should be continued.

NON-SPECIFIC CLINICAL PRESENTATION WITH CONSTITUTIONAL SYMPTOMS

Case vignette

A 53-year-old HIV-positive man presents with severe lethargy, odynophagia and significant weight loss (11 kg) over a period of 2 months. He was initially diagnosed with HIV 9 years ago. He was treated with several antiretroviral combination agent regimens. His CD4 count has been 500 and viral load undetectable 4 months ago. In the past he has suffered from CMV retinitis, oral thrush and *Pneumocystis carinii* pneumonia. He is homosexual and currently has no steady partner. He is occasionally sexually active. On examination the patient has generalised lymphadenopathy and evidence of significant wasting. He is afebrile.

1 What are your differential diagnoses for this presentation?
2 What investigations would you request?
3 Discuss your plan of management.

Approach to the patient

HIV can have various clinical presentations, and in each situation the candidate should judiciously estimate the clinical possibilities. A presentation with constitutional symptoms of fever, night sweats, weight loss and fatigue is common, and the possibilities that should be considered are:

- primary HIV infection itself
- lymphoma
- *Pneumocystis carinii* pneumonia
- infection with MAC
- toxoplasmosis
- bacterial pneumonia
- drug allergy
- bacterial sinusitis.

Investigations

The battery of investigations that should be performed in this situation includes:

1   Full blood count
2   Electrolyte profile
3   Liver function tests
4   Multiple blood cultures (at least three), including cultures for MAC
5   Cultures for acid-fast bacilli
6   Serology for syphilis, cryptococcosis (also test for the cryptococcal antigen) and toxoplasmosis
7   CT of chest and abdomen.

If the investigation is still inconclusive, perform a gallium scan (looking for foci of inflammation), a total body MRI scan, bone marrow biopsy (looking for MAC infection), a lumbar puncture and, if necessary, a liver biopsy.

The HIV patient can complain of chronic fatigue, and this presentation could be due to multiple causes. Some possible causes are infection, medication side effect, malnutrition, chronic pain and depression. Management in this setting is dependent upon the investigational results. Management objectives include aggressive therapy to control opportunistic infections (if detected), aggressive HAART regimen, proper nourishment, and antidepressant or psychiatric help if the patient is depressed.

CHRONIC ALCOHOLISM

Approach to the patient

History

Many long case patients may have chronic alcoholism as a significant factor contributing to the overall morbidity. Some important facts to remember in dealing with the problem of alcoholism are as follows:

1   There is a genetic predisposition to alcoholism, so the family history is important.
2   Twenty per cent of alcoholics can stop their habit without help.
3   Mortality in the alcoholic is commonly caused by heart failure (cardiomyopathy), ischaemic heart disease, stroke, cancer, accident or suicide.

In taking a history from patients who abuse alcohol, remember to obtain all relevant details of their habit. Pay particular attention to the amount and type of alcohol consumed each day, the duration of the habit, whether the patient has any drinking partners, how the patient finances their habit, how the family is coping and whether the patient has ever attempted to give up alcohol. Most alcoholics consume 8–10 standard drinks per day; however, this threshold may vary depending on the ethnicity and body habitus of the individual. Most patients may abuse multiple substances. Therefore it is important to ask about other recreational drug use and tobacco smoking. Remember: the patient may withhold the truth due to denial or confabulation. Ask about depression, suicidal ideation, sexual problems, family/marital issues and occupational problems.

The **C A G E** questionnaire is considered the standardised assessment of the severity of alcohol addiction. Ask the following questions of all suspected alcoholic patients:

C— Did you ever consider **cutting down** on the amount of alcohol you consume?
A— Do you feel **annoyed** when others criticise your drinking?
G— Have you ever felt **guilty** about your habit?
E— Do you consume alcohol as an **'eye opener'** in the morning?

The Michigan Alcohol Screening Test (MAST) can be used for a more formal assessment of the severity of alcoholism.

Examination

Signs of chronic alcoholism in the physical examination (Fig 11.1) are poor personal hygiene, obesity or malnutrition, multiple ecchymoses due to easy bruising, bilateral parotid gland swelling and Dupuytren's contracture. Look for atrial fibrillation and evidence of congestive cardiac failure due to alcoholic dilated

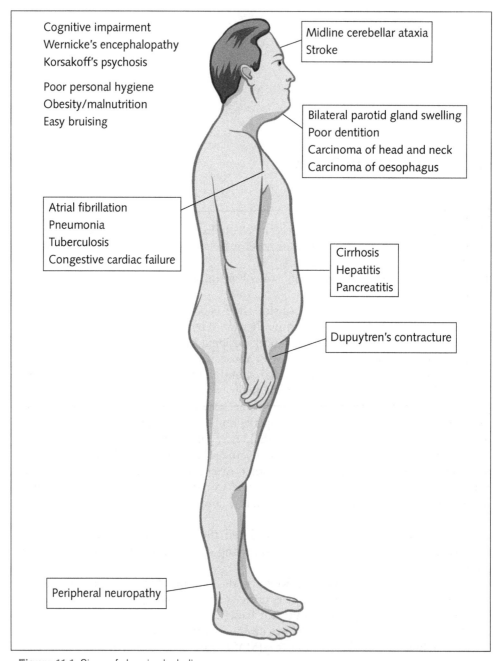

Figure 11.1 Signs of chronic alcoholism

cardiomyopathy. Perform a detailed neurological examination, looking for mid-line cerebellar ataxia, peripheral neuropathy and stroke. Examine the respiratory system, looking for evidence of pneumonia and tuberculosis. Gastrointestinal examination may reveal signs of alcoholic liver disease, alcoholic hepatitis and pancreatitis. Remember that chronic alcohol consumption is a risk factor for carcinoma of the head and neck and the oesophagus. Perform a cognitive assessment, looking for signs of alcoholic brain damage, Wernicke's encephalopathy and Korsakoff's psychosis.

Investigations

Do not be surprised to encounter denial of alcoholism, even in the most likely of patients. The following are some investigations that can be done to confirm chronic alcoholism:

1 Mean cell volume—this may be > 91 fL
2 Serum gamma-glutamyl transpeptidase (GGT) level—this may be > 30 mmol/L
3 Serum uric acid level—this may be elevated
4 Serum carbohydrate-deficient transferase level—this may be elevated
5 Serum triglyceride level—this may be elevated

Management

1 Acute management of the alcoholic patient includes the administration of oral vitamin B complex (with folic acid) and thiamine 100 mg daily. Alcohol withdrawal (see box) should be managed with diazepam orally, given in decremental doses over 3–5 days as guided by a standard alcohol withdrawal scale.
2 Rehabilitation and abstinence. Some useful steps that can be employed are:
   • education and motivation of the patient
   • eliciting family support to help stop the habit and to stop provision of alcohol to the patient
   • personal, sexual and vocational counselling.
3 Some patients may complain of persistent insomnia. This problem is better managed with behavioural methods, meditation and exercise than with medications.
4 Always offer the patient the option of group support in the form of Alcoholics Anonymous or institutions run by organisations such as the Salvation Army.
5 Discuss with the patient the options of pharmacological anti-craving agents, such as acamprosate and naltrexone. Cognitive behavioural therapy has also shown promise as a means of maintaining abstinence.

Symptoms and signs of alcohol withdrawal

1 Tremor
2 Tachycardia
3 Tachypnoea
4 Anxiety and panic

These features start appearing 5–10 hours after the last drink. They usually peak within the first 2–3 days and gradually improve through day 5. Alcoholic seizures occur within the first 48 hours and delirium tremens also occurs during this period. Delirium tremens is characterised by visual, auditory and tactile hallucinations. Some patients experience protracted abstinence syndrome and alcoholic hallucinosis, which can last as long as 6 months.

ALCOHOLIC/CHRONIC LIVER DISEASE

Case vignette

A 35-year-old man has been admitted with severe ascites and haematemesis in the background of chronic alcohol abuse and hepatitis C infection. Upper gastrointestinal endoscopy has revealed bleeding oesophageal varices, which was treated with banding. He has been experiencing increasing daytime somnolence. On examination he has finger clubbing and Dupuytren's contractures. He demonstrates asterixis and scleral icterus. His abdomen is tender and positive for shifting dullness. He has tense ascites and splenomegaly. His temperature chart demonstrates spiking fevers.

1   What investigations would you request to further work up this man?
2   What is your overall detailed assessment of this man's clinical status?
3   What immediate management plan would you consider?
4   What is his long-term prognosis?
5   What definitive management options are available to improve this man's outcome?

Approach to the patient

History

Ask about anorexia, abdominal pain and bloating. Obtain a detailed history on alcohol intake and also enquire into other risk factors for infective hepatitis. Intravenous drug abuse or previous tattoos may suggest hepatitic C infection, and unprotected sexual intercourse with multiple partners may suggest hepatitis B. Ask whether the patient has been tested for or diagnosed with viral hepatitis in the past. Obtain a detailed social history. Ask about the effects of hypogonadism in the male patient (lack of libido and impotence). Check whether the patient has had haemetemesis or melaena, which may be due to erosive gastritis, or oesophageal varicies due to portal hypertension. Perform a cognitive assessment to exclude hepatic encephalopathy.

Examination

1   Look for the sentinel features of chronic alcoholism as described above.
2   The patient may appear drowsy if encephalopathic (disturbed diurnal sleep pattern).
3   Observe for wasting and jaundice.

4 Commencing from the periphery, note finger clubbing, leuconychia, Terry's nails, palmar erythema, palmar crease pallor and Dupuytren's contractures. Check for asterixis, the flapping tremor of hepatic encephalopathy.

5 There may be proximal muscle wasting.

6 Note any tattoos that may suggest the possibility of associated hepatitic C infection.

7 Look in the eyes for scleral icterus and conjunctival pallor.

8 Do not forget to check for fetor hepaticus.

9 Examine the thoracic region for gynaecomastia and spider naevi.

10 Exclude the presence of a pleural effusion, especially in the right side.

11 Abdominal examination should be very detailed. In the distended abdomen, establish flank dullness and shifting dullness. Note caput medusae. Note the level to which the dullness persists when supine—this level may help decide on the access point for peritoneocentesis and also monitor the progression or regression of ascites. Check for abdominal tenderness. Palpate for hepatomegaly and splenomegaly and try to establish the length to which the organ edges extend below the costal margin. Cirrhotic liver is nodular and firm when palpable. Hard lumps or mass lesions in the liver may suggest the development of hepatoma or hepatocellular carcinoma, which is seen in those with cirrhosis (particularly viral). Auscultate for a Cruveilhier-Baumgarten murmur in the epigastrium, hepatic bruit and note the nature of bowel sounds.

12 In the male patient there may be testicular atrophy.

13 Examine the lower limbs for signs that mirror those of the upper limbs.

14 Check the tendon reflexes for exaggeration due to encephalopathy.

15 Note pitting oedema due to portal hypertension and hypoalbuminaemia.

16 Evidence of right heart failure may suggest the onset of portopulmonary hypertension. Observe the temperature chart or check the temperature for fevers associated with spontaneous bacterial peritonitis (particularly if the patient has abdominal tenderness).

17 Assess the urine output by studying the fluid balance chart. Significant oliguria may be indicative of dehydration or hepatorenal syndrome. The latter is a preterminal event.

Investigations

1 Full blood count—looking for evidence of anaemia (usually macrocytic), leucocytosis and thrombocytopenia (due to sequestration if there is significant splenomegaly). If there has been significant blood loss, the patient may have normocytic or even microcytic anaemia.

2 Coagulation profile—looking for prolonged prothrombin time/INR due to hepatic failure (decreased synthesis of clotting factors)

3 Serum electrolyte profile and renal function indices—looking for evidence of renal failure (hepatorenal syndrome) and hyponatraemia etc

4 Liver function indices including serum billirubin levels and albumin level. In cirrhosis, serum alkaline phosphatase (ALP), aspartate aminotransferase (AST), alanine aminotransferase (ALT) and GGT levels may be normal or abnormal. In alcoholic hepatitis or hepatitis due to other causes, these levels can rise to the thousands. There is a disproportionate elevation of AST relative to ALT in alcoholic liver disease. AST/ALT ratio is over 2 in this case. Patients also have hyperbilirubinaemia and hypoalbuminaemia.

5 Serum alpha-fetoprotein (AFP) level—high levels are seen with acute hepatitis and hepatocellular carcinoma. Progressive elevation of this marker is suggestive of hepatocellular carcinoma.

6 Ascitic fluid analysis for protein levels and microscopy and culture. An elevated (polymorphs) white cell count in the ascitic fluid may be due to spontaneous bacterial peritonitis.

7 Abdominal ultrasound—looking for evidence of portal hypertension, and also liver consistency and solid mass lesions that may suggest hepatocellular carcinoma, and fluid-filled masses that would suggest cysts. Doppler study helps identify portal vein thrombosis.

8 Measure arterial blood gases, especially if the patient is hypoxaemic on room air. Significant arterial deoxygenation may suggest hepatopulmonary syndrome.

9 Chest X-ray—looking for evidence of pleural effusion, pulmonary congestion (hepatopulmonary syndrome) or enlargement of pulmonary vasculature (portopulmonary hypertension)

10 Echocardiography if there are signs of right heart failure. Elevated pulmonary pressures and right heart strain is very suggestive of portopulmonary hypertension.

11 Measure the urine output—oliguria may suggest hypovolaemia or hepatorenal syndrome.

Causes of hepatitis

- Viral (hepatitis A/B/C, HIV, CMV)
- Alcohol
- Iatrogenic (statins, isoniazid, ketoconazole, halothane)
- Toxic (overdosing with paracetamol)
- Ischaemic
- Autoimmune

Causes of cirrhosis

- Chronic alcoholism
- Chronic viral hepatitis (B, C, D)
- Non-alcoholic steatohepatitis (NASH)
- Wilson's disease
- Hereditary haemochromatosis
- Alpha$_1$-antitrypsin deficiency
- Autoimmune hepatitis
- Primary biliary cirrhosis
- Budd-Chiari syndrome
- Drugs such as methotrexate

Other causes of liver disease

It is important to note that hepatitis, cirrhosis, chronic liver disease and hepatic failure can be due to causes other than chronic alcoholism. Where the aetiology is not clear, further diagnostic testing may be necessary. A hepatic disease screen should include the following battery of tests:

- Hepatitis B—HBsAg, HBeAg, HBV, DNA and antibodies to HB surface antigen, e antigen and core antigen
- Hepatitis C—HCV RNA, anti-HCV antibodies
- Hepatitis A—antibodies (IgM) to HAV
- Infectious mononucleosis—Paul-Bunnell test, Monospot test
- Autoimmune hepatitis—antinuclear antibody and antismooth muscle antibody (type 1), anti-LKM1 antibody (type 2), anti-SLP/LP (type 3)
- Hereditary haemachromatosis—serum iron indices, serum ferritin, transferring saturation
- Wilson's disease—serum copper, caeruloplasmin
- Alpha$_1$-antitrypsin deficiency—serum alpha$_1$-antitrypsin levels
- Liver ultrasound—looking for fatty infiltration, cirrhosis, nodularity and to examine portal veins (portal vein thrombosis), hepatic veins (hepatic vein thrombosis) and the biliary tract
- CT scan and/or MRI of liver
- Liver biopsy

Management

1   Alcoholism should be managed as per the discussion previously. Upon addressing and stabilising the withdrawal symptoms, the patient should be given supportive therapy and adequate nourishment. Another main objective of this strategy is to address complications and direct therapy at liver disease based on the stage viz. cirrhosis, hepatitis or fulminant hepatic failure. Associated other pathologies such as viral hepatitis may further influence the management approach.

2   Supportive measures include adequate IV hydration and nutrition. Vitamin supplementation (especially thiamine, pyridoxine and folic acid) is very important. Vitamin K injection may help address the coagulopathy.

3   Significant ascites should be tapped if necessary, with concurrent IV albumin infusion. Measures to treat portal hypertension and diuretic therapy with spironolactone help improve ascites.

4   Patients with hepatitis benefit from oral prednisolone therapy over periods of 4 or more weeks.

5   Abstinence from alcohol is a key objective and all measures to facilitate this should be put in place. Psychological support and counselling together with family or partner support should be provided. Detoxification under professional supervision should be organised.

6   End-stage cirrhosis in younger patients—consider referral for liver transplantation.

7   Management of portal hypertension—all patients with cirrhosis are at risk of portal hypertension. The dreaded complication of portal hypertension is bleeding oesophageal and/or gastric varices. Patients with portal hypertension should be treated with a non-selective beta-blocker such as propranolol. Patients with bleeding varices need upper gastrointestinal tract endoscopy for variceal banding or sclerotherapy. Patients may require repeat procedures in the event of rebleeding, which is not too uncommon. Measures to ease portal hypertension include transjugular intrahepatic portosystemic shunt (TIPS) and creation of a surgical portacaval shunt. Decompression by creating a portosystemic shunt has been observed to worsen hepatic encephalopathy. However, it is very effective at preventing and decreasing rebleeding.

8   Management of hepatocellular carcinoma—there is no consensus on the best approach to the management of this complication of cirrhosis. Some physicians promote watchful waiting if the tumour is not causing any complications. The behaviour of the tumour is highly variable and therefore so is the prognosis. However, as a general rule, life expectancy can vary from 6 months to 2 years from diagnosis. Large tumours can be treated with surgical resection and transplantation. Some centres offer cryoablation of the tumour. Hepatocellular carcinoma can also be managed with chemotherapy, radiotherapy, arterial chemoembolisation or alcohol ablation.

9   Management of hepatic encephalopathy—hepatic encephalopathy is believed to be due to increased blood ammonia levels generated in the intestines that cross the blood–brain barrier. Therefore the management strategy should first address the precipitating factors. Gastrointestinal bleeding and high protein intake have been associated with encephalopathy and therefore control of intestinal bleeding, gastric lavage and decreasing protein intake are important therapeutic steps. Other precipitants include constipation, sepsis and development of hepatocellular carcinoma. Sedative hypnotics such as benzodiazepines too can precipitate encephalopathy and should be withdrawn or withheld safely. Oral lactulose, lactitol or antibiotics such as oral neomycin also improve encephalopathy.

Child-Pugh classification of liver disease

Classification is based on:
- severity of ascites
- plasma albumin and bilirubin levels
- degree of coagulopathy (prothrombin time)
- severity of encephalopathy.

Child-Pugh score has three prognostic classes:
- Class A—well-compensated disease
- Class B—early decompensation
- Class C—decompensation.

Child-Pugh class correlates with patient mortality.

10 Patients with hepatitis C benefit from combination therapy with interferon and ribavirin. Acute exposure is treated with interferon monotherapy. Careful patient selection and close monitoring are important in instituting this therapy.

11 Patients with hepatitis B infection benefit from therapy with interferon and lamivudine.

HAEMOCHROMATOSIS

This is the most common autosomal recessive condition in the Caucasian population (affected frequency 1:400 and carrier frequency 1:10). Therefore, the chances of getting a patient with haemochromatosis in the examination are very high. Manifestations may vary from asymptomatic disease or diabetes mellitus to hepatocellular carcinoma associated with cirrhosis. This disease is associated with a mutation in the HFE gene in the short arm of chromosome 6. About 85% of cases manifest Cys 282 Tyr mutation, with 25% manifesting a second mutation, His 63 Asp.

Approach to the patient

History

Ask about:

- how the diagnosis was made
- any other illness that led to the diagnosis (such as diabetes)
- the family history and whether well family members have been screened
- alcohol intake—this can further compound the condition and cloud the initial diagnosis
- any liver biopsies performed.

The patient and the family may have been offered gene testing for the common mutations. Ask about the therapy received and ongoing monitoring of the disease. It is important to assess how the condition has affected the patient's personal, social, occupational and family life and to gauge the patient's insight into and knowledge of the condition.

Examination

Look for bronze pigmentation of the skin, which is more pronounced in the face, neck, extensor surfaces, genitals and scars, and for peripheral stigmata of chronic liver disease such as leuconychia, palmar erythema, jaundice, spider naevi, evidence of portal hypertension and hepatosplenomegaly. Check for gynaecomastia and lack of android hair distribution. Look for evidence of arthropathy, particularly in the second and third metacarpophalangeal joints and in the knees. Look for signs of congestive cardiac failure. Perform a detailed abdominal examination, looking for features of hepatic malignancy such as firm/hard hepatomegaly or mass lesion in the right upper quadrant. Check for lymphadenopathy and bony tenderness.

Investigations

1 Serum iron, transferrin saturation (> 50% is pathological), and serum ferritin concentration (> 500 mg/mL is pathological)

2 Liver biopsy and the hepatic iron index (normal index is < 1; in haemochromatosis it may be > 2). Liver biopsy may also show micro- or

macronodular cirrhosis. Biopsy is also important to exclude hepatocellular carcinoma in the cirrhotic patient.

3   If no liver biopsy has been performed, ask for abdominal MRI to look for the classic appearance of the iron-laden liver.

4   Genetic testing for Cys 282 Tyr mutation should be considered where necessary, if facilities are available.

5   All family members of the index patient should be screened for haemochromatosis by performing serum ferritin levels and transferrin saturations.

Management

1   Weekly or twice-weekly phlebotomy should be performed until the serum ferritin level and transferrin saturation becomes normal. From then onwards, phlebotomy can be performed at 3-monthly intervals or as necessary.

2   Male patients should be supplemented with testosterone to preserve libido and male sexual characteristics.

3   If the patient is anaemic for some reason, they cannot be treated with phlebotomy, and in this situation the treatment option is to use a chelating agent such as desferrioxamine. It should be remembered that phlebotomy has very little effect on joint pathology.

PEPTIC ULCER DISEASE

Case vignette

A 56-year-old man presents with severe nocturnal epigastric pain. The pain was initially relieved by food ingestion and antacids. However, lately the pain has been recalcitrant and progressive. He also complains of fatigue and exertional retrosternal discomfort. He is a heavy smoker and consumes alcoholic spirits on a regular basis. He is on aspirin. On examination there was tenderness to deep palpation in the epigastric region. He also had conjunctival pallor. His pulse rate was 110 bpm and irregularly irregular.

1 What are the main clinical issues in this man?
2 What investigations would you order to gain further insight into his condition?
3 Explain your management priorities and the overall strategy.

Approach to the patient

Peptic ulcer disease is a common associated morbidity in the long case.

History

Enquire about the initial presentation—the symptoms of epigastric pain, dyspepsia, reflux and anorexia. It is important to obtain details about any previous or current gastrointestinal bleeding. A medication history should be obtained, to exclude causative agents, such as aspirin or NSAIDs. Ask when and how the diagnosis was made and whether the patient has had a gastroscopy. Ask how the patient has been treated in the past and whether they have ever been tested for *Helicobacter pylori*. A history of gastrointestinal bleeding becomes an issue if the patient has a comorbid condition that would require anticoagulation or antiplatelet therapy, such as coronary stenting or AF. Be alert to features that may indicate the possibility of gastric carcinoma, such as significant weight loss, persistent vomiting or jaundice in the setting of liver secondaries.

Examination

The patient may have epigastric tenderness. A mass lesion in the abdomen should alert to neoplasia. Do not forget to look for signs of anaemia.

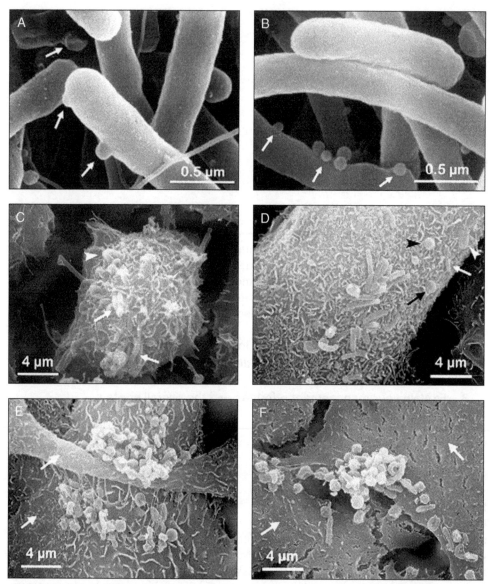

Figure 12.1 Scanning electron micrographs of a 48-h culture of *H. pylori* (A, B), and infection of cultured AGS cells for 24 h (C, D) or 48 h (E, F). A, blebs (→) protrude from the spiral-shaped bacterial body. B, numerous vesicles (→) are visible on the bacterial surface. C, bacteria are tightly embodied in a dense network of extended microvilli. Spirals are attached horizontally (→) or perpendicularly (arrowhead). D, *H. pylori* displays various shapes when attached to the cell surface: the spiral (white→), U-shaped (white arrowhead), doughnut (black→), or coccoid form (black arrowhead) (reprinted from Heczko U, Smith V C, Mark Meloche R et al 2000 Characteristics of *Helicobacter pylori* attachment to human primary antral epithelial cell. *Microbes and Infection* 2:8)

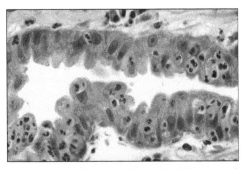

Figure 12.2 Foveolar cells with 'cobblestoning'. The changes are patchy and often mild. When the cells bulge out, resembling cobblestones, the appearance is almost always diagnostic of *H. pylori* infection (reprinted from Robin W J 2000 Gastric pathology associated with *Helicobacter pylori*. *Gastroenterology Clinics of North America* 29:47)

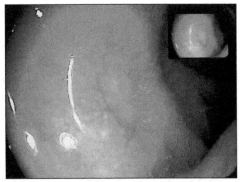

Figure 12.3 Duodenal ulcer (courtesy of Dr George Ostapowicz)

Investigations

All patients who present with symptoms suggestive of peptic ulcer disease or a diagnosis of peptic ulcer disease should be tested for *H. pylori* infection. This is achieved by performing the rapid urease test in those undergoing endoscopy and by serology. However, in individuals under age 50 without alarm symptoms, it is reasonable to treat without investigation and assess response (in both *H. pylori* positive and *H. pylori* negative individuals).

Negative tests can be confirmed with non-endoscopic tests, such as the urea breath test or the stool antigen test. The urea breath test can be accurately interpreted only if antisecretory therapy has been withheld for a minimum of 2 weeks prior to the test.

However, negative tests do not necessarily need confirmation (realising that serology may only be 70–80% accurate). In such situations it would be reasonable to treat with a proton pump inhibitor (PPI) initially. If there is no response or symptoms return, further investigation with gastroscopy is indicated.

If the patient has had an acute event, check the full blood count (looking for anaemia) and electrolyte profile (looking for an elevation in blood urea level that is disproportionate to the creatinine level). In this situation gastroscopy is definitely indicated.

Management

1   If the test is positive for *H. pylori* the patient has to be treated for 7–14 days with a triple-therapy combination. Currently prepared combinations include PPI (omeprazole or esomeprazole) together with amoxycillin and clarithromycin. Metronidazole is substituted in penicillin allergies. Bismuth is an agent only rarely used in resistant cases, generally as part of quadruple therapy.

2   The cure of infection is confirmed with a urease breath test performed 2 weeks after the completion of therapy. If there is ulcer disease without the presence of *H. pylori*, it is enough to treat with a PPI alone for 4–6 weeks. Therapy may be required for a longer period for large ulcers.

Be aware that ulcers may recur. High-risk individuals, such as those who have had a gastrointestinal bleed or require long-term aspirin or frequent NSAIDs therapy may require long-term acid suppression.

3   All gastric ulcers have to be biopsied during endoscopy, to exclude gastric carcinoma. The patient should be followed up with repeat gastroscopy a few weeks after the completion of the curative treatment, to confirm ulcer healing.

INFLAMMATORY BOWEL DISEASE

Case vignette

A 33-year-old female presents to hospital with high fevers and severe abdominal pain in the background of anorexia and weight loss. She was diagnosed with Crohn's disease 3 years ago upon investigation for chronic fevers, diarrhoea, weight loss, abdominal pain, nausea and vomiting. Her Crohn's disease is managed with long-term mesalazine therapy. She is also on cipramil for depression.

On examination she has tenderness with guarding in the left lower quadrant and aphthous ulceration in the oral mucosa. She is cushingoid. Investigations reveal a mild anaemia, leucocytosis, thrombocytosis and significantly elevated CRP. Abdominal CT reveals an abscess in the sigmoid region. She is commenced on high-dose antibiotics and steroids. The abscess is drained percutaneously under CT guidance.

While in hospital her symptoms improve. However, on the third day in hospital she develops severe retrosternal chest pain that radiates to the neck and jaw. ECG reveals ST segment elevation in the septal leads. She also complains of severe left calf pain and tenderness. She is commenced on a heparin infusion and subsequently taken to the cardiac catheterisation laboratory. Angiography shows evidence of slow coronary flow in the left anterior descending artery. Otherwise the coronary anatomy is normal with no evidence of any occlusive disease in any artery. She has a peak troponin I level of 20 and echocardiography shows significant hypokinesis of the anteroseptal region of the left ventricle, suggesting significant myocardial damage or stunning. Lower limb Doppler studies reveal DVT of the left leg.

1   How would you describe the interrelationship between the different aspects of her clinical picture?
2   What further investigations would you require to ascertain the certain aetiology of her myocardial infarction?
3   What is your comprehensive plan of management for this patient?
4   Describe your planned discussion with her about her prognosis, long-term management and available supportive care.

Approach to the patient (ulcerative colitis and Crohn's disease)

Knowledge of the basic principles of management of ulcerative colitis and Crohn's disease will be very useful because inflammatory bowel disease can make patients ideal long cases with multifaceted issues.

History

Ask when and how the initial presentation was made and what investigations led to the diagnosis. Take a detailed history of gastrointestinal symptoms, such as abdominal pain, diarrhoea, tenesmus, per rectum bleeding, rectal mucous discharge, anorexia, nausea and vomiting. Ask about constitutional symptoms and weight loss. The combination of symptoms such as per rectal bleeding and mucus together with tenesmus and constipation with the absence of systemic symptoms is very suggestive of ulcerative proctitis. Episodes of abdominal pain and bloating, together with vomiting a few hours after food ingestion are symptoms suggestive of small bowel involvement, especially terminal ileal Crohn's disease.

Ask about systemic features such as oral ulcers, arthritis, biliary colic (uncommon), pyoderma gangrenosum and erythema nodosum. Ask how often acute exacerbations happen and how they are treated. It is very important to obtain a detailed medication history, enquiring about current therapy as well as agents tried previously. Ask about adverse effects associated with medications, especially corticosteroids. Take a detailed smoking history, as smoking prevents exacerbation of ulcerative colitis but precipitates Crohn's disease. Check the family history, as Crohn's disease especially tends to be familial. The clinical features alone often may not differentiate between Crohn's disease and ulcerative colitis.

Once the precise disease entity is identified, it is important to localise the possible areas of involvement in the gastrointestinal tract. Ask about any diagnosis of gastrointestinal malignancy. Risk of malignancy, especially colorectal cancer, is increased in individuals with inflammatory bowel disease, especially ulcerative colitis.

The social aspects of inflammatory bowel disease are extremely important. Enquire about how the disease affects the patient's social, academic and occupational life. Ask about how it affects relationships, particularly with the patient's partner. Effects on sexual and reproductive function and cosmetic effects of surgery are key questions that should be addressed, particularly in the young patient. Ask about available social support and try to gain a good understanding of the level of insight the patient has into their condition, the treatment given and the side effects experienced. Depression is common among patients suffering from inflammatory bowel disease, and this should be enquired about. Pregnancy and management of inflammatory bowel disease is an important area, where many questions can be asked. Ask about how the patient is managing with the ileostomy or the colostomy (if they have had a colectomy). Some patients may have had an ileal pouch created after colectomy. In such patients, ask about symptoms of pouchitis and issues of continence. Ask whether the patient belongs to a support group such as a Crohn's or colitis association.

Examination

Look for wasting and stunted growth. Assess the level of hydration and nutrition. Note the signs suggestive of malnutrition if present. Look for peripheral stigmata such as finger clubbing, arthritis, oral ulcers, jaundice, pyoderma gangrenosum (Fig 12.4) and erythema nodosum (Fig 12.5). Do not miss uncommon signs such as iritis and jaundice (sclerosing cholangitis, though very rare), if present. Examine the abdomen, looking for surgical scars, colostomy or ileostomy bags, distension, right upper or lower quadrant tenderness, generalised abdominal tenderness, guarding and rigidity. A palpable mass lesion could suggest an abscess, a phlegmon (especially in the right lower quadrant) or a malignancy. Check the character of bowel sounds. Ask for the

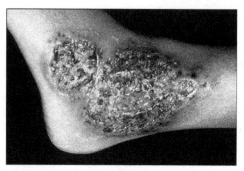

Figure 12.4 Pyoderma gangrenosum (reprinted from Hochberg M, Silman A, Smolen J et al 2003 *Rheumatology*, 3rd edn. Mosby, fig 26.21, p 288)

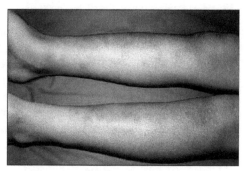

Figure 12.5 Erythema nodosum (reprinted from Mana J, Marcoval J 2007 Erythema nodosum, *Clinics in Dermatology* 25:7)

findings of the per rectum examination. Per rectal examination may show perianal skin tags (Crohn's disease especially), discharging sinuses or fistulae (Crohn's disease) and blood.

Differential diagnoses in inflammatory bowel disease

- Infective colitis (*Shigella, Salmonella, Campylobacter*) (CMV colitis in the immunocompromised)
- Ulcerative colitis
- Crohn's disease
- Pseudomembranous colitis (*Clostridium difficile* colitis)
- Radiation colitis
- Ischaemic colitis—especially in older individuals and/or those with vascular disease

Ulcerative colitis

Investigations

1 Stool microscopy—looking for white and red cells, organisms, parasite ova or cysts, and the results of stool culture
2 Full blood count—looking for anaemia and leucocytosis (and rarely haemolysis)
3 Electrolyte profile—looking for hypokalaemia, and elevated levels of urea and creatinine if the patient has lost body fluids (only relevant if significant diarrhoea present but always useful in establishing a baseline)
4 Liver function test results once again—to establish the baseline and monitor regularly (patients with ulcerative colitis can rarely develop primary sclerosing cholangitis and very rarely develop cholangiocarcinoma)
5 Iron studies—looking for iron deficiency
6 Results of sigmoidoscopy and biopsy and the result of colonoscopy

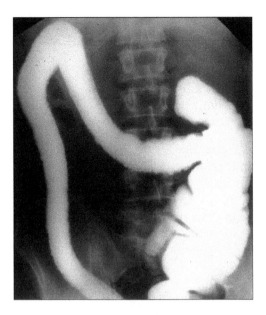

Figure 12.6 Barium enema of ulcerative colitis showing pseudopolyposis, lack of haustral markings and straightening of ascending and transverse colon (reprinted from Kanski J, Pavesio C, Tuft S 2005 *Ocular inflammatory disease*, Elsevier, fig 8.41)

7   Plain X-ray (both supine and erect views)—useful in acute colitis to check for colonic oedema (thumb-printing) and to exclude megacolon, or to assess for proximal constipation in proctitis
8   Abdominal CT may be useful in acute presentations with unusual features (such as severe pain, high fever and abdominal signs) to exclude complications

Management

Acute ulcerative colitis

The management objective is to induce remission.

1   Mild to moderate pancolitis (or subtotal colitis)—treat with oral aminosalicylic acid (ASA) agents. Specific agents used for the purpose of disease control include sulfasalazine, olsalazine and mesalazine. All three agents can be used to treat active disease as well as to maintain remission. Olsalazine and mesalazine are prescribed for patients who cannot tolerate the sulfa component of sulfasalazine. Olsalazine is made up of two molecules of aminosalicylic acid combined, and mesalazine is a coated aminosalicylic acid preparation that releases the active ingredient in the terminal ileum.
2   Severe pancolitis—treat with prednisone (prednisolone). However, if the patient is severely ill, treatment with IV hydrocortisone is indicated.
3   Antibiotics (e.g. metronidazole) may be a useful adjunct therapy, especially if there is a suspicion of sepsis.
4   Steroid enemas can also be used in this setting.
5   Patients admitted to hospital require prophylactic anticoagulation (unfractionated heparin or low molecular weight heparin).
6   Ulcerative proctitis is treated with mesalazine suppositories, foam or enemas, or with steroid foam or enemas, depending on the extent of the disease.

Maintenance of remission

1 Steroids should be weaned over 8–12 weeks upon achieving remission. Long-term or frequent steroid use should be avoided.
2 ASA agents have been shown to decrease the risk of relapse in ulcerative colitis and should be used in all confirmed cases for at least a few years.
3 In individuals who relapse on ASA, a second-line agent such as azathioprine or 6-mercaptopurine should be used (or this option should at least be discussed with the patient).

Advanced management of severe acute ulcerative colitis resistant to IV corticosteroids (upon being treated for at least 7 days)

1 IV cyclosporin infusion (continuously for 10–14 days)—in some patients infliximab may be used instead to prevent or delay the need for colectomy.
2 Azathioprine can also be commenced but in itself is not useful as its effect is delayed for 6–8 weeks or longer.
3 Patients with severe ulcerative colitis require close monitoring with daily or twice-daily medical reviews, daily FBC, electrolytes and abdominal X-ray.
4 A surgical review is recommended, and surgeons should be notified of the patient. Any significant deterioration or development of toxic megacolon, even if within the first few days of IV steroid therapy, requires urgent surgical assessment and possible emergency colectomy.
5 Toxic megacolon is a medical and surgical emergency, and treatment should be commenced with IV corticosteroids and IV antibiotics. The patient should be kept 'nil by mouth'. They should be rolled to the prone position regularly and urgent referral should be made to the surgeon to assess the need for colectomy.
6 Because of their propensity to develop colonic carcinoma, patients who have had ulcerative colitis for more than 10 years should be screened for malignancy every 2 years with colonoscopy and multiple biopsies. Strong consideration should be given to colectomy in patients whose biopsy shows mucosal dysplasia.
7 Patients need emotional and social support to cope with this chronic and distressing condition.
8 Patients with a stoma need counselling and the help of a qualified stoma nurse or therapist.

Crohn's disease

Investigations

1 Stool investigation for microscopy and culture—looking for white and red cells, pathogenic bacteria, parasitic ova and cysts
2 Full blood count—looking for anaemia and leucocytosis and inflammatory markers (CRP, ESR)
3 Liver function tests, serum vitamin B_{12} levels and iron studies
4 Colonoscopy with terminal ileal cannulation/intubation (with segmental biopsies) is the definitive investigation for diagnosis and assessment of disease activity and extent.

5 Individuals with known (terminal ileum abnormal on colonoscopy) or suspected small bowel disease should undergo small bowel imaging, including small bowel series or enema (this is of relatively low sensitivity), CT or MRI enteroclysis. Wireless capsule endoscopy can show small bowel mucosal abnormalities (see box) suggestive of Crohn's disease but should be avoided if strictures are suspected (where capsule may not pass through, necessitating surgical removal).

6 Sigmoidoscopy and biopsy may be of use on specific occasions. This is not generally used in the initial approach, as disease is frequently proximal to the sigmoid colon. It is of use occasionally to reassess activity of known distal disease.

7 Abdominal X-ray (with barium), CT of the abdomen—abdominal CT may show areas of small bowel inflammation, phlegmon or other complications. This is useful in acute and non-acute settings.

8 Immunological markers—ANCA and anti-saccharomyces cerevisiae antibody (ASCA) (occasionally used to help differentiate between ulcerative colitis and Crohn's)

Endoscopic features in Crohn's disease

- Cobblestone lesions
- Skip lesions (areas of mucosal ulceration interspaced between normal mucosa)
- Pseudopolyps (also seen in ulcerative colitis)
- Mucosal strictures
- Aphthous ulcers, linear ulcers, serpiginous ulcers
- Thickening of mucosal folds

Note: 5–10% of cases remain indeterminate colitis.

Differential diagnoses of Crohn's disease

- Infective colitis, enteritis
- *Yersinia* ileitis
- Diverticulitis
- Appendicitis (Crohn's ileitis)
- Ischaemic colitis
- Lymphoma of small bowel

Management

The hallmark feature of Crohn's disease is transmural inflammation. Mucosal changes are typically patchy in distribution. Histopathology also may reveal granulomatous lesions seen in < 50% of cases.

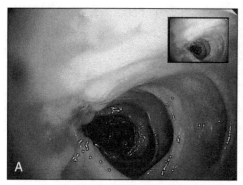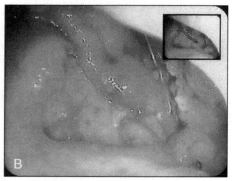

Figure 12.7 Colonic Crohn's disease (courtesy of Dr George Ostapowicz)

Acute luminal disease

The primary objective is to induce remission. Also ensure rehydration, restoration of electrolytes, and adequate nutrition.

1   Mild Crohn's—oral ASA agents as outlined above may be of some help. Note that in suspected ileal disease, mesalazine should be used, as the other agents are released only in the colon.
2   Moderate to severe Crohn's—oral prednisone (or prednisolone) is indicated. If the patient is significantly ill, requiring hospital admission, therapy with IV hydrocortisone should be considered. Antibiotics (e.g. metronidazole) may be a useful adjunct, especially if there is suspicion of infection or mass/phlegmon. In resistant disease, tumour necrosis factor antibody (TNF Ab) such as infliximab may be tried.
3   An elemental or semi-elemental diet may help achieve better disease control.
4   Complications such as collections or phlegmons may require surgical treatment.

Maintenance of remission

1   Steroids should be weaned over 8–12 weeks. Long-term or frequent steroid use should be avoided as they do not maintain remission.
2   ASA agents may be of some benefit in mild cases but the overall evidence for their benefit is dubious. In individuals who relapse on ASA (this is quite likely) or present with severe disease, especially if complications are involved, a second-line agent such as azathioprine or 6-mercaptopurine should be offered—this is effective in maintaining remission or decreasing disease activity in a significant percentage of patients.
3   Patients with luminal disease in whom second-line agents are ineffective can be treated with methotrexate or TNF Ab such as infliximab.
4   Perianal disease may require the use of antibiotics such as metronidazole and ciproflaxacin (4–6 weeks). Surgical involvement is necessary and specific treatment may include drainage of collections or more involved surgical procedures. Treatment with second-line agents such as azathioprine may result in fistula closure. In resistant cases, TNF Ab such as infliximab may be effective (50–60%).
5   Similarly in fistulising disease elsewhere (e.g. enterocutaneous), second-line agents such as azathioprine may also result in fistula closure. In resistant cases, TNF Ab such as infliximab may be effective (50–60%).

6 Surgery is not curative, but ultimately many patients require a surgical procedure. Surgery has a role in the treatment of complications: stricture(s), masses/phlegmons, collections, fistulae, severe perianal disease. May involve hemicolectomy, total colectomy, small bowel resection and 'ostomy' or pouch creation.

Complications of Crohn's disease

- Oral mucosa—aphthous ulcers, gum and mouth pain, cheilitis, sialadenitis
- Skin—erythema nodosum, pyoderma gangrenosum
- Joints—seronegative spondyloarthropathy, large joint arthritis in the periphery, ankylosing spondylitis, sacroilitis
- Eyes—uveitis, episcleritis, iritis
- Vascular system—thromboembolism (venous as well as arterial, as was the case in the above case vignette—a DVT and paradoxical embolism via a possible patent foramen ovale (PFO))
- Abdominal—abscess, draining sinuses, fistula formation, perforation, peritonitis, obstruction, cancer (small bowel, colon)
- Kidneys—amyloidosis and associated renal failure
- Liver—primary sclerosing cholangitis
- Skeletal system—osteoporosis
- Respiratory—pulmonary embolism
- Haematological—haematinic deficiency anaemia, autoimmune haemolytic anaemia

Microscopic colitis: lymphocytic, collagenous

This is a relatively uncommon condition that occurs more frequently in older patients.

Presentation

Usually painless chronic diarrhoea. Sometimes diarrhoea is severe.

Aetiology

Unknown, but could be associated with some drugs, especially NSAIDs.

Diagnosis

Colonoscopy and biopsy. Macroscopic appearance of the large bowel is normal.

Management

Treatment is often suboptimal and the exact duration unknown. Suspected precipitants should be withdrawn. Therapeutic agents used include antidiarrhoeals (loperamide), ASA agents and cholestyramine. Budesonide can be effective but has potential adverse effects, especially if long term. Azathioprine has rarely been used but can only be justified in very severe diarrhoea.

COELIAC DISEASE

Approach to the patient

History

This is familial enteropathy due to hypersensitivity to the gliadin component of gluten. Ask about initial diagnosis and age of diagnosis. Most often coeliac disease manifests and is diagnosed in childhood and early adulthood. Presenting symptoms could be abdominal pain, anorexia, diarrhoea, constipation, bloating, steatorrhoea and constant flatulence. Ask about growth failure during childhood. Patients may also have weight loss and pallor, fatigue and/or dyspnoea due to anaemia. Ask about associated conditions such as IgA deficiency, diabetes mellitus, autoimmune thyroid disease and rare associations such as pernicious anaemia and liver disease. Gastrointestinal lymphoma is a very rare but dreaded complication. If any of these conditions are present, you should enquire about therapy and the response to therapy.

A pathological fracture due to metabolic bone disease (osteopenia and osteoporosis), though not very common, should not be overlooked. Ask about arthritis and, if present, the details thereof. Ask about problems with fertility and menstrual irregularities in the young female. Some patients may have had recurrent spontaneous abortions. Ask about neurological symptoms such as ataxia and epilepsy. Some patients may have anxiety and/or depression. Ask whether the patient has sought help for the psychological manifestations. Check the patient's family history. Ask how the disease has been treated and the response to therapy.

Examination

In the physical examination look for evidence of malnutrition and short stature. Conjunctival, palmar crease or mucosal pallor may suggest anaemia. Examine the skin and mouth for the classic rash of dermatitis herpetiformis. Examine the abdomen for tenderness or masses.

Investigations

1 Serological tests for auto antibodies—IgA antihuman tissue transglutaminase and IgA-endomysial antibody. Always check IgA levels, as a deficiency will give a false negative result.
2 Small bowel biopsy—looking for the histological features of villous atrophy (Fig 12.8) (blunted villii), hyperplastic crypts, loss of height in the surface enterocytes. There is infiltration of the epithelium by lymphocytes. These changes improve once the patient is commenced on a gluten-free diet.
3 Renal function indices—looking for chronic renal failure due to IgA nephropathy (uncommon)
4 Full blood count—looking for anaemia. If anaemia is present, check the haematinics for Fe deficiency, B_{12} deficiency (this is uncommon, as the terminal ileum is not typically affected) and folate deficiency. Also consider serum levels of calcium, parathyroid hormone (PTH), vitamin D, vitamin A.
5 Liver function indices—looking for mild elevation of liver enzyme levels
6 Bone densitometry—looking for osteoporosis

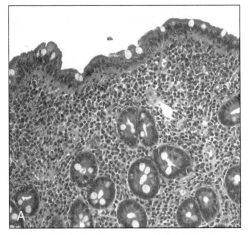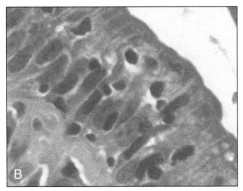

Figure 12.8 Coeliac disease (A) total villous atrophy with crypt hyperplasia (H&E × 100). (B) Intraepithelial lymphocytes (H&E × 400) (courtesy of Dr George Ostapowicz)

Management

1   The mainstay of treatment is a gluten-free diet. The patient should be referred to a qualified dietitian, and given ample education and counselling.
2   Haematinic replacement and replacement of other nutrients.
3   Prophylactic immunisation against meningococcus and pneumococcus is indicated in patients who have hyposplenism, which is not too uncommon with coeliac disease.
4   Non-responders to a gluten-free diet may require corticosteroid therapy.

RHEUMATOID ARTHRITIS

Case vignette

A 44-year-old female presents with severe depression. She was diagnosed with rheumatoid arthritis 3 years ago. She has experienced painful upper- and lower-extremity small joint arthritis despite therapy with multiple agents. The disease has progressed despite therapy, leading to deformed fingers, and she has had to give up her job as a designer. Lately she has experienced extreme fatigue and progressive dyspnoea. In the wake of these symptoms she has gone through the break-up of her 10-year marriage.

On examination the patient appears cushingoid and has a flat facial affect. Upper limb examination shows mild ulnar deviation of her fingers bilaterally. Proximal interphalangeal joints and metacarpophalangeal joints are tender, warm and boggy to palpation. On auscultation of her lung fields there are fine crepitations distributed widely. Her JVP is elevated and she has peripheral oedema.

1   What is your assessment of this woman's current clinical status?
2   What investigations would help you with her work-up?
3   What are the management objectives in this case, in order of priority?
4   What is your plan of management in detail?

Approach to the patient
History
Ask about:
- joint pain, stiffness, swelling and tenderness
- distribution of the joint symptoms
- onset, duration and frequency of symptoms—age of onset is important
- pain on moving the neck—would suggest involvement of the cervical spine, particularly the upper segment
- early-morning stiffness lasting more than 1 hour—highly suggestive of rheumatoid arthritis

- whether the patient has experienced any neurological deficit in the way of localised weakness and/or sensory loss
- dyspnoea or exertional dyspnoea
- any extraarticular features (as listed in the box below)
- whether the patient suffers from any constitutional symptoms, such as lethargy/fatigue, anorexia, weight loss or fever
- the impact of the disease on the patient's social life, occupational life, finances and overall quality of life
- the various treatment modalities tried, and their effects and side effects
- toxicities the patient has experienced with NSAIDs and slow-acting anti-rheumatoid arthritis drugs (SAARD)—should be especially enquired into
- detailed history of the psychosocial impact of the disease.

Examination

The examination needs to be detailed and meticulous. Look for wasting or cushingoid body habitus. Note any skin bruises, oral ulcers, oral candidiasis or surgical scars. Look for features that are characteristic of rheumatoid arthritis, such as symmetrical distribution of deforming arthropathy, involvement of the proximal interphalangeal joint, metacarpophalangeal joint and the wrist (Fig 13.1, overleaf), Baker's cyst of the popliteal fossa, and involvement of the upper cervical spine and the joints of the feet. Warm, tender and stiff joints may suggest active arthritis.

Assess the JVP and feel the precordium for a right ventricular heave. Auscultate the lung fields for fine crepitations of fibrosis. Listen to the heart for muffling of heart sounds due to pericardial effusion and loud P_2 due to pulmonary hypertension. Palpate the abdomen, looking for splenomegaly. Perform a detailed eye examination and a neurological examination.

Hand examination is important. The following features should be looked for:
- radial deviation of the wrist
- ulnar deviation of the digits, swan-neck deformity and boutonnière deformity of the fingers, palmar subluxation of proximal phalanges
- 'Z' deformity of the thumb
- wasting of intrinsic musculature
- Tinel's sign and neurological deficit in the distribution of the median nerve.

Assess the manual functional ability by asking the patient to pick up a pen and write their name, hold a cup, button and unbutton a shirt, and comb their hair.

Examination of the foot is also significant. Features to look for include:
- plantar subluxation of the metatarsal heads
- hallux valgus
- eversion of hind foot at the subtalar joint
- neurological deficit (foot drop, peripheral neuropathy).

Extraarticular manifestations of rheumatoid arthritis

- Rheumatoid nodules in the elbow, Achilles tendon and the occiput (Fig 13.2)
- Vasculitic features, such as nailfold infarcts (Fig 13.3), necrotic leg ulcers, mononeuritis multiplex

- Pleural effusion and bibasilar fine crepitations of pulmonary fibrosis (Fig 13.4)
- Signs of pericardial effusion—elevated JVP, peripheral oedema etc (Fig 13.5)
- Ocular signs of scleritis, episcleritis, scleromalacia perforans (Figs 13.6–13.8)
- Splenomegaly, if Felty's syndrome is suspected

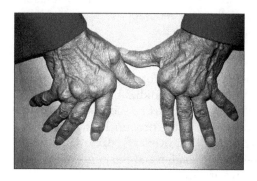

Figure 13.1 Rheumatoid hand signs: view of the hands showing swelling of metacarpophalangeal (MCP) and proximal interphalangeal (PIP) joints (reprinted from Hochberg M, Silman A, Smolen J et al 2003 *Rheumatology*, 3rd edn. Mosby, p 770, fig 68.6)

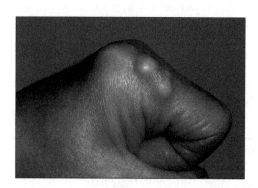

Figure 13.2 Rheumatoid nodules (reprinted from Hochberg M, Silman A, Smolen J et al 2003 *Rheumatology*, 3rd edn. Mosby, p 288)

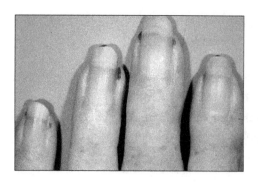

Figure 13.3 Vasculitic features: nailfold infarcts (reprinted from Hochberg M, Silman A, Smolen J et al 2003 *Rheumatology*, 3rd edn. Mosby, p 790, fig 69.28)

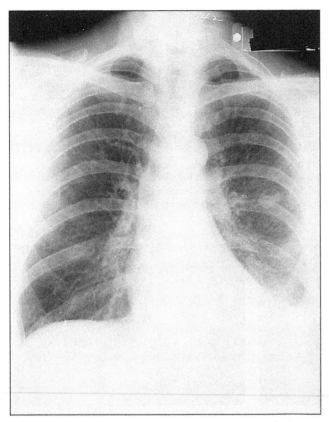

Figure 13.4 Pleural effusion and bibasilar fine crepitations of pulmonary fibrosis (reprinted from Hochberg M, Silman A, Smolen J et al 2003 *Rheumatology*, 3rd edn. Mosby, p 784, fig 69.9)

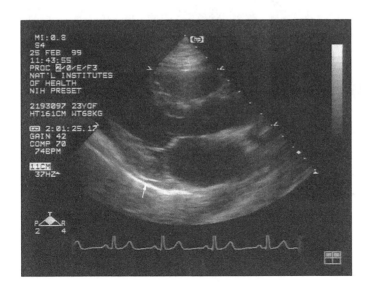

Figure 13.5 Signs of pericardial effusion: elevated JVP, peripheral oedema (reprinted from Hochberg M, Silman A, Smolen J et al 2003 *Rheumatology*, 3rd edn. Mosby, p 1719, fig 158.1)

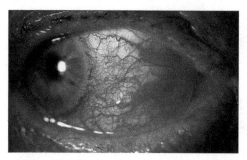

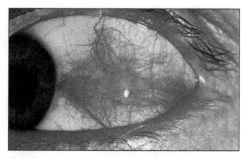

Figure 13.6 Ocular signs of scleritis (reprinted from Hochberg M, Silman A, Smolen J et al 2003 *Rheumatology,* 3rd edn. Mosby, p 786, fig 69.16)

Figure 13.7 Ocular signs of episcleritis (reprinted from Webb L A 2004 *Manual of eye emergencies:* diagnosis and management. Elsevier, p 24, fig 2.15a)

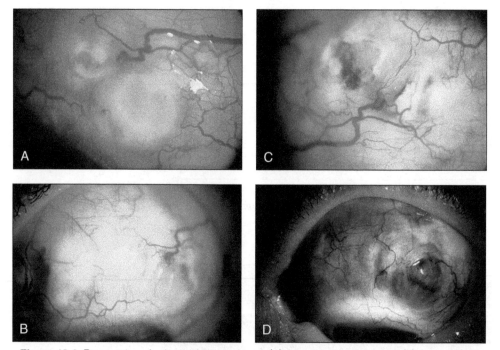

Figure 13.8 Progression of scleromalacia perforans (A) Scleral necrotic patches (B) Extension of scleral necrosis (C and D) Progressive scleral thinning and exposure of underlying sclera (reprinted from Kanski J, Pvesio C, Tuft S 2005 *Ocular inflammatory disease,* Elsevier, fig 5.26)

Neurological associations of rheumatoid arthritis

- Peripheral neuropathy
- Mononeuritis multiplex
- Entrapment syndrome
- Cervical myelopathy

Investigations

1   Serum rheumatoid factor—this is present in only two-thirds of patients suffering from rheumatoid arthritis. It has more prognostic than diagnostic value, in that rheumatoid factor positivity is associated with more severe disease and the development of extraarticular manifestations. Human leucocyte antigen (HLA) haplotyping may have diagnostic and prognostic utility. Anti-CCP (anti-citrullinated cyclic peptide) is a very important disease-specific marker and may be detected several years prior to disease onset.

2   Full blood count—looking for anaemia of chronic disease or iron deficiency anaemia associated with NSAID therapy and/or thrombocytopenia and leucopenia of Felty's syndrome. Anaemia and thrombocytosis correlate with disease activity.

3   Inflammatory markers such as ESR and C-reactive protein level—to monitor disease activity

4   Synovial fluid analysis—looking for features that suggest active arthritis, such as low viscosity, white cell count 20 000–50 000/mL with a predominance of polymorphs

5   X-rays of involved joints—looking for periarticular soft tissue swelling, joint deformity, joint space narrowing, juxtaarticular osteopenia, loss of articular cartilage and bony erosions, in chronic cases (Fig 13.9, overleaf)

6   Chest X-ray—looking for pleural effusion, rheumatoid nodules, features suggestive of pulmonary fibrosis and cardiomegaly suggesting pericardial effusion

7   Echocardiogram—looking for pericardial effusion, pulmonary hypertension (usually secondary), right heart strain and any suggestion of tamponade, which is a particularly rare phenomenon

8   Urine analysis—looking for proteinuria, and renal function indices looking for evidence of renal failure due to therapy-related toxicity

9   Liver function indices—looking for evidence of methotrexate or sulfasalazine toxicity

---

Differential diagnoses of rheumatoid arthritis

- Psoriatic arthritis
- Postviral arthritis
- Arthritis of inflammatory bowel disease
- Systemic lupus erythematosis

Management

Management of rheumatoid arthritis has three objectives: 1) control the symptoms, 2) optimise function and 3) retard progression.

Symptom control

This requires an interdisciplinary approach. Pain and stiffness can be managed with physical therapeutic modalities, antiinflammatory agents such as aspirin, NSAIDs, cyclo-oxygenase-2 inhibitors and parenteral glucocorticoid injections. Systemic

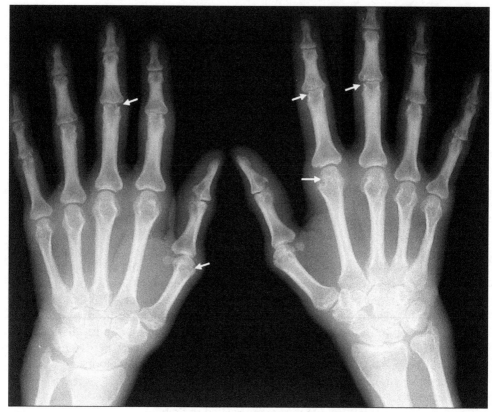

Figure 13.9 X-ray of rheumatoid joint: bilateral hand radiographs demonstrate multiple erosions involving predominantly the proximal interphalangeal (PIP) and metacarpophalangeal (MCP) joints (reprinted from Hochberg M, Silman A, Smolen J et al 2003 *Rheumatology,* 3rd edn. Mosby, p 253, fig 25.1)

glucocorticoid therapy is helpful in high-dose pulses at times of severe exacerbation and in low doses for the maintenance of remission. Severe deformity may need corrective surgery. The patient may need physical therapy for joint stiffness, and occupational therapy to improve functionality. Psychological and social help should be facilitated as required.

Disease-modifying agents

These drugs prevent disease progression and joint damage. They should be commenced early in the disease for maximum benefit. However, their onset of action is usually delayed by about 2–4 months. Some commonly used agents are as follows:

1 Methotrexate—given at weekly doses that vary between 7.5 mg and 25 mg per week. The maximum benefit may take up to 6 months to manifest. Patients should be monitored for the side effects of oral ulcers, hepatotoxicity, pneumonitis, lung fibrosis, anaemia and bone marrow suppression. Patients should be administered folic acid supplements concurrently. As this agent is teratogenic, female patients of reproductive age should take contraceptive measures while being treated.

2 Sulfasalazine (in male patients this agent can cause mild azoospermia)
3 Hydroxychloroquine—be aware of ocular complications
4 Gold
5 Leflunomide
6 Anti-tumour necrosis factor (TNF) agents play a major role in the management of rheumatoid arthritis—infliximab, an antibody against TNF-alpha, or etanercept, a soluble TNF receptor/F_c fusion protein. These agents are expensive and also have the side effects of tumour formation, sepsis and precipitating tuberculosis in susceptible individuals.
7 Anti-CD 20 agent—rituximab (selectively depletes CD 20+ B cells), for those not responding to anti-TNF therapy, usually given with methotrexate
8 T-cell modulator (costimulation modulator agent)—abatacept, for those not responding to anti-TNF therapy. Be cautious: in lung disease, it can worsen chronic obstructive pulmonary disease.

Combination therapy

Methotrexate can be given in combination with infliximab, etanercept or rituximab. Other effective combinations include methotrexate and leflunomide or methotrexate and sulfasalazine together with hydroxychloroquine. The latter triple combination is becoming popular.

SYSTEMIC SCLEROSIS

Case vignette

A 55-year-old woman with a background history of systemic sclerosis presents with progressive exertional dyspnoea of 1 month's duration. She complains of significant debilitation recently—she can barely walk up a flight of stairs without experiencing significant dyspnoea. On examination there is evidence of sclerodactyly and pitting scars on her fingerpads. Tightness and cutaneous fibrosis is also evident in her face, with loss of skin creases and microstomia. There is a parasternal heave. On auscultation of the precordium there is a significant systolic murmur and a loud P_2. Fine crepitations are audible all over the lung fields.

1 What is your assessment of this woman's current clinical picture?
2 What further investigations would you organise?
3 Discuss the different management options and the relevance thereof.
4 Explain how you would discuss the patient's prognosis with her.

Approach to the patient

There are two forms of this condition, according to the anatomical distribution of the disease:

• *Limited cutaneous systemic sclerosis*—with skin thickening limited to hands, face and neck. Limited systemic sclerosis is associated with CREST syndrome. CREST syndrome consists of calcinosis, Raynaud's phenomenon, oesophageal dysmotility, sclerodactyly (Fig 13.10) and telangiectasia.

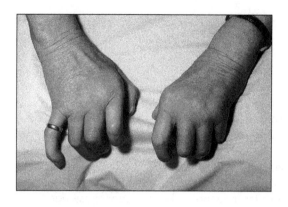

Figure 13.10 Sclerodactyly: creaseless skin with slightly swollen and clawed fingers (reprinted from Kanski J, Pavesio C, Tuft S 2005 *Ocular inflammatory disease,* Elsevier, fig 5.10)

- *Diffuse cutaneous systemic sclerosis*—with diffuse involvement of the skin and other organ systems such as the lungs, heart and kidneys. Use history and examination to determine the specific nature of the disease.

Skin thickening (without organ disease) limited to two or three anatomical sites is termed *morphoea.*

History
Ask about:
- onset of symptoms
- duration and frequency of exacerbation—get the patient to describe the progression of the disease
- common symptoms—including swelling of fingers, forearm, feet and face, arthralgias, swelling and stiffness of the joints
- symptoms of Raynaud's phenomenon (see box and Fig 13.11)
- skin thickening, hardening and the formation of contractures
- upper extremity pain and numbness due to carpal tunnel syndrome and weakness of proximal musculature (consider overlap syndrome)
- dyspareunia in the female patient due to vaginal dryness
- reflux and dysphagia associated with oesophageal dysmotility syndrome
- weight loss and diarrhoea due to malabsorption associated with intestinal dysmotility and bacterial overgrowth
- respiratory symptoms of dyspnoea and cough
- progressive and debilitating exertional dyspnoea—may suggest pulmonary hypertension

Raynaud's phenomenon
Raynaud's phenomen is a combination of symptoms: digital pallor (due to vasoconstriction) followed by cyanosis (due to stasis) and subsequent hyperaemia (due to reactive vasodilation). This reaction is triggered by cold and relieved by heat. There may be associated paraesthesias and pain. In severe forms, digital infarction can occur. Causative associations include systemic sclerosis, SLE peripheral vascular disease, ergot, beta-blockers and smoking. When it occurs de novo it is termed *Raynaud's disease.*

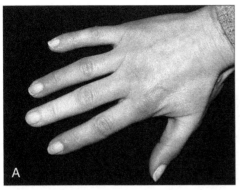
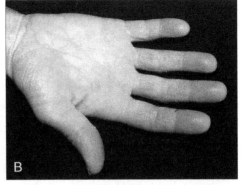

Figure 13.11 Raynaud's phenomenon (reprinted from Gayraud N 2007 Raynaud's phenomenon. *Joint, Bone and Spine* 74:1)

- specific and supportive/symptomatic therapy—its efficacy and the patient's tolerance
- the socioeconomic impact of the disease, occupational difficulties, depression and the support available

Examination

The patient may demonstrate the classic 'bird-like' facies and evidence of malnutrition and wasting. Examine the extremities for shiny muscle wasting and joint contractures. A patient who has developed renal failure may have an AV fistula or a vascular access device for dialysis. Observe skin changes of shiny tightness, hypopigmentation, hyperpigmentation, hair loss, dryness, telangiectasis and thickening etc. Perform a detailed hand examination, looking for nailfold infarcts, nail dystrophy, pulp loss in the fingers, sclerodactyly, calcinosis, evidence of carpal tunnel syndrome (confirm with Tinel's sign) and arthritis. Facial signs found in systemic sclerosis include beak-like nose, microstomia, lack of wrinkles, flat affect and poor dental hygiene.

Perform a detailed joint examination, looking for changes similar to that in rheumatoid arthritis. Assess the degree of proximal muscle weakness and perform an abdominal examination, looking for distension and the absence of bowel sounds due to paralytic ileus. Respiratory examination may show bibasilar crepitations of pulmonary fibrosis. Check the blood pressure for hypertension. In the cardiovascular examination look for elevated JVP with a prominent Q wave, a parasternal heave and a loud pulmonary component of the second heart sound, features that suggest the presence of pulmonary hypertension. Look for evidence of congestive cardiac failure due to cardiomyopathy, and features of chronic systemic hypertension. A 6-minute walk test is a functional assessment with prognostic significance.

Investigations

1 Full blood count—looking for anaemia, which could be multifactorial. The possible contributory causes are: anaemia of chronic disease, renal anaemia, gastrointestinal blood loss, vitamin B_{12} and folate deficiency due to malabsorption, and haemolytic anaemia due to microangiopathic haemolytic anaemia (MAHA).

2 Serum protein electrophoresis, looking for hypergammaglobulinaemia.

3 Autoimmune serology—rheumatoid factor (this is positive in almost 25% of patients), ANA (positive in almost 95% of patients). Specific markers of systemic sclerosis, such as: antitopoisomerase antibody (Scl-70), anti-RNA polymerase antibody (predominant in diffuse disease), anticentromere antibody and antiribonuclear protein antibody (more prevalent in the limited disease).

4 Anti-PM/Scl (polymyositis/scleroderma) is a marker of the overlap syndrome with associated polymyositis.

5 Electrolyte profile and renal function indices—looking for evidence of renal failure.

6 Chest X-ray—looking for cardiomegaly, pleural effusion and features that would suggest pulmonary fibrosis.

7 High-resolution CT scan of the lung—looking for pneumonitis/alveolitis or fibrosis. Active alveolitis is amenable to therapy, and therefore classic CT findings may require confirmation with bronchoalveolar lavage (BAL) or lung biopsy.

8 ECG—looking for left ventricular or right ventricular hypertrophy.

9 Transthoracic echocardiogram—looking for pulmonary hypertension and pericardial effusion. Right heart catheterisation with vasodilator challenge is indicated in patients with pulmonary hypertension.

10 Faecal fat quantification—looking for evidence of malabsorption.

11 Microscopy and culture of duodenal aspirate—looking for bacterial overgrowth.

12 Upper gastrointestinal endoscopy and biopsy—to exclude reflux oesophagitis, Barrett's oesophagitis and peptic ulcer disease.

13 Oesophageal motility studies.

Management

Major objectives in the management of patients with systemic sclerosis are: 1) control symptoms, 2) improve functional capacity, and 3) treat organ-specific disease.

Skin thickening (in limited disease) may respond to UV rays, topical steroids or methotrexate; d-penicillamine therapy is no longer considered because of lack of supportive clinical evidence and substantial toxicity.

The fundamentals of medical management are as follows:

1 Topical and low-dose systemic corticosteroid therapy (with immunosuppressant combinations in resistant cases)—for skin, arthritis, myositis, pericarditis and early pneumonitis. *Caution*: Systemic steroids can precipitate renal crisis.

2 Physical therapy and avoidance of cold—for Raynaud's phenomenon. Calcium channel blockers/ACE inhibitors provide symptom relief. Bosentan and iloprost may be useful too. Resistant cases may require surgical sympathectomy. Severe recalcitrant and painful limb ischaemia or infarction may require surgical therapy.

3 Proton pump inhibitors and prokinetic agents—such as erythromycin and metoclopramide, for oesophagitis and oesophageal dysmotility. *Caution*: These agents cause QT prolongation.

4 Bacterial overgrowth in the small intestines and malabsorption can be treated with rotating antibiotics. Severe cases may require parenteral nutrition. Intestinal pseudo obstruction may require surgical referral.

5 Active alveolitis is treated with steroids and immunosuppressants.

6 Low-flow oxygen is indicated for patients with persistent respiratory failure due to pulmonary fibrosis.

7 ACE inhibitor therapy is of significant benefit to the patient suffering from hypertension, proteinuria and renal failure.

8 Renal dialysis for patients with end-stage renal failure. Because the disease is complicated and systemic, these patients are not usually considered for renal transplantation.

9 Patients with pulmonary hypertension benefit from therapy with calcium channel blockers (those who respond to vasodilator therapy during right heart catheterisation), endothelin receptor blockers such as bosantan (oral), prostacyclins (IV or subcutaneous), and sildenafil.

10 Extreme disease may require referral for heart–lung transplantation.

11 Myocarditis is treated with low-dose corticosteroids and pericarditis with NSAIDs or corticosteroids when resistant.

Mixed connective tissue disease

This disorder manifests as an overlap of clinical features of systemic lupus erythematosus, systemic sclerosis, polymyositis and rheumatoid arthritis. Anti-U1RNP antibody is a specific marker for this condition.

SYSTEMIC LUPUS ERYTHEMATOSUS

Case vignette

A 37-year-old woman presents with left-sided hemiparesis. She experienced sudden-onset weakness of the left upper limb and lower limb. The weakness has progressed over a few hours. She cannot identify any associated precipitating events. She denies headache or trauma. She denies smoking or illicit drug use. She has been married for 5 years and has had two pregnancies spontaneously aborted. Her background history is also remarkable for seizure disorder and distal upper extremity arthritis over a long period, during which she self-medicated with paracetamol. Her seizures have been controlled with valproate.

On examination she has 3/5 motor weakness at all levels in the upper limb and the lower limb on the left side. There is also sensory impairment to touch in the affected half of the body. The reflexes are diminished correspondingly. She also has an erythematous rash in the malar region bilaterally.

1 What are the possible differential diagnoses in this patient's case?

2 What battery of tests would you request, to further work up this patient?

3 What are the management priorities in this case?

4 Discuss your therapeutic plan.

Approach to the patient

Systemic lupus erythematosus (SLE) is a multisystem disorder with manifold presentations, and the severity may vary at different times.

History

Enquire about constitutional symptoms of lethargy, fatigue, fever and weight loss. Most patients suffer from arthralgias, myalgias, rash with associated photosensitivity and patchy alopecia. Ask about hip pain due to ischaemic necrosis of the head of the femur (usually due to high-dose steroids). Discoid skin lesions with scarring may suggest discoid lupus. Ask about seizures, psychotic episodes, headache and peripheral sensory impairment. Some patients may present with oedema due to nephrotic syndrome or dyspnoea and pleuritic chest pain due to pulmonary or cardiac involvement. Check whether the patient has had spontaneous abortions or recurrent thromboembolic disease (myocardial infarction, ischaemic stroke, pulmonary embolism, hepatic vein thrombosis). Some patients experience eye irritation and visual disturbance. Remember that antiphospholipid syndrome can also occur in isolation.

Take a drug history to exclude exposure to agents such as procainamide, hydralazine, isoniazid, D-penicillamine and alpha-methyldopa, which are known to cause drug-induced lupus.

Examination

In the examination look for wasting or cushingoid body habitus.

A detailed joint examination should be performed, and the features to look for are spindle-shaped fingers and swelling and tenderness of proximal interphalangeal, metacarpophalangeal and wrist joints. Arthritis of SLE is usually non-deforming, but rarely a deforming but non-erosive form called Jaccoud's arthropathy is seen. Examine the hip and knee joints for pathology.

Note malar rash (butterfly rash), discoid lesions, scarring, patchy alopecia and panniculitis (Figs 13.12–13.15). Examine the eyes carefully. There will be conjunctival pallor, conjunctivitis, cytoid bodies and cataracts caused by steroid therapy. Note oral ulcers, lymphadenopathy and splenomegaly.

Neurological examination may reveal peripheral neuropathy and proximal weakness.

Cardiovascular examination may reveal features of pulmonary hypertension, cardiac failure or endocarditis (Libman-Sacks). In the respiratory tract examination, look for signs of pleural effusion and bibasilar crepitations of lung fibrosis. Do not miss oedema due to nephrotic syndrome and any lymphadenopathy.

Investigations

1   Full blood count—looking for anaemia, lymphopenia and thrombocytopenia. Ask for a haemolytic screen, and iron studies if there is anaemia.
2   Autoimmune serology relevant to systemic lupus—such as antinuclear antibody titre, anti-double-stranded DNA antibody and anti-Sm antibody. The latter two are relatively specific for SLE. If there is a history of recurrent thromboembolism or fetal loss, check for the presence of antiphospholipid antibody, anticardiolipin antibody and the lupus anticoagulant.

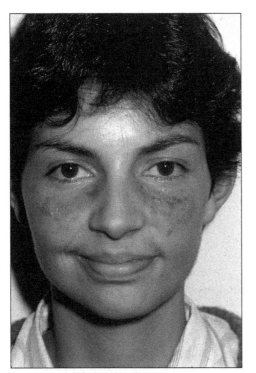

Figure 13.12 Malar rash (butterfly rash) (reprinted from Hochberg M, Silman A, Smolen J et al 2003 *Rheumatology*, 3rd edn. Mosby, p 1361, fig 122.2)

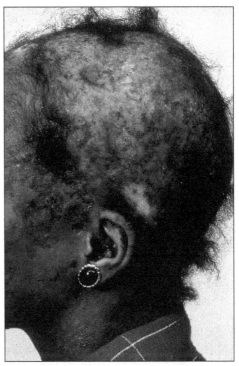

Figure 13.13 Patchy alopecia (reprinted from Hochberg M, Silman A, Smolen J et al 2003 *Rheumatology*, 3rd edn. Mosby, p 1362, fig 122.5)

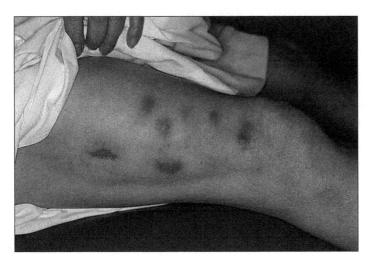

Figure 13.14 Panniculitis (reprinted from Hochberg M, Silman A, Smolen J et al 2003 *Rheumatology*, 3rd edn. Mosby, p 1685, fig 154.4)

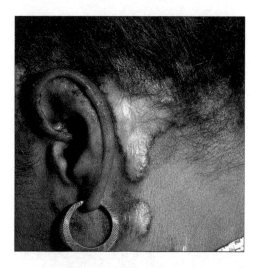

Figure 13.15 Discoid lesions (reprinted from Kumar V, Abbas A, Fausto N 2005 *Robbins and Cotran pathologic basis of disease,* 7th edn. Elsevier, p 1258, fig 25.31a)

3 C3, C4 levels and total haemolytic component (CH50)—these may be low, suggesting complement consumption. Some may have genetic complement deficiencies such as C1q and C2.

4 Electrolyte profile and renal function indices—looking for evidence of renal failure.

5 Urine analysis for proteinuria and haematuria, followed by urine microscopy— looking for red cell casts. If there is proteinuria, it should be quantified with a 24-hour collection.

6 Chest X-ray—for pleural effusion and features of fibrosis. High-resolution CT scan of the lungs to further characterise the pulmonary parenchyma.

7 Echocardiogram—looking for pericardial effusion and valvular vegetations.

Management

Management of SLE has three objectives: 1) control acute exacerbations and disease flare-ups, 2) control the symptoms of the chronic disease and 3) manage organ-specific diseases.

1 Inflammatory manifestations such as arthritis, myalgias and constitutional symptoms can be managed with NSAIDs or cyclo-oxygenase-2 inhibitors. Dermatitis and arthritis can be managed with antimalarial agents, such as hydroxychloroquine given in a dose of 400 mg/day for 3 months followed by a maintenance dose of 200 mg/day. This therapy should be carried out with annual review by the ophthalmologist to monitor for retinal toxicity. The patient should be advised to wear complete sun block to circumvent photosensitivity and prevent the resultant dermatitis or SLE flare-ups.

2 Severe disease is managed with high-dose systemic corticosteroids. Severe acute flare-ups, lupus nephritis and central nervous system involvement should be treated with 3–5 days of IV pulsed methylprednisolone in a dose of 500 mg/ day. In the treatment of glomerulonephritis, addition of cyclophosphamide to corticosteroid therapy has been shown to be significantly beneficial. Mycophenolate mofatil, azathioprine, cyclosporine and methotrexate are other agents that have been useful in the treatment of these patients.

3   For patients who suffer from recurrent thromboembolic disease, lifelong anticoagulation with warfarin is indicated. The INR should be maintained at 2.5–3.5.
4   Psychological and social support, and physical and occupational therapy, should be incorporated into the overall management plan.

SJÖGREN'S SYNDROME

Approach to the patient

History
Ask about dry, gritty eyes and the details thereof. Fatigue is a very common complaint. Enquire about dry mouth, dental disease and difficulties associated with dysphagia and odynophagia. Patients may also have arthralgia and Raynaud's phenomenon. Some patients may also have neurological complications such as peripheral neuropathy and poly- or mononeuropathy. Enquire about bladder symptoms. Ask about the onset of the disease and how it affects the patient's daily life.

Examination
Look in the eyes for conjunctival desiccation and in the mouth for dry mucosae and decreased salivary pool. Examine the mouth closely for poor dental hygiene, buccal hypertrophy and dental caries. Feel the parotids, looking for tenderness and enlargement. Examine the extremities for weak distal pulse, cold peripheries and digital infarcts. Perform a detailed neurological examination. Check for lymphadenopathy. These patients can develop type I renal tubular acidosis, and they have a propensity to develop B-cell lymphomas.

Investigations
1   Full blood count—looking for anaemia and leucopenia
2   ESR—looking for elevation
3   Serum rheumatoid factor, antinuclear antibodies (with speckled pattern), and anti-Ro (SSA)and anti-La (SSB) antibodies. Note that, in pregnant females, anti-Ro antibodies can cross the placenta and cause congenital heart block in the baby.
4   Serum amylase levels—looking for elevation. The clinical utility of this test, however, is dubious.
5   Serum protein electrophoresis and immunoelectrophoresis—looking for hypergammaglobulinaemia
6   Schirmer's test (Fig 13.16), fluoroceine ocular stain (Fig 13.17) and biopsy of the minor salivary glands (Fig 13.18) in the lower lip—to confirm the diagnosis)
7   Renal function indices—to check for renal failure

Management
1   Artificial tears for dry eyes and regular ophthalmic review
2   Dentist review, meticulous dental care and maintenance of oral hygiene. Patients benefit from artificial saliva and oral pilocarpine or cevimeline (not available in Australia) to stimulate salivary secretion.

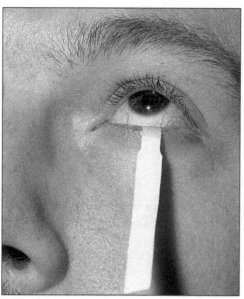

Figure 13.16 Schirmer's test (reprinted from Batterbury M, Bowling B 2005 *Ophthalmology: an illustrated colour text*, 2nd edn, Elsevier p 30, fig 1)

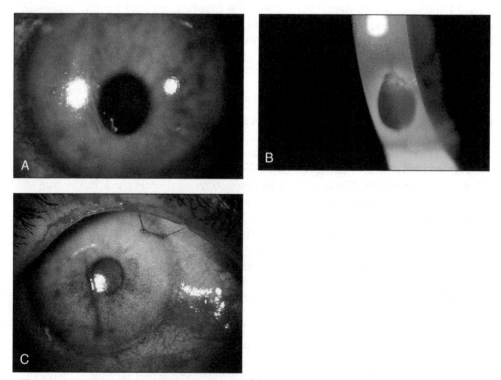

Figure 13.17 Signs of keratoconjunctivitis sicca (A) Mucous debris in the tear film (B) Dry spot in a fluorescein-stained tear film (C) Mucous plaques stained with rose bengal (reprinted from Kanski J, Pavesio C, Tuft S 2005 *Ocular inflammatory disease*, Elsevier, figs 2.1, 2.6, 2.9)

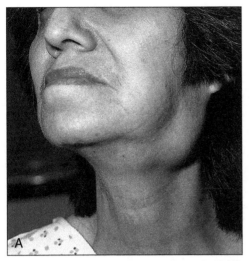
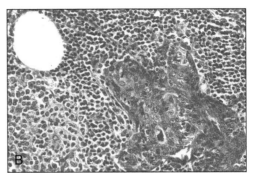

Figure 13.18 Enlargement of salivary gland (A) and salivary gland biopsy (B) in Sjögren's disease (reprinted from Kumar V, Abbas A, Fausto N 2005 *Robbins and Cotran pathologic basis of disease,* 7th edn. Elsevier, p 236, fig 6.38)

3 Immunomodulators such as corticosteroids/cyclophosphamide for systemic vasculitis
4 Hydroxychloroquine for arthralgias
5 Sodium bicarbonate for renal tubular acidosis

MONARTHRITIS
Approach to the patient
Monarthritis can present as the sole complaint or as a comorbidity in a patient admitted for another pathology.

History
Ask about the onset and the progression of symptoms. Duration of symptoms should help distinguish between acute monarthritis and chronic monarthritis. Causes of acute monarthritis can differ from those of chronic monarthritis (see box). Check whether the patient has had previous episodes and, if so, ascertain the details of the diagnosis and the management. Enquire about precipitating and relieving factors such as alcohol, food with high purine content such as shellfish or offal. Check the medication list and ask about recent alcohol binges (gout). Ask about other associated conditions such as chronic renal failure, penetrating joint trauma, diabetes etc.

Causes of monarthritis

Acute
* Crystal-induced arthritis
* Monosodium urate (gout)
* Calcium pyrophosphate dihydrate (pseudogout)

- Calcium oxalate (especially in renal dialysis)
- Haemarthrosis
- Septic arthritis
- Osteoarthritis
- Osteomyelitis
- Trauma
- Avascular necrosis of bone

Chronic
- Haemarthrosis
- Septic arthritis
- Charcot's joint (neuropathic)
- Sarcoidosis
- Pigmented villonodular synovitis
- Osteochondritis dissecans

Examination

Perform a detailed joint examination without causing distress to the patient, who may have an inflamed, painful and swollen joint (Fig 13.19). Check the mobility of the joint, both active and passive. Check the temperature chart. Perform a systemic examination to identify other pertinent features such as gouty tophy, peripheral neuropathy etc.

Investigations

1 Joint aspiration of synovial fluid—for white cell count and differential, Gram stain, cultures and an examination for crystals
2 Blood cultures if the patient is febrile

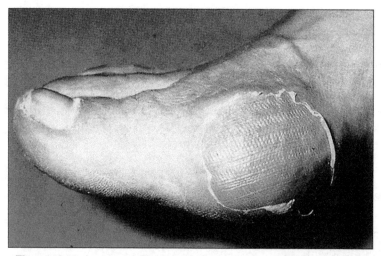

Figure 13.19 Acute gout. The first metatarsophalangeal (MTP) joint is involved at some time in approximately 75% of patients. Desquamation of the skin often occurs. (reprinted from Hochberg M, Silman A, Smolen J et al 2003 *Rheumatology*, 3rd edn. Mosby, p 194, fig 19.3)

3   Radiographs of the joint
4   Occasionally, a radionuclide scan, CT or MRI may be required

Management

1   Consider septic arthritis until proved otherwise.
2   If there is a history of previous episodes that resolve spontaneously, a diagnosis of crystal-induced arthritis is likely.
3   Septic arthritis should be treated promptly with antibiotics upon joint washout.
4   Acute crystal-induced arthritis can be managed with analgesics, NSAIDs, corticosteroids or, rarely, colchicine.
5   Acute gout is treated with NSAIDs or colchicines. Allopurinol is given for long-term prevention once the patient has settled.

OSTEOARTHRITIS

Approach to the patient

History

Osteoarthritis is the most common form of arthritis. Patients usually present with chronic joint pain and loss of functionality or mobility. Osteoarthritis usually affects the feet, knees, hips, spine and hands, but other joints can also be affected, especially the shoulders, ankles and wrists. If there is involvement of uncommon sites (second, third metacarpophalangeal joints) think of secondary causes such as calcium pyrophosphate dihydrate (CPPD) or haemochromatosis. Ask about joint pain and transient morning stiffness, and evening stiffness. Ask what factors precipitate the pain. Secondary osteoarthritis can set in due to overuse or previous joint injury, and therefore it is important to enquire about such associations.

Check how the disease has been managed and any side effects associated with therapy. Ask about physical therapeutic modalities that have been tried and the success thereof. Ask about surgical interventions and joint replacements in detail. Some genetic associations have been identified, and so enquiring about the family history is of value. Ask how the arthritis and the pain and loss of mobility have affected the patient's occupation and daily life.

Examination

Perform detailed examinations of the joints involved. Define the pattern of distribution of the disease. Assess joint movement actively and passively. In the hands, look for Heberden's nodes in the distal interphalangeal joints and Bouchard's nodes in the proximal interphalangeal joints. Feel for joint tenderness. Look for joint crepitus and also any evidence of joint effusion. Assess muscle strength to check for any muscle wasting.

Investigations

1   Joint X-ray—looking for subchondral sclerosis, subchondral cysts, joint space narrowing, osteophytes
2   MRI of the joint if required
3   Markers of inflammation—ESR, CRP (which should be normal)
4   Joint aspirate and microscopy in the setting of effusion
5   Arthroscopy for complicated cases

Management

1 Physical therapeutic modalities are very important in relieving joint pain as well as improving functionality.
2 Analgesics and NSAIDs, COX-2 inhibitors
3 Local injection of steroids or hyaluronic acid
4 Joint replacement surgery
5 Address the precipitating factors—weight loss etc.

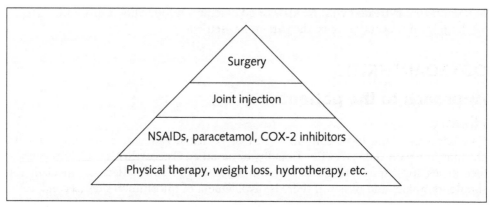

Figure 13.20 Pyramid of therapy for osteoarthritis

Classification of osteoarthritis

1 *Primary/idiopathic*—age-related and may be associated with degeneration
2 *Secondary*—due to another pathology affecting the joints, such as:
   • previous joint injury/insult
   • joint instability (ligamentous laxity)
   • congenital disorders
   • diabetes
   • obesity
   • pregnancy
   • haemachromatosis
   • Wilson's disease
   • acromegaly
   • hypothyroidism
   • neuropathy—Charcot's joint
   • other joint disorders—calcium pyrophosphate crystal-induced arthritis (pseudogout), gout, Paget's disease of the bone, rheumatoid arthritis

Part

02

Clinical investigations and interpretations

14

Clinical investigations
and interpretations

ESSENTIALS OF ELECTROCARDIOGRAM READING

There are a few common electrocardiogram (ECG) abnormalities that can be encountered in the long case setting. It is very important to be able to identify such abnormalities and interpret them accurately. On many occasions the candidate will be presented with a normal ECG and asked for an opinion. Therefore, you should not always expect abnormal ECGs or be surprised to see a normal ECG at the examination. Candidates should have the audacity to decide that the ECG is normal and not to fabricate findings.

The major components to observe in the interpretation of an ECG are the rhythm, rate, axis and morphology, as shown by the P wave, P-R interval, QRS complex, ST segment, T wave and Q-T interval (see box).

Interpretation of ECG

1 Confirm the name and the date of birth/age of the patient and the date on which the ECG was recorded.

2 Ascertain the number of leads on display (usually 12 leads).

3 Check the calibration: standard paper speed is 25 mm/s (where each small 1 mm square denotes 0.04 s or 40 ms horizontally); vertically each 1 cm square denotes 1 mV.

4 Check the rate.

5 Check the rhythm (regular, irregular): this is best seen in lead II—the rhythm strip.

6 Check the axis (normal axis is between −30° and +120°; if between −90° and −30° it is left-axis deviation and if between +120° and +180° it is right-axis deviation).

7 Analyse the P wave (morphology, regularity and relationship to the QRS complex).

8 Assess the P-R interval (normal is 200 ms).

9 Analyse the QRS complex: morphology (e.g. presence of delta waves), width (normal is 120 ms), height of R wave and depth of S wave, presence of Q waves and R wave progression in the precordial leads.

---

10 Analyse the ST segment: depression and elevation in relation to the isoelectric line and its significance according to the context.

11 Check the Q-T interval (this is a rate-dependent phenomenon; < 430 ms is normal for the adult male, < 450 ms for the adult female).

12 Study the T wave: height and morphology.

13 Look for special features (e.g. bundle branch block) and possible diagnosis according to the clinical context.

It is not necessary to describe the ECG in the traditional and pedantic way, opening with the rate, rhythm and axis and then going on to describe the rest if they are normal. At the examination this may sound superfluous, and there is no time to waste! Candidates should identify the name of the patient and the date the ECG was done, and immediately start describing the abnormalities with references to the clinical findings. The following is a discussion of the various ECG findings commonly encountered in the long case examination.

Acute (transmural) myocardial infarction

ST elevation of more than 1 mm in two contiguous leads. In anterior infarcts this would be in the chest leads V_2–V_6. Left heart infarcts show this in leads I, II and aVL. In inferior infarcts it is seen in leads II, III and aVF. Posterior infarctions show up as reciprocal changes in the anterior leads, and the classic findings include R waves, ST segment depression or tall T waves in leads V_1 and V_2. Acute myocardial infarction can sometimes present as a new bundle branch block.

Q waves are pathological if they are broader than 1 mm or deeper than 2 mm (or > 25% of the height of the following R wave).

Subendocardial ischaemia

ECG changes consistent with subendocardial ischaemia (acute coronary syndrome) are ST segment depression of 1 mm or more, 0.08 seconds after the J point and corresponding T wave changes. The slope of the ST segment may provide some clues to the severity of the ischaemic phenomenon. Upward sloping indicates less severe disease, horizontal sloping indicates more severe disease, while downward sloping is usually considered the most significant and severe. The T wave changes include T wave flattening and T wave inversion.

Left ventricular hypertrophy

Left ventricular hypertrophy is described according to voltage criteria and strain/repolarisation criteria.

Voltage criteria

1 Length of the deepest S wave in leads V_1 or V_2, or height of the tallest R wave of lead V_5 or V_6 > 25 mm

2 Sum of the lengths of the S wave of V_1 and the R wave of either V_5 or V_6 > 35 mm

3 Height of the R wave in aVL > 12 mm and height of the R wave in aVF > 20 mm

4 Sum of the lengths of the S wave in lead III and R wave of lead I > 25 mm

Repolarisation criteria
1   Non-specific ST segment depression and T wave inversion in the left precordial leads
2   Incomplete or complete left bundle branch block

Right ventricular hypertrophy

This may be associated with pulmonary stenosis or pulmonary hypertension.
1   Tall R wave in leads V_1 and aVR (the height of the R wave exceeds the length of the S wave)
2   Right axis deviation
3   Prominent S waves in leads V_5 and V_6
4   Poor R wave progression

Left atrial hypertrophy/strain

1   Biphasic P waves in lead V_1
2   Notched P waves in the limb leads

Right atrial hypertrophy/strain

This is associated with right atrial overload, as in pulmonary hypertension and right heart failure.
1   P waves taller than 2.5 mm, best seen in leads II and V_1

Right bundle branch block

This is seen in right heart strain associated with pulmonary hypertension, chronic lung disease, pulmonary emboli and mitral valve pathology. Some people may have non-pathological right bundle branch block, which is of no significance.
1   Broad QRS complex
2   Right axis deviation
3   rSR pattern in lead V_1 with a smaller r wave followed by a broad and deep S wave and a dominant R wave
4   qRS pattern in V_6 with a small q wave followed by a broad and tall R wave and deep S wave

Left bundle branch block

This is seen in ischaemic heart disease, hypertension, aortic stenosis and cardio-myopathy. Features to notice:
1   Broad QRS complex
2   Notched R waves in leads I, II, aVL, aVF, V_5 and V_6
3   R waves may be tall in the left precordial leads (V_5, V_6)
4   Deep S waves and Q waves in the right precordial leads (V_1)
5   The ST segment and T wave changes are non-specific in this setting.

Left anterior hemiblock

This is the most common cause of left-axis deviation. There is marginal prolongation of the QRS complex with left-axis deviation. Also notice terminal R waves in leads aVR and aVL, deep S wave in lead II, and RSR pattern in leads II, III and aVF. This feature is commonly seen in anterolateral or inferior myocardial infarcts.

Left posterior hemiblock

This abnormality is associated with right-axis deviation of about 120°, Q waves in leads II, III and aVF, R waves in leads I and aVL. When left posterior hemiblock is present it is almost always associated with right bundle branch block. This combination has a poor prognosis, and progression to complete heart block needing a pacemaker is the likely eventuality.

Bifascicular block

Right bundle branch block in combination with a left-sided hemiblock or left bundle branch block. There is a high likelihood of progression to complete heart block requiring a permanent pacemaker.

First-degree heart block

The rate is usually normal and the main abnormality is a prolonged P-R interval (> 200 msec or 5 mm).

Second-degree heart block

Type I (Wenckebach phenomenon)

The sinus rate is normal but the ventricular rate is slower than normal. The main abnormality is the gradual prolongation of the P-R interval until one P wave is not conducted to the ventricles. A new cardiac cycle begins following the non-conducted P wave. Rhythm is usually irregular. This pattern has an association with inferior myocardial infarctions.

Type II

The sinus rate is normal but the ventricular rate is a definite fraction of the sinus rate. There are more P waves than QRS complexes, as only one P wave is conducted for several subsequent P waves. Note the block, which is 2:1, 3:1 or more. This condition is usually associated with anterior myocardial infarctions.

Complete heart block

The sinus rate is normal but the ventricular rate is much slower. The ventricular rate is dependent on the site of the escape pacemaker (if it is in the AV junction, the rate would be around 40–60 bpm; if ventricular, the rate would be < 30 bpm). The P-R interval changes constantly and the P wave has no relationship to the QRS complex (AV dissociation).

Tachyarrhythmias

Ventricular tachycardia

A broad complex tachycardia with a rate exceeding 100 bpm. In practice, however, it is common to see the rate at 140–200. The rhythm is regular. It is called *sustained ventricular tachycardia* if it persists beyond 30 seconds. The QRS complex is longer than 140 milliseconds. There is evidence of AV dissociation, fusion beats and variable retrograde conduction. QRS pattern of all precordial leads should be in concordance. There may be features of left-axis deviation in the presence of right bundle branch block. A broad complex ventricular rhythm at a rate of less than 100 bpm is called *accelerated idioventricular rhythm*.

Atrial tachycardia

The rhythm is regular and the rate is 140–280 bpm. QRS complex follows each P wave, but the P wave may also be buried in the QRS complex or the T wave and not be visible.

Atrial flutter

The rhythm is most often regular but may vary if the degree of AV nodal block changes. Ventricular rate may vary between 60 and 150, again depending on the block. There are characteristic atrial oscillations described as 'sawtooth'-shaped flutter waves. These flutter waves occur regularly at a rate of 250–300 per minute. Depending on the block, the rhythm should be described as atrial flutter with 2:1, 3:2 or 4:1 block.

Junctional tachycardia (AV nodal re-entry tachycardia)

The rhythm is regular and the rate is 100–200 bpm. The P wave appears inverted and is located immediately before or after the QRS complex due to retrograde conduction.

Wolff-Parkinson-White syndrome

This conduction defect occurs due to ventricular pre-excitation due to the presence of an accessory AV conduction pathway. The P-R interval is shorter than 110 milliseconds and the QRS complex has a slurred upstroke (delta wave). The patient may be in atrial fibrillation. A negative delta wave in lead V_1 suggests a right-sided bypass tract.

Hypertrophic obstructive cardiomyopathy

Patients with hypertrophic obstructive cardiomyopathy may show non-specific ECG features. Evidence of left ventricular hypertrophy and diffuse, widespread, deep and broad Q waves are some commonly seen abnormalities.

HAEMATOLOGICAL STUDIES

Blood test results encountered in the examination include the full blood count, electrolyte profile, renal function indices, liver function studies, endocrine studies and serology. Serological tests can be either infective or autoimmune serology.

Full blood count

Here the focus should be on haemoglobin level, haematocrit, mean cell volume, mean cell haemoglobin concentration, and white cell count with differential and platelet count.

Candidates should know the normal values of all the above so that an abnormal value can be spotted immediately and interpreted accurately. When an abnormality in the blood count is present, ask for the report of the blood film for further clarification and, if appropriate, ask for other tests such as the results of the bone marrow biopsy, haemolytic screen, iron studies and vitamin B_{12} and folate levels in anaemia, results of the blood culture in the setting of significant leucocytosis and febrile illness, and antiplatelet antibodies in idiopathic thrombocytopenia.

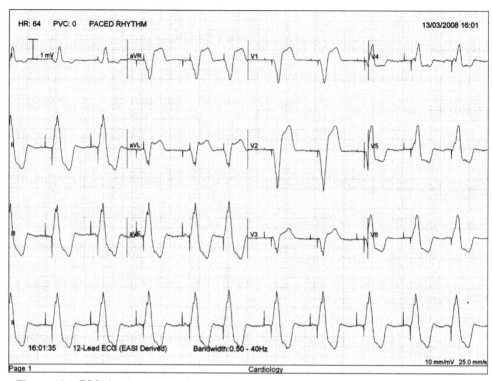

Figure 14.1 ECG showing atrial and ventricular paced rhythm with pacing spikes clearly visible before each atrial and ventricular complex. Also note the left bundle branch block (LBBB) pattern due to the early stimulation of the right ventricle by the pacing lead located there.

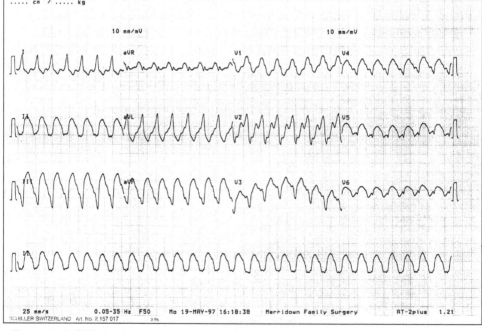

Figure 14.2 ECG showing ventricular tachycardia

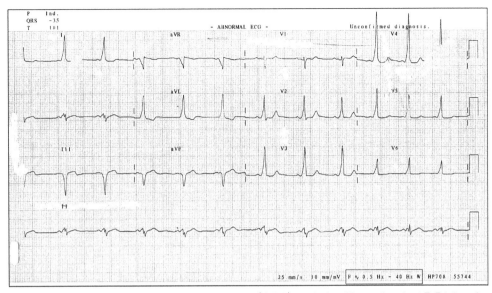

Figure 14.3 ECG showing Wolff-Parkinson-White (WPW) syndrome. Notice the short P-R interval and the delta wave visible in most QRS complexes.

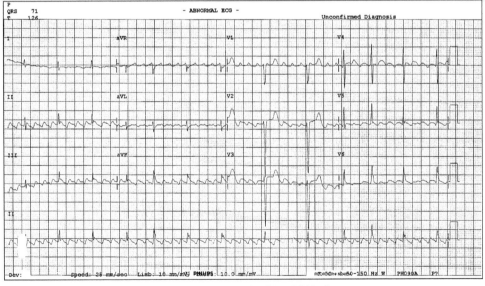

Figure 14.4 ECG showing atrial flutter with variable AV nodal block

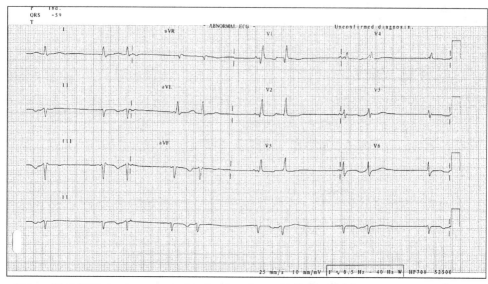

Figure 14.5 ECG showing supraventricular bigeminy and left axis deviation

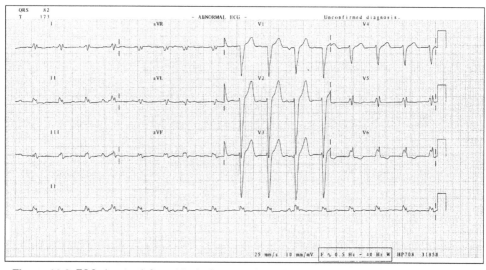

Figure 14.6 ECG showing left ventricular hypertrophy with non-specific ST–T changes

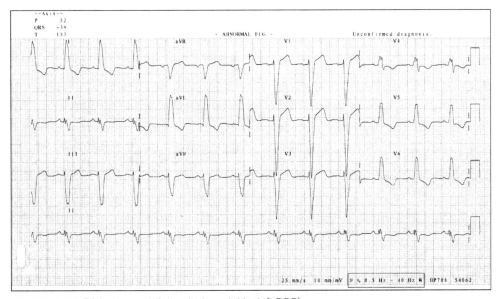

Figure 14.7 ECG showing left bundle branch block (LBBB)

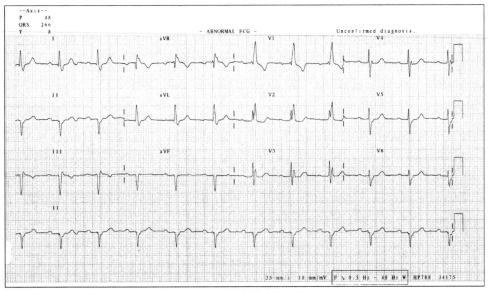

Figure 14.8 ECG showing right bundle branch block (RBBB)

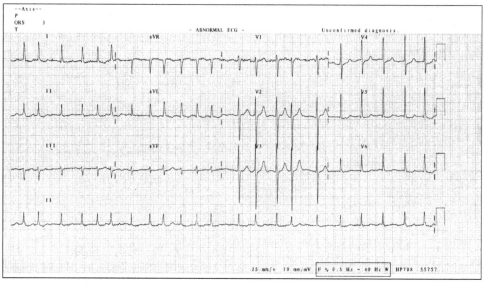

Figure 14.9 ECG showing atrial fibrillation

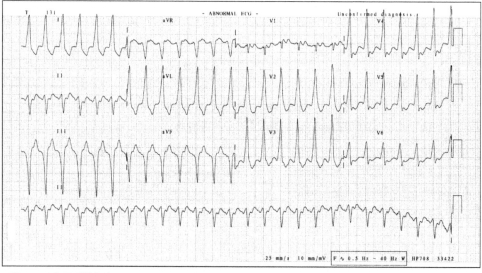

Figure 14.10 ECG showing supraventricular tachycardia with aberrancy

Neutrophilia

Neutrophilia is diagnosed when the neutrophil count is elevated above 7.5×10^9/L. The possible causes are:

1 Bacterial sepsis
2 Inflammatory conditions (as guided by the clinical setting)
3 Tissue damage due to infarction or trauma

4   Glucocorticoid excess
5   Haematological malignancy—chronic myeloid leukaemia, polycythaemia rubra
    vera and myelofibrosis.

Lymphocytosis

Lymphocytosis is diagnosed when the lymphocyte count is elevated above $4 \times 10^9/L$. The possible causes are:
1   Viral sepsis
2   Intracellular bacterial sepsis
3   Lymphoma
4   Chronic lymphocytic leukaemia.

Eosinophilia

Eosinophilia is diagnosed when the eosinophil count is elevated above $0.5 \times 10^9/L$. The possible causes are:
1   Parasitic infestation
2   Allergic disorders and atopy
3   Vasculitic conditions such as polyarteritis nodosa
4   Addison's disease
5   Eosinophilic-myalgic syndrome
6   Hypereosinophilic syndrome
7   Acute interstitial nephritis.

Basophilia

Basophilia is diagnosed when the basophil count is elevated above $0.1 \times 10^9/L$. The possible causes are:
1   Chronic myeloid leukaemia
2   Polycythaemia rubra vera
3   Myelofibrosis
4   Ulcerative colitis.

Leucopenia

Leucopenia is diagnosed when the white cell count is less than $4 \times 10^9/L$. The possible causes are:
1   Viral sepsis
2   Drugs—chloramphenicol, carbimazole, propylthiouracil, chlorpromazine,
    ganciclovir, myelosuppressive agents
3   Felty's syndrome
4   SLE
5   Bone marrow infiltration by sepsis and malignancy.
    Microangiopathic haemolytic anaemia (MAHA) should be suspected in an anaemic and coagulopathic patient if the blood film report shows fragment cells, helmet cells, polychromasia and reticulocytosis. The possible causes include:
1   Disseminated intravascular coagulation due to severe sepsis, severe organ failure
    (liver, heart and kidney), massive trauma and disseminated malignancy
2   Haemolytic-uraemic syndrome (ask for renal function indices)
3   Thrombotic thrombocytopenic purpura
4   Malignant hypertension.

Blood film
Red cell morphology:
1 Pencil cells—in iron deficiency anaemia
2 Teardrop poikilocytosis—in myelofibrosis
3 Spherocytes—in hereditary spherocytosis, autoimmune haemolytic anaemia
4 Target cells—in liver disease, iron deficiency, thalassaemia
5 Polychromasia—reflects a high reticulocyte count.

Thrombophilic screen
This should be performed in cases of thromboembolic disease with a strong family history or recurrent spontaneous venous thrombosis in any patient, arterial thrombosis in a patient aged under 30 years, and venous thrombosis in a patient aged under 40 years without a predisposing condition.

Thrombophilic screen involves testing for the following:
1 Lupus anticoagulant and antiphospholipid antibody
2 Factor V Leiden
3 Protein C and S levels, looking for deficiency
4 Antithrombin III levels, looking for deficiency
5 Dysfibrinogenaemia
6 Prothrombin gene mutation.

Electrolyte profile
Look at the sodium level, potassium level, chloride level, bicarbonate level and the renal function indices. If any abnormality is noticed, try interpreting it in the context of the clinical setting or a causative medication.

Sodium
The normal serum sodium level is 136–144 mmol/L.

Hypernatraemia
This can be caused by hypovolaemia and dehydration as well as primary hyperaldosteronism, Cushing's syndrome and excess salt intake. Patients present with lethargy, irritability, fever, nausea, vomiting and confusion. Management is with controlled hydration using 4% dextrose with 1/5 normal saline or 5% dextrose solution together with judicious diuretic therapy.

Hyponatraemia
This can be caused by inappropriate secretion of antidiuretic hormone (SIADH), congestive cardiac failure, severe hepatic failure, Addison's disease, aldosterone insufficiency, hypothyroidism, diuretic therapy, salt-losing nephropathy, renal tubular disorders and water retention.

SIADH can be due to small cell lung cancer, central nervous system disorders such as meningitis and subarachnoid haemorrhage, lung disease such as asthma, pneumonia and tuberculosis, and drug therapy with tricyclic antidepressants, carbamazepine and monoamine oxidase inhibitors. The phenomenon of pseudohyponatraemia occurs in hyperglycaemia, alcohol excess and hyperuricaemia. Significant hyponatraemia (serum sodium of < 125 mmol/L) presents with lethargy, confusion, convulsions and coma. Management of severe symptomatic hyponatraemia uses controlled infusion

(1–3 mL/kg/h) of hypertonic saline (3% NaCl) with judicious diuretic therapy. Chronic, asymptomatic hyponatraemia can be well managed with fluid restriction to 1 L/day. Resistant hyponatraemia due to SIADH can also be treated with regular oral demeclocycline.

Potassium

The normal serum potassium level is 3.5–5.0 mmol/L.

Hyperkalaemia

This can be caused by ACE inhibitor therapy, potassium-sparing diuretics, inadvertent potassium supplementation, acidosis, blood transfusion, haemolysis, severe renal failure, rhabdomyolysis and hypoaldosteronism.

Patients present with severe muscular weakness, paralytic ileus, symptomatic bradycardia and heart block. Management of hyperkalaemia includes administration of 10 mL 10% calcium gluconate if there are electrocardiographic changes of hyperkalaemia (peaked T waves, small P waves and wide QRS complexes). Rapid reversal of potassium levels can be achieved by giving 50% glucose with insulin infusion, but the levels may rise again in a few hours. Concurrently administer oral or per rectum resonium 15–30 g and repeat administration as guided by subsequently measured serum potassium levels. Hyperkalaemia of severe renal failure needs haemodialysis.

Hypokalaemia

Causes of hypokalaemia include loop diuretic therapy, primary hyperaldosteronism, Cushing's syndrome, renal tubular disease, alkalosis and hyperthyroidism. Therapy with drugs such as verapamil, beta-agonists and amiodarone should be excluded.

Hypokalaemia presents with muscle weakness or tetany. Significant hypokalaemia can lead to rhabdomyolysis. To manage hypokalaemia, usually oral supplementation alone will suffice. If the level is < 2.9 mmol/L, parenteral supplementation with KCl 10 mmol/L over an hour through a central venous line is indicated. The patient's cardiac function should be monitored during this infusion. It should be repeated as guided by the subsequently performed serum potassium levels.

Calcium

The normal serum calcium level is 2.2–2.5 mmol/L. The serum calcium level varies with the serum albumin level, and the correction can be made using the following formula:

$$\text{Corrected serum Ca level (in mmol/L)} = \text{Measured serum Ca level} + 0.02 \times (40 - \text{serum albumin level}) \text{ (in g/L)}$$

Hypercalcaemia

This can be caused by primary hyperparathyroidism, squamous cell carcinoma of the lung, cancer with bony metastases, multiple myeloma, sarcoidosis, vitamin D intoxication, milk-alkali syndrome and thiazide diuretics.

Significant hypercalcaemia presents with anorexia, nausea, vomiting, constipation, polyuria, severe weakness, stupor and eventually coma.

Steps in the management of hypercalcaemia include, first, hydration with adequate amounts of normal saline, together with loop diuretic therapy. More severe hypercalcaemia needs treatment with a bisphosphonate such as etidronate or pamidronate. Calcitonin injected subcutaneously or intravenously (200 units, 6-hourly) has a short-lived effect. Hypercalcaemia due to multiple myeloma, sarcoidosis or vitamin D toxicity can be treated also with glucocorticoids. Oral phosphate is useful when there is hypercalcaemia together with hypophosphataemia.

Hypocalcaemia

Causes of hypocalcaemia include hypoparathyroidism, vitamin D deficiency, osteomalacia, acute pancreatitis, chronic renal failure, malignancy with osteoblastic metastases, and pseudohypoparathyroidism.

Patients present with circumoral and distal limb paraesthesias, painful muscle cramps, tetany and seizures. Patients may also have Chvostek's sign and Trousseau's sign.

Symptomatic hypocalcaemia and corrected serum levels of < 1.88 mmol/L should be treated with parenteral calcium in the form of 10% calcium gluconate.

Acid–base status

Metabolic acidosis

This diagnosis should be suspected when plasma bicarbonate (HCO_3) is less than 10 mmol/L and $PaCO_2$ is low with a low pH (a low HCO_3 value can be seen in respiratory alkalosis as well as in metabolic acidosis). The anion gap helps the interpretation of metabolic acidosis in more detail, and is calculated as follows:

$$\text{Anion gap} = ([Na] + [K]) - ([HCO_3] + [Cl])$$

The normal value is 10–14 mmol/L. Metabolic acidosis could be with a normal or increased anion gap.

Metabolic acidosis with a normal anion gap is due to an associated loss of HCO_3 molecules from the body. The possible causes are:

1   HCO_3 loss from the gut due to diarrhoea, ureterosigmoidostomy, ileal conduit, pancreatic drainage or biliary drainage
2   HCO_3 loss from the kidney due to the use of carbonic anhydrase inhibitor, urinary diversion, renal tubular acidosis (proximal or distal), early renal failure or interstitial nephritis.

This condition is managed with volume repletion and correction of associated hypokalaemia with potassium supplementation.

Acidosis with an increased anion gap is due to the presence of non-volatile acids in the body. The possible causes are:

1   Diabetic ketoacidosis
2   Lactic acidosis
3   Severe renal failure with uraemia
4   Salicylate poisoning
5   Severe hepatic failure.

Metabolic alkalosis

This is caused by excess HCO_3 or alkali or the loss of H^+ due to metabolic causes. A high HCO_3 level and an elevated $PaCO_2$ level together with a high pH characterises metabolic alkalosis. The serum chloride level would give further clues to its aetiology.

Hyperchloraemic metabolic alkalosis is seen in primary hyperaldosteronism, glucocorticoid excess, hypercalcaemia, Liddle's syndrome and Bartter's syndrome. Hypochloraemic metabolic alkalosis is seen in gastrointestinal fluid loss (vomiting), diuretic therapy and after hypercapnoea.

Respiratory acidosis

This is caused by alveolar hypoventilation and associated hypercapnoea. A high HCO_3 and a high $PaCO_2$ with a low pH is suggestive of respiratory acidosis.

Respiratory alkalosis

This is caused by alveolar hyperventilation. A low HCO_3 level and a low $PaCO_2$ with an elevated pH is suggestive of respiratory alkalosis.

Be alert to mixed disorders, where the pH value does not correlate very well with the HCO_3 or the $PaCO_2$ level.

RENAL FUNCTION INDICES

Any elevation of the blood urea or serum creatinine level is suggestive of renal failure. Ask for the previous levels, to ascertain whether the renal impairment is acute or chronic and to ascertain whether it is progressive or stable. If the renal impairment is new, further tests should be carried out to find out the cause (as described in Ch 6).

LIVER FUNCTION TESTS

Aminotransferases (ALT/AST)

This enzyme has two isoforms: alanine aminotransferase (ALT) and aspartate aminotransferase (AST). Massive elevation of the serum levels of this enzyme is seen in severe viral hepatitis, hepatotoxic-induced liver injury and ischaemic liver injury. Moderate elevations are characteristic of mild acute viral hepatitis, chronic active hepatitis, alcoholic hepatitis, cirrhosis and hepatic metastases.

Usually the ALT elevation parallels AST elevation, but in alcoholic liver disease AST elevation far exceeds that of ALT. The ratio of AST/ALT in this setting is > 2.

Alkaline phosphatase (ALP)

A striking elevation of this enzyme is seen in cholestatic disorders. Moderate and transient elevations are seen in all types of liver pathology, including hepatitis, metastatic disease and hepatic infiltrative conditions such as lymphomas, leukaemia and sarcoidosis.

Gammaglutamyl transpeptidase (GGT)

The level of this enzyme correlates with that of ALP. Its level also goes up in alcoholism, diabetes mellitus, cardiac failure, pancreatic disease, fatty liver and renal failure. Elevation of the level of this enzyme is often non-specific.

Prothrombin time (PT) and international normalised ratio (INR)

Elevation of the PT level and the INR is seen when hepatic synthetic function is impaired. All clotting factors except factor V are synthesised in the liver.

Serum albumin level

This marker also reflects the hepatic synthetic capacity, and hence it is low in significant liver disease.

Bilirubin

The conjugated (direct) bilirubin level is elevated in cholestasis. Unconjugated (indirect) hyperbilirubinaemia is seen in haemolysis, ineffective erythropoiesis, Gilbert's syndrome and the rare Crigler-Najjar syndrome.

Autoimmune markers of liver disease

- Antimitochondrial antibody (AMA)—seen in primary biliary cirrhosis and autoimmune chronic active hepatitis
- Antinuclear antibody (ANA)—seen in autoimmune hepatitis
- Antismooth muscle antibody—seen in autoimmune hepatitis
- Anti-liver kidney microsomal antibody (anti-LKM)—seen in autoimmune hepatitis type II.

ENDOCRINOLOGICAL STUDIES

Thyroid function tests

Commonly performed thyroid function tests include serum free T3, free T4 and thyroid-stimulating hormone (TSH) levels. The most sensitive assay of thyroid function is the serum TSH level (normal range for TSH is 0.3–3 mU/L).

Direct test of thyroid function

Hyperthyroidism is defined as hyperactivity of the thyroid gland. Thyrotoxicosis by definition is excess thyroid hormone due to any cause.

A technetium-99 (Tc99) scan helps to identify the cause of thyrotoxicosis. Causes of thyrotoxicosis include Graves' disease, toxic nodular goitre, initial phase of Hashimoto's thyroiditis, excess iodine intake, thyrotoxicosis factitia and subacute thyroiditis. Radioactive iodine uptake is another test that can be performed to assess the activity of the thyroid gland. In the latter three conditions, the uptake of radioactive iodine is reduced. Thyroid scintigraphy using radioactive iodine or Tc99 pertechnetate is also useful for the assessment of hot and cold spots in a goitre.

Autoimmune markers relevant to thyroid disease should be requested in appropriate situations. Antithyroid peroxidase antibody, antimicrosomal antibody and antithyroglobulin antibody are seen in Hashimoto's thyroiditis and Graves' disease. In addition, in Graves' disease, thyroid-stimulating antibodies are encountered.

Ultrasonography of the thyroid gland is done to distinguish between cystic nodules and solid nodules.

In the sick euthyroid syndrome, free T4 levels would be high, low or normal, T3 levels would be low and TSH levels would be low or normal.

Amiodarone causes an elevation in free T4 levels, decrease in T3 levels and an elevation in TSH levels.

In thyrotoxicosis (non-pituitary) the TSH level will decrease to undetectable levels (< 0.1 mU/L).

Adrenal function tests

Cushing's syndrome (excess secretion of corticosteroids)

Screening tests for Cushing's syndrome are the measurement of 24-hour urinary free cortisol or the overnight dexamethasone suppression test.

Confirmatory for the diagnosis of Cushing's syndrome is a low-dose dexamethasone suppression test (0.5 mg dexamethasone every 6 hours for 48 hours).

To determine the aetiology of the Cushing's syndrome, a high-dose dexamethasone suppression test can be performed (2 mg dexamethasone every 6 hours for 48 hours). If there is suppression of cortisol secretion, the likely diagnosis is that of an adrenocorticotrophic hormone (ACTH)-secreting pituitary tumour. If there is failure of suppression, the aetiology is likely to be adrenal neoplasia or ectopic secretion of ACTH.

The plasma ACTH level may also give clues to localising the focus of hypersecretion. An elevated plasma ACTH level may suggest a pituitary or an ectopic origin. To localise the pituitary tumour, imaging studies with cranial CT or MRI should be done. But for the localisation of pituitary microadenomas that do not manifest in the imaging studies, selective venous sampling of the inferior petrosal sinus is necessary.

A suppressed plasma ACTH level is highly suggestive of an adrenal neoplasia and should be followed up with pelvic imaging studies such as CT.

Tests for adrenal insufficiency

In patients presenting with symptoms of weakness, anorexia, weight loss, hypotension, postural drop in blood pressure, syncope and vitiligo as well as investigational findings of hyperkalaemia, hyponatraemia, hypercalcaemia and low bicarbonate levels, adrenal insufficiency should be considered as a top differential diagnosis. Screening for adrenal insufficiency involves performing a short Synacthen® test. This test involves checking the plasma cortisol level 30–60 minutes after an injection of 250 mg cosyntropin.

To localise the level where the secretory function is defective, plasma ACTH should be checked 30 minutes after the injection of 250 mg cosyntropin. If the ACTH shows an elevatory response, the likely site is the adrenal gland, and if there is no elevation the likely site is the pituitary.

Test for hyperaldosteronism

When a patient presents with diastolic hypertension, headache, muscle weakness with fatigue and if there is associated hypokalaemia in the electrolyte profile, consideration should be given to the possible diagnosis of hyperaldosteronism. The first test to be performed is the plasma renin/aldosterone ratio. If it is normal or elevated, go on to measure the plasma aldosterone level before and after saline loading. If there is no suppression of aldosterone secretion with a salt load, consider aldosterone-secreting adrenal tumour and perform relevant imaging studies of the abdomen and pelvis in the form of CT and MRI.

Test for phaeochromocytoma

Phaeochromocytoma should be considered in hypertensive patients presenting with a history of headache, profuse sweating, palpitations, anxiety and weight loss. The screening test for phaeochromocytoma is the assessment of the levels of metanephrines and free catecholamines in a 24-hour urine collection. If there are excess levels of the above markers, abdominopelvic imaging studies and an MIBG scan should be done to localise the tumour.

Parathyroid hormone tests
Test for hyperparathyroidism
This condition is commonly diagnosed incidentally in middle-aged women who are discovered to have hypercalcaemia. However, in any patient with hypercalcaemia it is important to exclude metastatic malignant disease, squamous cell carcinoma, multiple myeloma, chronic renal failure, hypocalciuric hypercalcaemia, thyrotoxicosis, multiple endocrine neoplasia (MEN) type 1 and MEN type 2A.

The initial test for suspected hyperparathyroidism is the serum parathyroid hormone assay. If this is elevated, surgical exploration by a skilled surgeon is the best way of localising the involved parathyroid adenoma or the hyperplastic gland. Remember to exclude chronic renal failure, as there is hyperparathyroidism associated with autonomously hypersecreting parathyroid glands in tertiary hyperparathyroidism of chronic renal failure.

Pituitary function tests
In suspected growth hormone excess, the best initial tests are:
1   Measurement of the plasma growth hormone level 3 hours after a glucose challenge, where the normal response would be the suppression of growth hormone secretion.
2   Measurement of the serum level of insulin-like growth factor, which is elevated in growth hormone excess.

When inadequate secretion of growth hormones is suspected, the best initial test is to assess the growth hormone response to insulin, levodopa or L-arginine challenge.

In both the above situations, an abnormal test should be followed up with pituitary imaging studies in the form of MRI.

In suspected prolactin excess, the best test is the assessment of serum prolactin level.

LUNG FUNCTION TESTS
Formal lung function studies include a flow–volume curve demonstrating the inspiratory flow rate in litres per second as depicted by the curve below the meridian, and the expiratory phase as depicted by the curve above the meridian. The candidate should be able to interpret the curve to diagnose obstructive lung pathology, restrictive lung pathology, the severity of each condition, large airway obstruction and its exact location, as well as mixed airway disease.

The other component of the lung function study is the carbon monoxide diffusion capacity. This would indicate whether the lung pathology is confined to the airways alone where the diffusion capacity is normal, or whether the pulmonary parenchyma is affected where the diffusion capacity is reduced.

By combining the two sets of information, the candidate should be able to make a diagnosis of the lung condition as guided by the clinical findings. The FEV_1/FVC ratio is an age-related phenomenon. However, a ratio less than 75% in a young individual or less than 60% in an older individual is considered consistent with obstructive airway disease. An FEV_1/FVC ratio of 80% or more with both FEV_1 and FVC values being very low is suggestive of restrictive lung pathology.

Following are some possible patterns of lung function study findings that can be expected at the examination:

1 Severe obstructive lung disease (FEV_1/FVC ratio < 50%) without impairment of the carbon monoxide diffusion capacity—likely diagnosis is asthma
2 Severe obstructive lung disease with significant impairment of the carbon monoxide diffusion capacity—likely diagnosis is emphysema
3 Severe restrictive lung disease (FEV_1/FVC ratio > 90%) with impaired carbon monoxide diffusion capacity—likely diagnosis is pulmonary fibrosis.

NUCLEAR IMAGING

Lung scan

Lung scans are performed to confirm or exclude a clinical diagnosis of pulmonary embolism or to ascertain lung function (gas exchange).

Ventilation-perfusion (V/Q) scan

This is performed to confirm or exclude a clinical diagnosis of pulmonary embolism. It is of further help in the follow-up of treatment for pulmonary embolism. Radioactive Xe133 or Xe127 gas is used for the ventilation scan. Perfusion is assessed with injection of Tc99m macroaggregated albumin (MAA). A plain chest X-ray should be obtained before or soon after the scan, for reference purposes. Mismatched areas show normal ventilation with impaired perfusion. A patient whose V/Q scan has a reported high probability of pulmonary embolism should be treated with therapeutic anticoagulation, first with IV heparin and then with oral warfarin for a total of 6 months.

The finding of a high probability scan has high correlation with the findings of pulmonary angiography, which is the gold standard test. Scans reported as being of intermediate probability should be followed up with a pulmonary angiogram to confirm the diagnosis. If a scan is reported as low probability, the likelihood of pulmonary embolism is remote and other possible diagnoses should be looked for.

Follow-up scans should be performed several weeks or months after the initial study. Follow-up scans may show resolution of the initial defects as well as recurrent pulmonary embolism. A normal perfusion scan with impaired ventilation is usually due to atelectasis. Chronic airflow limitation and emphysema manifest as matched defects.

Thyroid scan

A thyroid scan is used to assess global as well as differential activity (e.g. hot or cold nodules). Scans are performed using radioactive iodine (I^{123}) or Tc^{99}.

Increased uptake of the nuclear marker is seen in:
- hyperthyroidism/Graves' disease
- thyroiditis (early stages of Hashimoto's thyroiditis)
- iodine deficiency
- lithium therapy
- toxic nodules (there is low uptake in the background).

Decreased uptake is seen in:
- hypothyroidism
- malignant nodularity
- iodine excess
- some forms of thyroiditis (late in Hashimoto's thyroiditis).

Adrenal scan

Metaiodobenzylguanidine (MIBG) is a neurotransmitter precursor that is taken up by the diseased adrenals and the thyroid gland. This agent is used to image the adrenals on blocking its uptake by the thyroid by administering Lugol's iodide solution. A normal gland shows minimal or no uptake. Uniform increased uptake bilaterally is seen in adrenal hyperplasia. Unilateral increased uptake is suggestive of neuroectodermal tumours such as carcinoid, phaeochromocytoma and neuroblastoma. Distant metastases of these tumours can also be identified by their increased activity.

Renal scans

Tc99m DMSA is used to assess the renal cortical anatomy. Tc99m DTPA or Tc99m MAG3 is used to assess renal dynamics—perfusion and function. These are technetium-labelled radiopharmaceutical agents with low toxicity and low radiation.

These tests are useful in the assessment of renal artery stenosis in the hypertensive or vasculopathic patient. Other uses include assessment of the effects of renal revascularisation therapy, assessment of differential renal function prior to nephrectomy, assessment of glomerular filtration, and ascertaining the aetiology of transplant failure (rejection, tubular necrosis, cyclosporin toxicity).

Administration of captopril 50 mg (captopril-perfusion scan) increases the diagnostic accuracy of renal artery stenosis. The stenotic kidney shows decreased or delayed perfusion and delayed clearance of nuclear contrast. Substitution of captopril with high-dose aspirin has been shown to be equally efficacious with less toxicity.

Delayed images visualise the distal drainage system. Obstructive uropathy should be suspected if there is:
- dilated renal collecting system
- delayed parenchymal clearance of nuclear contrast
- impaired visualisation of the ureters.

Cardiac scans

Nuclear scans are useful in the assessment of cardiac perfusion abnormalities and dynamic function. The nuclear test is more sensitive than the standard exercise stress (ECG) test for ischaemia, but has similar specificity. Agents commonly used in the assessment of the heart are thallium (Tl201) chloride and technetium (Tc99m) sestamibi. Tc99m sestamibi gives images with better resolution and has better tissue penetration, and is therefore useful in obese subjects.

Perfusion imaging

Differential perfusion of myocardium at rest and with increased activity (after exercise) or vasodilator administration (pharmacological stress test) is indicative of significant coronary artery stenosis. When the coronary artery is stenosed less than 90% but more than 50% (considered significant), perfusion during rest is preserved. But with activity or administration of vasodilator, there is relative impairment of the perfusion to the areas supplied by the relevant artery. For impairment of perfusion at rest, the artery should be narrowed by more than 90%. This differential perfusion is suggestive of significant coronary artery disease.

For the exercise stress study, the patient is exercised on a treadmill or a bicycle ergometer. The patient should be exercised to the maximum stress according to the protocol used, or to a heart rate of ≥ 85% of the maximal predicted. Fatigue, dyspnoea, angina, hypotension, arrhythmia and significant ECG changes suggestive of ischaemia are indications to terminate exercising. Nuclear agent is injected at peak exercise to obtain the initial 'stress' image. Imaging is repeated after 4 hours of rest to look for redistribution of the coronary flow. Beta-blocker or calcium channel blocker therapy should be withheld for at least 12 hours prior to the study.

Pharmacological stress testing with the use of a vasodilator agent is used for those who cannot perform physical exercise. This test has similar sensitivity and specificity to the exercise test. Commonly used vasodilator agents are dipyridamole, adenosine and dobutamine. Coronary flow usually increases with the administration of the vasodilator agent in the normal arteries. But in stenotic vessels this change is not significant, so there is differential distribution of the nuclear agent, highlighting coronary ischaemia. Patients should not consume any caffeine or xanthine-containing food material for 24 hours before the study. A resting study is performed later to assess redistribution.

Reversible areas of hypoperfusion indicate significant coronary artery disease. Fixed defects highlight areas of previous myocardial infarction. False-positive results are seen in cardiomyopathy.

Acute myocardial infarction

Tc99m pyrophosphate is used to diagnose subacute myocardial infarction. But this test is not commonly used because ECG and cardiac enzyme or troponin assessment is readily available.

Gated heart pool scan

This study is used to assess ventricular systolic function. Tc99m-labelled red blood cells are used to image the blood pool. Imaging is gated according to the sequence of cardiac cycle. This test also allows the assessment of segmental wall motion in the ventricle. A gated heart pool scan is of value in the assessment of myocardial damage due to ischaemia, cardiomyopathy, and cardiotoxins such as anthracyclines.

RADIOLOGICAL IMAGING STUDIES

Chest X-ray

Interpretation of the patient's chest X-ray is almost an integral part of the long case. Candidates should be able to identify and interpret the most obvious and most striking abnormality in the radiograph immediately. The most commonly encountered conditions are consolidation, pulmonary oedema (alveolar or interstitial), bronchiectasis, hyperinflation associated with emphysema, pneumothorax and mass lesions. An ideal approach is as follows:

1 Start by giving the name of the patient and the date of the investigation as mentioned on the film.
2 Name the projection (frontal or lateral).
3 Identify the abnormality and describe its appearance in detail.
4 Give a comprehensive list of differential diagnoses relevant to the clinical picture of the patient.
5 If relevant, ask for other imaging to further clarify the lesion.
   Following are some examples of commonly encountered X-ray abnormalities.
• *Opacification of a section of the lung field*—Describe the nature of the opacification (confluent, patchy, homogeneous, heterogeneous) and the exact distribution

(mention the possible lobes involved). Identify additional features (air bronchograms, miliary seeding etc). Ask for a lateral projection to define the exact distribution of the lesion.

- *Cystic lesions*—These may be due to cystic bronchiectasis, lung abscess (notice air-fluid level) or emphysematous bullae. Request a high-resolution CT scan to further clarify the lesion.
- *Mass lesions*—Consider primary or secondary malignancies, progressive massive fibrosis or benign tumours. Request a chest X-ray done at least 3 months previously to look for the presence of the same lesion, again asking for the CT scan with lung windows to further clarify the lesion and mediastinal windows to look for any lymphadenopathy.
- *Bronchogenic carcinoma*—This appears as a solitary mass lesion in the central or peripheral lung field. Look for cavitation. If present, it is more suggestive of squamous cell carcinoma. Look for hilar enlargement and mediastinal widening due to lymphadenopathy. There may be segmental or lobar atelectasis due to airway obstruction by the mass. Check for the presence of any post-obstructive pneumonia. The presence of asymmetry of the diaphragmatic shadows may suggest involvement of the phrenic nerve.
- *Cardiac failure*—A cardiothoracic ratio of more than 50% is suggestive of cardiomegaly. The hilar shadows may appear prominent due to congestion of the large arteries. Vascular shadows directing to the upper lobes may appear prominent (upper lobe diversion). These vessels seem as thick as or thicker than those vessels supplying the lower zones.
- *Pulmonary oedema*—In addition to upper lobe diversion, look for cuffing of the walls of the bronchi. This is due to the accumulation of interstitial fluid around the bronchi, and is a sign of interstitial oedema. Further progression of cardiac failure can lead to alveolar oedema, which manifests as patchy and diffuse opacifications. Septal oedema gives rise to Kerley B lines, which appear as horizontal linear opacifications in the lung peripheries that extend perpendicularly to the pleura, and Kerley A lines, which appear as long, fine linear shadows that radiate up from the hilar regions in the upper lung zones.
- *Bronchiectasis*—There may be increased lung markings due to retained secretions. Look for cystic spaces due to dilatation of bronchi and loss of definition of lung markings due to peribronchial fibrosis. Severe cases may also have the appearance of 'honeycombing'. There may be compensatory hyperinflation of the uninvolved lung in cases with unilateral disease.
- *Interstitial lung disease*—Manifests as linear and/or nodular opacifications. In the acute setting there may be peribronchial cuffing, blurring of hilar shadows and blurring of vascular shadows. In the chronic setting look for fine reticulations, an appearance that suggests potentially reversible active pneumonitis. Coarse reticulations and honeycombing (nodular radiolucencies with background opacity) suggest progression to potentially irreversible fibrosis.
- *Emphysema*—Look for hyperinflation of the lung with flattening of the diaphragmatic shadows. There may be pulmonary vascular pruning and peripheral bullae. Cardiac shadow is likely to demonstrate right heart enlargement. If the height of the anterior border of the cardiac shadow in the lateral view chest X-ray is more than one-third the height of the sternum, it may suggest right heart enlargement.

- *Cystic fibrosis*—Look for longitudinal shadows of mucous plugging, tramline appearance with surrounding cystic bronchiectasis, areas of atelectasis and large pulmonary arteries suggesting pulmonary hypertension.
- *Bronchiolitis obliterans with organising pneumonia (BOOP)*—Manifests as unilateral or bilateral patchy consolidation of air spaces. There may be widespread nodularity and irregular linear opacifications. Also look for pleural thickening and effusion.

CT scan of the chest

Computed tomography (CT) of the chest is necessary to further clarify information gathered from the chest X-ray. There are different types of chest CT scan—the high-resolution scan, the helical scan, the scan with lung windows and the scan with mediastinal windows. The candidate should be familiar with the different types so that the scan most appropriate to the clinical setting can be requested.

High-resolution CT scan

Slices of the images are 1 mm thick and are made 1 cm apart. These scans can demonstrate fine changes in the parenchymal architecture. This helps examine the lung parenchyma in more detail to better define interstitial lung pathology. It is indicated in parenchymal lung disease, alveolar disease, emphysema, pneumonitis, drug effects, BOOP and small airway disease.

It is most useful in the diagnosis of interstitial pneumonitis and lung fibrosis. If the pneumonitis shows a 'ground glass' appearance, this is consistent with an active inflammatory process progressing to fibrosis. Some reversibility may be achieved in this situation, and a trial of systemic corticosteroid therapy is indicated. If the picture is that of 'honeycombing', the fibrosis has progressed beyond reversibility.

Normal-resolution CT scans

These images are of 1 cm slices taken in a contiguous run. They give a good overall impression of the lung architecture.
- *Lung windows*—This setting is indicated for the diagnosis of lung masses, abscesses, bullae, consolidation, and pleural diseases such as plaques and mesothelioma. In the lung window the air spaces appear black and the tissue appears white.
- *Mediastinal windows*—These pictures better define mediastinal anatomy and differentiate between fat, blood vessels and solid structures such as lymph nodes. They are indicated in the study of mediastinal mass lesions, lymphadenopathy and for visualisation of the mediastinal vessels.

Helical CT scan

This scan looks at the pulmonary vasculature, and the indication is for the diagnosis of pulmonary thromboembolism, particularly involving larger arteries. Contemporary radiography involves helical or spiral scanning on all occasions.

The following are some commonly encountered conditions where CT scan of the lung may be indicated.
- *Interstitial lung disease*—Look for sharp interstitial nodules, 'ground glass' opacifications or 'honeycombing' that appear in the subpleural region as a reticular pattern with small cystic changes. Ground glass appearance is a manifestation of acute or subacute pneumonitis and is consistent with potential reversibility. Honeycombing is associated with (irreversible) fibrosis.

- *Bronchiectasis*—In the high-resolution CT scan, look for tramline opacities and signet-ring sign of thickened bronchi in end-on profile.
- *Emphysema*—Look for discrete, well-demarcated areas of radiolucency and pulmonary vascular pruning.
- *Lung tumours*—To better define the anatomy and characteristics of the mass lesion and look for metastases.
- *Post-primary tuberculosis*—To better define the lesion and look for necrosis, and to distinguish from an apical tumour with secondary pneumonia.

Abdominal imaging

Abdominal imaging should be requested when there is suspicion of abdominal malignancy, intestinal obstruction, organomegaly, liver disease, pancreatitis, septic collections or biliary obstruction.

Abdominal ultrasound

Look at the hepatic parenchyma, gallbladder, cystic duct, hepatic duct and common bile duct. Dilatation of the common bile duct (> 6 mm diameter) suggests possible obstruction. Ultrasound can show hepatic mass lesions, stones in the gallbladder, stones in the duct system, chronic cholecystitis and tumour of the gallbladder or the bile duct. To further clarify the above lesions, ask for the abdominal CT scan or the result of endoscopic retrograde cholangiopancreatography (ERCP) or magnetic resonance cholangiopancreatography (MRCP), depending on the clinical setting.

Abdominal X-ray

This is indicated in the setting of intestinal obstruction (look for air-fluid levels in the erect film), suspected intestinal perforation (look for gas under the diaphragm), chronic pancreatitis (pancreas appears calcified), gastric dilatation and megacolon.

Barium swallow

This is performed to assess mechanical or functional obstruction of the oesophagus.

Abdominal CT scan

This is usually performed with oral as well as IV contrast. Look at the hepatic parenchyma, porta hepatis, stomach, duodenum, gallbladder, bile duct, portal vein, small and large intestines, abdominal aorta, inferior vena cava, pancreas, kidneys, pelvic organs and retroperitoneum as clinically indicated.

Abdominal MRI scan

This is used to define the anatomy of abdominal and pelvic organs and vasculature with better resolution and definition. It is a preferred imaging modality to better identify pathology.

Cranial imaging

Cranial imaging is done to look for intracranial mass lesions, intracranial haemorrhage, cerebral oedema, cerebral atrophy and hydrocephalus. Investigations for suspected intracranial or intracerebral haemorrhage should be done without the injection of radiocontrast media, as fresh blood is highlighted in white.

Cranial CT scans

Following are some common conditions encountered in cerebral CT scans.

- *Subarachnoid haemorrhage*—In the cranial CT scan, look for white opacifications (hyperdensity) in the subarachnoid space around the brain (around sulci and gyri), sylvian fissure, the basal cisterns, superior cerebellar cistern and the ventricles. Look for evidence of obstructive hydrocephalus.
- *Epidural haemorrhage*—This lesion appears as a biconvex (lenticular) extraaxial fluid collection. Also look for the mass effect that manifests as an anatomical shift in the intracranial content and effacement of gyri and sulci.
- *Subdural haemorrhage*—This lesion manifests as an extraaxial peripheral crescentic fluid collection with concavity in the inner margin. A convex outer margin follows the contour of the cranial vault. The lesion appears as a hyperdensity in the first week, with transformation to isodensity around the second week. It becomes hypodense from the third week onwards (chronic subdural).
- *Metastatic lesions*—These appear as haemorrhagic, cystic or calcified space-occupying lesions. Most often the cerebral metastases are located in the corticomedullary junction, but remember to look in the subarachnoid space, subependymal space and the skull. They manifest as hyperdense lesions when imaged without injection of radiocontrast material and as hypervascular lesions when imaged with contrast.
- *Primary brain tumours*—Glioblastoma multiforme accounts for almost 50% of intracranial tumours. In the contract-enhanced CT scan it appears as a homogeneous or non-homogeneous mass lesion with ring enhancement. Request MRI scan for further clarification.
- *Ischaemic stroke*—Acute stroke (within the first 24 hours) appears as a localised hypodensity in the basal ganglia region or the grey–white matter junction. In the subacute stage (at 1–7 days), its appearance takes a wedge-shaped hypodensity with the base facing the cerebral cortex. Note the localisation to a vascular distribution and the manifestation of mass effect with sulcal effacement and/or transtentorial herniation due to the surrounding oedema.
  - *Basal ganglia infarct*—Manifests as a dense homogeneous enhancement outlining caudate nucleus, putamen, globus pallidus or thalamus.
  - *Lacunar infarct*—Manifests as a discrete area of hypodensity between 3 and 15 mm. The usual area of location in the order of frequency is the upper two-thirds of putamen, caudate nucleus, thalamus, pons and internal capsule.
- *Binswanger's disease*—This condition is due to arteriosclerosis of the poorly collateralised distal penetrating arteries, and it correlates with hypertension and ageing. The CT scan shows multifocal hypodense lesions in the periventricular white matter. There may be evidence of lacunar infarctions in the basal ganglia. There is sulcal enlargement and dilated lateral ventricles, signifying brain atrophy.
- *Multiple sclerosis*—In the CT scan there is non-specific atrophy of the brain. Foci of active demyelination may appear as areas of hyperdensity in the contrast-enhanced CT scan during acute attacks.

Cranial MRI

- *T1-weighted scans*—Cerebrospinal fluid appears dark and fat-containing tissue (brain tissue) appears bright white. Brain white matter appears brighter than grey matter.

- *T2-weighted scans*—Cerebrospinal fluid appears white. Oedema and fluid accumulations also appear white. This weighting helps to better identify abnormalities, so it is important to look at the T2-weighted image first.
- *Diffusion scans*—This scan helps identify acute stroke as early as within 2 hours of onset. The infarcted tissue appears white, and it is important that all images highlight the relevant area to diagnose stroke conclusively.
- *Perfusion scans*—Segmental images are made with the injection of gadolinium contrast. There is evidence of decreased perfusion in areas of ischaemic stroke.

The following are some conditions in which MRI scan of the brain is indicated.

- *Multiple sclerosis*—MRI is the imaging modality of choice in this condition, with 95% specificity. Areas of demyelination are usually distributed in the undersurface of the corpus callosum, the periventricular region and the brainstem. They appear as well-demarcated, discrete foci of increased signal intensity on the T2-weighted and proton density scans. These foci are hypodense in the T1-weighted scans. However, there is gadolinium-DTPA enhancement of the lesions in the T1-weighted scans.
- *Stroke*—Lesions appear as described above.

Skeletal imaging and arthritis

It is appropriate to ask for skeletal and joint imaging in patients with arthritis, joint pain or back pain, if the condition is relevant and important in the current clinical setting. Rheumatoid arthritis, chronic or acute backache, seronegative arthropathy, Paget's disease and crystal-induced arthropathy are some of the more commonly encountered conditions in the long case examination where the candidate should consider skeletal and joint imaging as appropriate to clarify the diagnosis and assess the disease severity.

The following are some common radiological appearances with which the candidate needs to be thoroughly familiar.

- *Rheumatoid hand*—Describe the apparent deformities, such as ulnar deviation of the fingers, 'Z' deformity of the thumb, and swan-neck and boutonnière deformity of the fingers. Other common radiological abnormalities in the rheumatoid hand are joint space narrowing, subluxation of the metacarpophalangeal joints, periarticular erosions, juxtaarticular demineralisation, evidence of previous joint surgery or replacement, soft tissue masses suggestive of pannus formation or periarticular oedema and absence of the ulnar styloid.
- *Osteoarthritis*—Look for joint space narrowing, periarticular osteosclerosis, subchondral cysts and marginal osteophyte formation.
- *Ankylosing spondylitis*—Look for the loss of definition of the sacroiliac joints due to erosion and sclerosis. Later this may progress to joint fusion. The vertebral column may lose its curvature (loss of lumbar lordosis and thoracic kyphosis) and manifest syndesmophytes (vertical bony bridging between vertebrae). Individual vertebrae become square-shaped. Look for calcification of the longitudinal ligaments and fusion of the facet joints. These changes together with syndesmophytes give rise to the characteristic 'bamboo spine'.
- *Diffuse idiopathic skeletal hyperostosis* (DISH)—This disorder manifests radiologically as flowing ossification of the anterior and lateral aspects of the vertebral column due to bony overgrowths and ligamentous calcification. Similar

changes may be seen in the extraspinal locations, particularly in the lower limbs. Clinical manifestation of this condition is relatively silent.

The following pages contain some radiographic imaging studies commonly encountered in the examination. The text underneath each image gives an example of the way in which it needs to be interpreted.

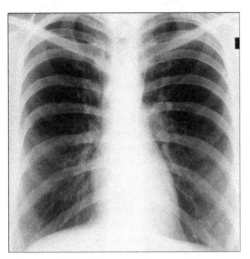

Figure 14.11 This is a frontal projection, postero-anterior view chest X-ray. It is of normal appearance.

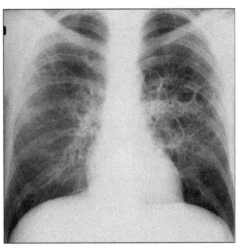

Figure 14.13 There is a coarse interstitial pattern with central and basal predominance. Cystic spaces are a prominent feature. Apices are relatively spared. Mediastinum is normal. Appearance of this chest X-ray is consistent with *Pneumocystis carinii* pneumonia in a patient with HIV infection.

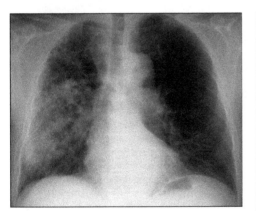

Figure 14.12 Diffuse alveolar opacification of the right lung with evidence of preexisting CAL and normal heart size. The appearance is consistent with atypical pneumonia, especially due to *Legionella*. Other differential diagnoses include unilateral pulmonary oedema, pulmonary haemorrhage and unilateral bronchiolitis obliterans with organising pneumonia (BOOP).

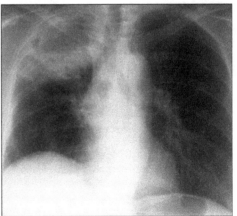

Figure 14.14 Extensive irregular opacity in the right lung apex, with cavitation and a fluid level. This has the appearance of a cavitating abscess. There is elevation of right hemidiaphragm. Other differential diagnoses include post-primary tuberculosis of right apex, *Klebsiella pneumonia,* and right apical malignancy with cavitation.

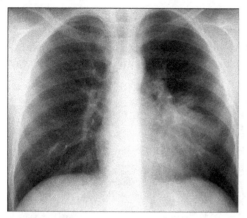

Figure 14.15 There is obliteration of the upper segment of the left heart border and opacification of the mid-segment of the left lung. There are air bronchograms. This is consolidation of the lingula.

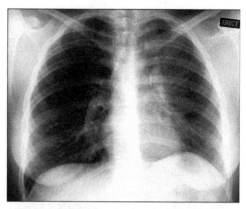

Figure 14.17 There is a band of opacification behind and running parallel to the sternum, thicker superiorly. There is slight elevation of the left hemidiaphragm and mediastinal shift to the left. These features suggest left upper lobe collapse.

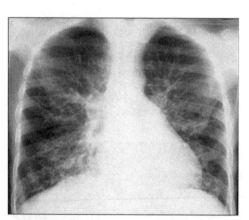

Figure 14.16 There is hyperinflation of both lung fields and increased lung markings. Multiple cystic areas are present in both lungs, suggesting bronchiectasis. Appearance of a large main pulmonary artery segment suggests pulmonary arterial hypertension. This picture shows diffuse bronchiectasis consistent with cystic fibrosis.

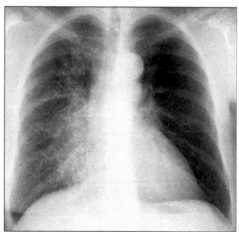

Figure 14.18 There is absence of the left breast shadow. There is a coarse reticular pattern throughout the right lung with perihilar predominance. The left lung is clear. This picture is highly suggestive of lymphangitis carcinomatosis in a patient who has had left-sided mastectomy for cancer of the breast.

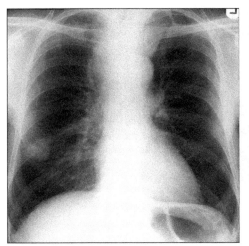

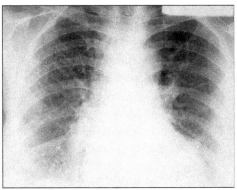

Figure 14.21 There are reticulonodular markings in the lower zones bilaterally. This is the honeycomb pattern of pulmonary fibrosis. The differential diagnoses include rheumatoid arthritis, asbestosis, scleroderma, idiopathic pulmonary fibrosis and chronic aspiration with fibrosis.

Figure 14.19 This chest X-ray shows a mass in the lateral basal segment of the right lower lobe with widening of the upper mediastinum and irregularity of the outline of the trachea. This appearance is consistent with metastatic carcinoma of the lung.

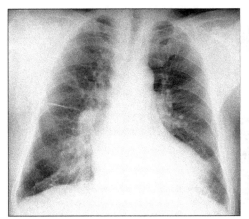

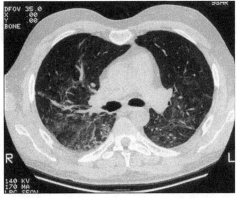

Figure 14.22 This high-resolution CT scan of the lung shows widespread air space opacification bilaterally. This opacification has the ground glass appearance suggestive of active interstitial inflammation.

Figure 14.20 This chest X-ray shows an interstitial pattern throughout the lung fields with septate lines (Kerley A and B) and perihilar haze. There is interstitial oedema, suggesting high left atrial pressures. There are widespread areas of confluence, suggesting alveolar pulmonary oedema, and therefore left atrial pressure should be above 40 mmHg.

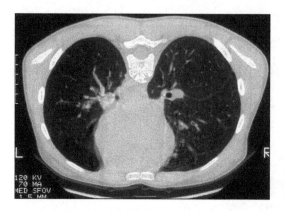

Figure 14.23 This high-resolution CT scan of the lung shows asymmetrical transradiancy between the two lungs. There are peribronchial cuffing, tramline markings and cystic spaces. This is bronchiectasis of the left lower lobe.

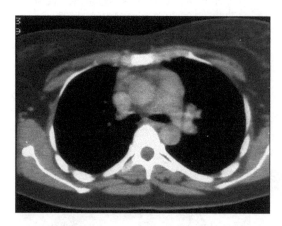

Figure 14.24 This thoracic CT scan performed in the mediastinal window shows mediastinal lymphadenopathy in both preaortic and aortopulmonary areas. The differential diagnoses include soft tissue malignancy, metastatic lung cancer and lymphoma.

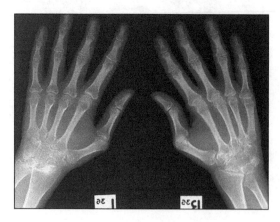

Figure 14.25 This X-ray of left and right hands shows periarticular osteopenia, ankylosis and deformity of the carpus, subluxation and deformity of the radiocarpal and distal radioulnar joints. There are periarticular erosions and erosion of the ulnar styloid. There is loss of joint space at the first metacarpophalangeal joint. This picture is consistent with rheumatoid arthritis of the hands.

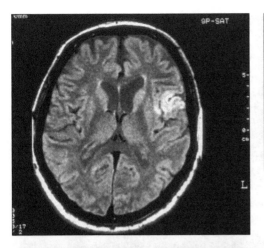

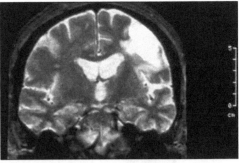

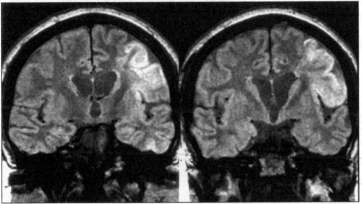

Figure 14.26 The MRIs show an area of abnormality in the left parietal lobe. There is a wedge-shaped area that is slightly hypointense on the T1-weighted picture and hyperintense on the T2-weighted picture. This is consistent with an area of infarction. In addition there are areas that are hyperintense on T1-weighted, T2-weighted and intermediate images consistent with extracellular methaemoglobin. This picture is consistent with subacute haemorrhage.

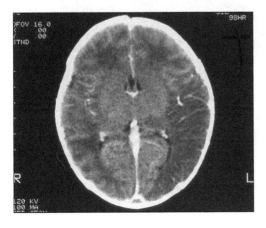

Figure 14.27 There are moderately well-defined low-density areas in the left posterior temporal, parietal and occipital cerebral lobes and similar smaller areas in the right posterior parieto-occipital regions. This picture is consistent with areas of watershed infarction.

239

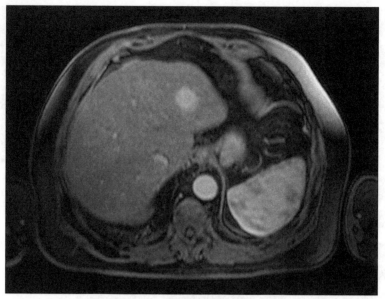

Figure 14.28 Cirrhotic liver with a contrast enhancing mass lesion

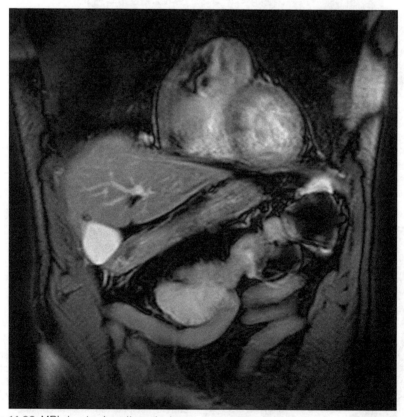

Figure 14.29 MRI showing hepatic metastases

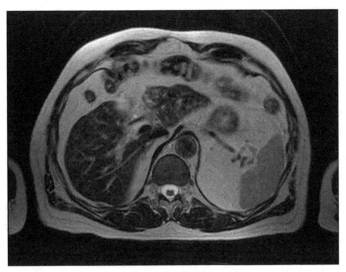

Figure 14.30 MRI of primary sclerosing cholangitis

CORONARY AND CARDIAC IMAGING

Coronary angiography

Study the left coronary tree first. Notice the calibre of the vessels along their length and estimate the percentage stenosis of the diameter of narrowed segments due to atherosclerosis. Define the left main segment and the left anterior descending artery (LAD) (the artery that spans all the way to the cardiac apex) and the left circumflex (LCX) artery. The LAD has diagonal and septal branches arising from it. The LCX has obtuse marginal branches and posterolateral branches originating from it. Then go on to examine the right coronary artery and the posterior descending branch (PDA) arising from it. In 10% of the population the PDA arises from the LCX and this is described as left coronary dominance. If the patient has had coronary artery bypass grafts, study the graft angiograms for any stenoses or disease. The grafts could be vein (saphenous) grafts, radial arterial grafts, or left or right internal mammary artery (LIMA or RIMA) grafts. Usually the LIMA is grafted to the LAD.

Echocardiogram

Study the echo images or the report first, looking at left ventricular dimensions and the contractility. Check the ejection fraction. Look at the sizes of the four chambers and left ventricular wall and septal thickness. Then study the valves for stenosis and regurgitation. In the febrile patient look for valvular vegetations. Study the septi for any left/right communications or shunts. If there is a septal defect, note the direction of blood flow. Read the pressure gradient across the stenotic valve. Study the chamber pressures and the estimated pulmonary pressure. In the patient with atrial fibrillation look for intracardiac thrombi, particularly in the left atrial appendage. Examine the pericardial space for any effusion and the pericardium for calcification.

241

Coronary CT

Coronary CT is gaining rapid popularity as a less invasive imaging modality of the coronary arterial anatomy. The study is useful as a screening test for coronary or vein graft stenosis. It is useful in the investigation of patients who are stable and in an intermediate risk category. Calcification of the arteries and metallic stents can cause interference and shadows, compromising its definition. The images are acquired during diastole in the cardiac cycle, and therefore heart rate needs to be slow for satisfactory results. If the heart rate is too rapid, beta-blocker administration is indicated.

Cardiac MRI

Useful in defining cardiac anatomy. Motion artifacts compromise the quality of images.

Intracoronary ultrasound

Useful in studying the cross-section of a coronary artery by introducing a rotating ultrasound transducer into the coronary artery. This is more sensitive at detecting and measuring coronary stenosis. This modality is useful in studying stent apposition to the vessel wall after coronary stent deployment.

Intracardiac ultrasound

This imaging technology facilitates a closer scrutiny of the cardiac chambers by introducing an ultrasound probe into the right atrium via the inferior vena cava. The access is from a femoral vein. This modality is particularly useful in the device closure of intracardiac shunts and in performing septal puncture to access the left atrium from the right-sided circulation.

Electrophysiological study/RF ablation

These studies are done to identify and isolate aberrant conduction pathways in the heart that create rhythm disturbances. Catheters are introduced into the heart and placed in the areas of interest, which may include the cardiac chambers, bundle of His, coronary sinus (allows access to conduction pathways to the left ventricle) and pulmonary veins (to study atrial fibrillation). When the culprit pathways have been identified and isolated, they can be ablated with radiofrequency energy (RF ablation) and thus, on most occasions, cure the patient of the rhythm disorder.

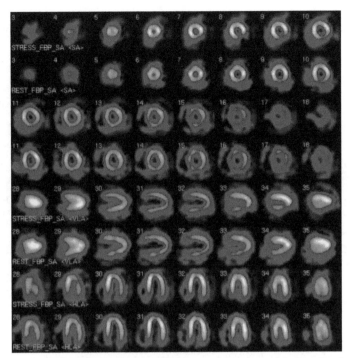

Figure 14.31 Technetium-sestamibi scan showing normal coronary perfusion at rest and impaired perfusion during stress. The top row of each view depicts perfusion during activity and the bottom row depicts perfusion at rest. In this scan the stress images show a defect in the left ventricular wall that normalises during rest (reprinted from Niederkohr R D, Daniels C, Raman S V 2008 Concordant findings on myocardial perfusion SPECT and cardiac magnetic resonance imaging in a patient with myocarditis. *Journal of Nuclear Cardiology* 15(3):466–8).

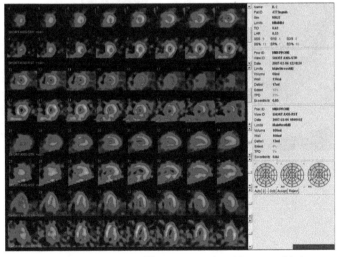

Figure 14.32 An abnormal sestamibi scan. The stress and rest tomographic images are labelled and the equivalent stress views are above the corresponding resting views. In this scan there is reversible ischaemia in the anterior wall. (Image courtesy of Dr P Sullivan)

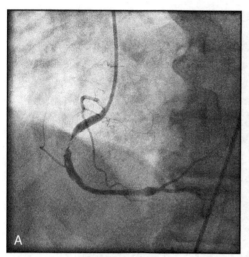 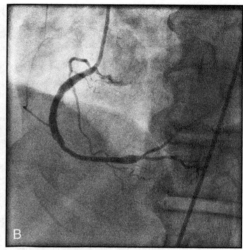

Figure 14.33 A 65-year-old man presented with exertional angina with a background history of hypertension and hypercholesterolaemia. His exercise stress test was positive for reversible coronary ischaemia. (A) Subsequent coronary angiography showed a significant stenosis of the right coronary artery. (B) This lesion was treated with angioplasty and stent placement.

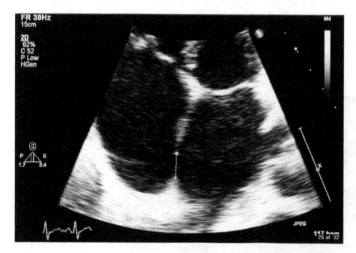

Figure 14.34 A 31-year-old woman presented with exertional dyspnoea. On examination she had fixed splitting of the second heart sound. On echocardiography there was a septum secundum type atrial septal defect (ASD). She was treated with percutaneous closure of the defect.

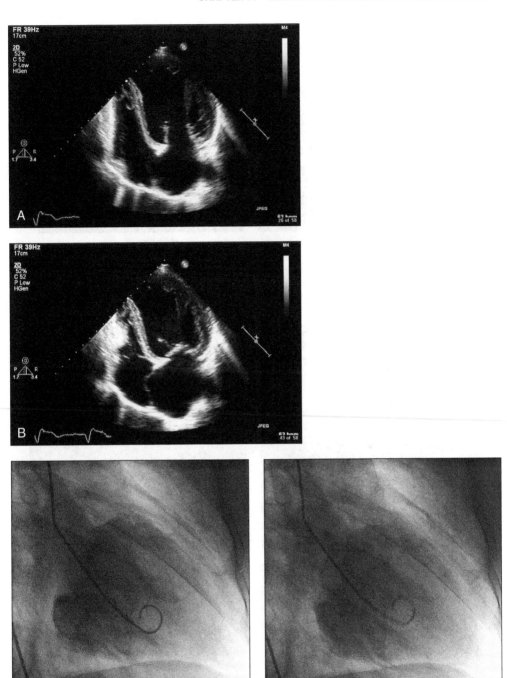

Figure 14.35 A 44-year-old man presented with progressive dyspnoea and peripheral oedema in the background of chronic alcoholism. On examination there was bilateral pitting oedema of the ankles and an elevated JVP. There was an audible S3 gallop in the precordium. There were bibasilar crepitations in the lung fields. Echocardiogram showed (A) left ventricular dilation and (B) impairment of systolic function. His coronary angiography was normal. (C and D) Left ventriculography showed severe impairment of systolic function.

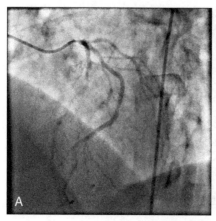
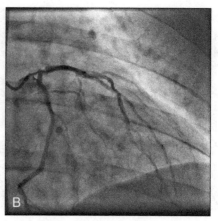

Figure 14.36 A 71-year-old man was brought in by ambulance after a cardiac arrest and successful resuscitation in the local shopping mall. Upon presentation the ECG showed deep T wave inversion in the septal and left lateral leads. Urgent coronary angiography showed significant narrowing at the osteum of the left main coronary artery (A and B). The patient was referred to the cardiac surgeon for urgent coronary artery bypass surgery, and in the meantime was anticoagulated with heparin.

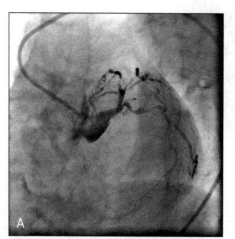
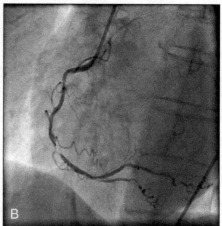

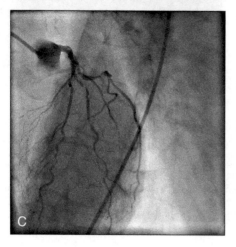

Figure 14.37 A 75-year-old woman with diabetes presented with 2 hours of retrosternal ache radiating down the right arm. She also complained of nausea. Her ECG showed ST segment depression of 2 mm in the inferior leads. She had cardiac biomarker positivity. Coronary angiography showed diffused, critical stenoses in all three coronary arteries (triple vessel disease). The patient was referred to the cardiac surgeon for coronary artery bypass surgery.

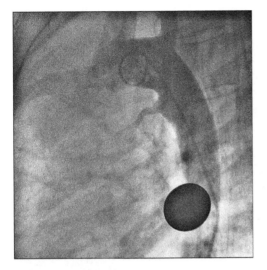

Figure 14.38 A 20-year-old woman was referred by the family practitioner upon the incidental finding of a machinery murmur heard all over the precordium. The murmur was loudest in the left subclavian region. Echocardiography showed a patent ductus arteriosus (PDA). This was confirmed by ascending aortography. Note the 10-cent coin placed over the patient's chest during aortography to help estimate the size of the PDA. This PDA was closed percutaneously with a ductal occluder.

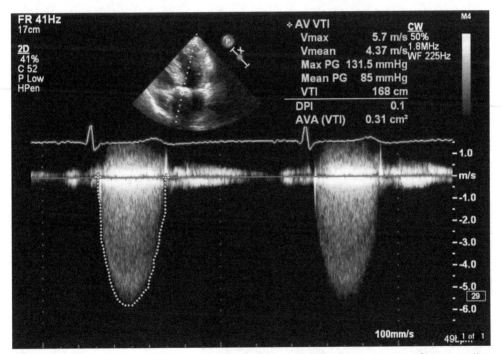

Figure 14.39 An 86-year-old woman presented with sudden loss of consciousness. On examination she had a slow rising pulse and a harsh ejection systolic murmur that radiated to her carotids bilaterally. Echocardiography demonstrated a calcified aortic valve with a critical gradient on Doppler assessment. Note the maximum and mean pressure gradients of significance. She was referred to the cardiac surgeon for valve replacement.

247

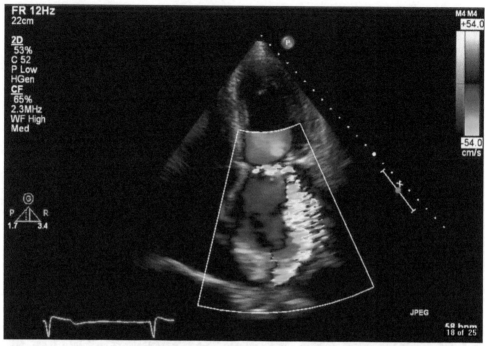

Figure 14.40 A 60-year-old man who presented with retrosternal chest pain was diagnosed with acute coronary syndrome. There were deep T wave inversions in the lateral lead in the ECG. He had significant troponin level elevation. He subsequently developed an apical systolic murmur that radiated to his left axilla. Echocardiography showed an eccentric jet of mitral regurgitation on colour flow Doppler assessment. Coronary angiography showed a tight stenosis of the large left circumflex coronary artery. This lesion was treated with angioplasty and stent placement. Subsequent echocardiography showed significant improvement of the mitral regurgitation. The valve defect was due to papillary muscle ischaemia associated with the circumflex artery stenosis.

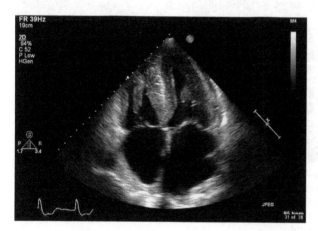

Figure 14.41 A 74-year-old man presented with dyspnoea, orthopnoea and paroxysmal nocturnal dyspnoea. On echocardiography there was severe hypertrophy of the left ventricle with impaired diastolic filling.

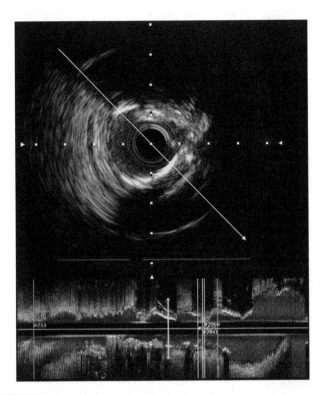

Figure 14.42 A 60-year-old smoker presented with angina on exertion. Coronary angiography showed stenosis of the left anterior descending (LAD) artery. This lesion was further characterised and measured with intravascular ultrasound (IVUS) imaging. The lesion was subsequently treated with a coronary stent.

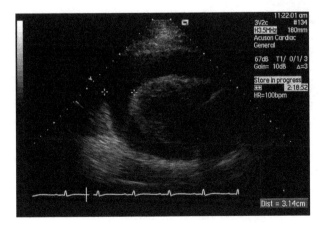

Figure 14.43 A 47-year-old woman with a past history of breast cancer presented with syncope. On examination she was hypotensive at 80/40 mmHg and her pulse rate was 120 bpm. Her JVP was elevated with evident Kussmaul's sign. There was pulsus paradoxus. Echocardiography revealed a significant pericardial effusion with evidence of cardiac tamponade. Note the large collection of fluid around the left ventricle.

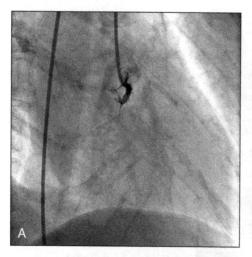

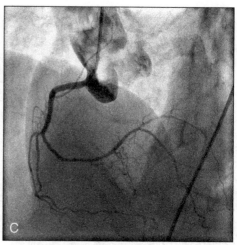

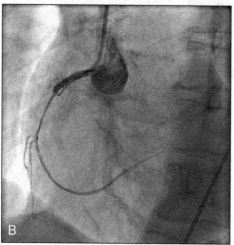

Figure 14.44 A 46-year-old heavy smoker presented with severe retrosternal chest tightness, nausea, vomiting and diaphoresis of 1 hour's duration. He was hypotensive on assessment. The 12-lead ECG showed ST segment elevation of 2 mm in leads II, III and AVF, confirming the diagnosis of ST elevation myocardial infarction (STEMI) (see figure D). The patient was referred to the interventional cardiology team for primary percutaneous intervention (primary PCI). Angiography revealed an occluded right coronary artery (RCA) which was reopened with balloon angioplasty and stenting.

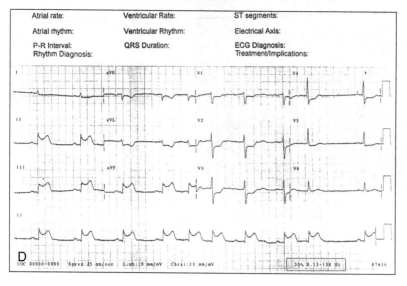

Atrial rate:	Ventricular Rate:	ST segments:
Atrial rhythm:	Ventricular Rhythm:	Electrical Axis:
P-R Interval:	QRS Duration:	ECG Diagnosis:
Rhythm Diagnosis:		Treatment/Implications:

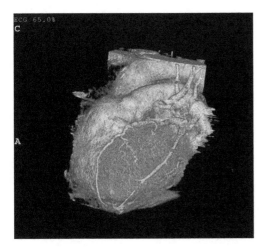

Figure 14.45 CT coronary angiogram

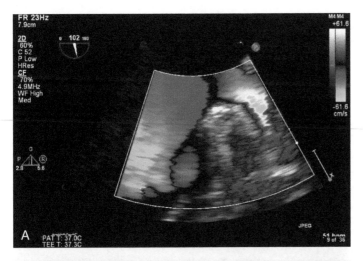

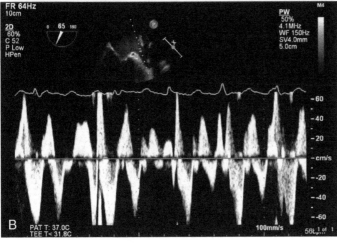

Figure 14.46 A 52-year-old man with new-onset atrial fibrillation underwent transoesophageal echocardiography (TOE) prior to direct current cardioversion. There was no thrombus seen within the left atrial appendage and the Doppler flow assessment ruled out stasis in the vicinity.

251

Part

03

Long case discussions

This part of the book contains eight sample cases for the purpose of introducing to the candidate the 'prototype long case'. Most cases discussed here have been encountered in the real examination by the author and colleagues. The Q&A sections give an overview of the types of questions and expected answers in the real examination situation. Some conditions not discussed in the previous section of the book are discussed in the following case discussions.

15

INTRODUCTION

RW is a 40-year-old man presenting with recurrent and resistant Hodgkin's disease, the course of which has been complicated by significant chemotherapy-associated side effects. He is also a single parent with financial difficulties.

CASE IN DETAIL

RW's problems started 11 years ago when he was incidentally diagnosed with Hodgkin's disease when admitted to hospital with a traumatic injury related to a motor vehicle accident. His Hodgkin's disease was treated with mantle radiotherapy alone on subsequent biopsy and staging. He denies any side effects associated with this treatment.

He was well until 7 months ago, when he presented to his general practitioner with retrosternal discomfort. He could recall experiencing drenching night sweats over the days preceding his presentation, but denied fevers or known weight loss. Chest X-ray performed subsequently showed mediastinal widening suggestive of mediastinal lymphadenopathy and he was referred to a haematologist, who diagnosed recurrent Hodgkin's disease. He has had multiple investigations, including lymph node biopsy, CT of thorax and abdomen, a gallium scan and bone marrow biopsy. He was immediately commenced on the ABVD (doxorubicin, bleomycin, vinblastine and dacarbazine) combination chemotherapeutic regimen. He showed good disease response, with disappearance of symptoms as well as lymphadenopathy on follow-up imaging. His treatment was prematurely terminated after three cycles (5 months ago) due to his developing bleomycin-associated pneumonitis. At this stage he denied any respiratory symptoms. The lung toxicity was discovered on routine screening with the carbon monoxide diffusion capacity test.

Four and a half months ago he was commenced on the MOPP (mechlorethamine, vincristine, procarbazine, prednisone) combination chemotherapy regimen. He suffered side effects of nausea, vomiting and alopecia associated with this treatment. He also experienced easy bruising and oral candidiasis associated with the steroid use, but denied any mood swings or insomnia. He has not been investigated for diabetes or osteoporosis. After three cycles of therapy, 2 months ago he was admitted to hospital with high fevers and was diagnosed with febrile neutropenia. During this admission he was also treated in the intensive care unit for 5 days. He could not recollect in detail the events surrounding this episode and the treatment he received. After 2 weeks in hospital he was discharged on prophylactic trimethoprim and sulfamethoxazole one tablet daily. He has been compliant with this treatment and denies any associated side effects.

He had his fourth cycle of chemotherapy without any complications. He is currently waiting for his fifth and final cycle of MOPP, the administration of which has not been planned as yet. He has had a PET scan 1 week ago and has been told by the haematologist that he still has some residual disease activity. He currently suffers from extreme lethargy, weakness and exertional dyspnoea on walking 100 metres on flat ground. He has lost a total of 10 kg over the past 7 months.

His medication summary includes trimethoprim/sulfamethoxazole and occasional paracetamol. He denies any known allergy to medications.

His father is alive at the age of 71 and suffers from ischaemic heart disease. His mother is 69 and suffers from severe rheumatoid arthritis. He has only one sister, who is well at the age of 36. He has no family history of malignancy.

He worked as a private security guard until 6 months ago. He is currently unemployed and survives on a single-parent benefit from the government. He finds it difficult to meet his and his family's needs with this income.

He has never smoked. He previously consumed 100 g of alcohol per day in the form of beer and did so for approximately 10 years. He has not consumed any alcohol during the past 7 months. Prior to his current diagnosis he denies experiencing any lymph node pain associated with alcohol consumption.

He separated from his wife 2 years ago. Before that he was married for 3 years. He has two children, a boy aged 5 and a girl aged 4, both of whom live with him. His mother looks after his children when he is in hospital. She finds it difficult to continue supporting him due to her debilitating arthritis.

He is independent with daily activities and drives too. He lives in a house for which he is paying off a mortgage.

He has never been depressed, even with the current diagnosis and the stormy course he has had. He is very positive about the future. His main problem, as he identifies it, is finding enough finances to support his family and to pay off the mortgage. His only social support is his ailing mother.

The dietary history suggests satisfactory nutrition. He has good insight into his disease and the chances of survival and cure as well as the toxicities associated with his treatment.

ON EXAMINATION

RW was alert and cooperative. He was alopecic and cushingoid. He had a portacath in the inner aspect of his left forearm and the site was not inflamed.

His pulse rate was 50 beats per minute and was regular in rhythm and normal in character. His blood pressure was 125/80 mmHg and there was no postural drop. His respiratory rate was 12 per minute at rest. He was afebrile. His estimated body mass index was 28 and his cognition was intact, with a Mini-Mental State score of 30/30.

He did not have any palpable lymphadenopathy. There was no mucositis or mucosal pallor. He had multiple ecchymoses, particularly in the dorsal aspects of his forearms and the thighs. He had a buffalo hump, but there was no bony tenderness or kyphoscoliosis.

His respiratory system examination showed reduced but symmetrical expansion of the upper and lower thorax. His lung fields were resonant throughout and the breath sounds were vesicular. There was fine early inspiratory crepitation in the lower zones bilaterally that did not clear with coughing.

In his cardiovascular system examination, the jugular venous pressure was not elevated. He had two heart sounds of normal intensity and no third heart sound or pericardial rub. There was no peripheral oedema.

His gastroenterological system examination was remarkable for oral thrush but his abdomen was soft, not distended and non-tender. There was no organomegaly or palpable mass.

Neurological examination showed normal visual acuity and normal fundoscopy bilaterally. The rest of the cranial nerve examination was unremarkable. His upper limb motor examination showed normal tone, power (surprisingly, even in the proximal musculature) and coordination. His reflexes were depressed at all levels symmetrically. Sensory function was intact.

Lower limb examination showed proximal weakness of 4/5 bilaterally with depressed reflexes at all levels. His coordination and sensation to all modalities were preserved. His plantar reflexes were flexor bilaterally and his gait was normal. However, he was unable to stand up from the squatting position without assistance.

His musculoskeletal examination was unremarkable.

He belongs to stage 1 of the ECOG (Eastern Cooperative Oncology Group) performance scale.

In summary, this is a 40-year-old man with recurrent Ann Arbor stage 4 Hodgkin's disease, with poor tolerance to first-line chemotherapy and inadequate response to second-line therapy, of which the course was complicated by a serious episode of febrile neutropenia. He also has significant social problems, including financial difficulties. Although his prognosis appears to be guarded, he is optimistic.

The main issue with this man is achieving disease remission and addressing the complications of chemotherapy.

To approach the management of this man I have identified three acute medical problems and one social problem. I have also identified two long-term medical problems and a social problem:

- **Acute medical problems**
  1 Decide on the best treatment protocol to achieve disease remission.
  2 Prevent further organ damage due to chemotherapy and identify and remedy, as much as possible, the damage done so far.
- **Acute social problem**
  – Find ways of helping this man meet his financial needs.
- **Long-term medical problems**
  1 Maintenance of disease remission once achieved, and surveillance for recurrence of lymphoma or secondary malignancies due to cytotoxic chemotherapy.
  2 Maximise his functional capacity.
- **Long-term social problem**
  – Address the issue of the care of his two young children if he succumbs to his illness or becomes incapacitated to any significant extent.

To decide on the best treatment protocol to achieve disease remission, I would like to look at the histology report of the lymph node biopsy he had during the initial work-up, and also the results of the staging investigations, including the bone marrow biopsy and the most recent gallium scan, to see where the residual disease activity is localised.

According to the history, I believe that this man has presented with Ann Arbor stage 4 disease. He has not tolerated first-line chemotherapy with the ABVD combination. He has incomplete response to the conventional MOPP combination.

The mainstay of his management now is to restage the disease and decide on salvage therapy. Salvage therapeutic options to be considered include alternative chemotherapy regimens such as the BEAM (carmustine, etoposide, cytarabine and melphalan) or BEACOP (bleomycin, etoposide, adriamycin, cyclophophamide, vincristine, predniso-lone) combinations or autologous or allogenic bone marrow transplantation. The main concern here is whether this man would be able to tolerate such aggressive therapy given his compromised organ function and physical status.

To restage his disease I would do the following investigations:

1 Full blood count
2 Liver function tests
3 Electrolyte profile and renal function indices
4 Erythrocyte sedimentation rate
5 Chest X-ray
6 CT of chest, abdomen and pelvis
7 Bone marrow biopsy.

I would also like to see the results of his recent PET scan.

To address the issue of organ damage, I would like to assess his current functional status by looking at the results of the following:

1 Gated heart pool scans, to ascertain the degree of cardiac damage secondary to anthracycline therapy
2 Formal lung function tests, looking for a restrictive pattern with impaired diffusion capacity.

If the degree of organ damage is significant, further therapy with agents having similar toxicity is absolutely contraindicated. This poses the challenge of looking for suitable chemotherapeutic agents for ongoing therapy. This is especially important if the option of myeloablative therapy with stem cell infusion is to be considered.

To prevent further cardiac damage it is important to identify and strictly control RW's coronary risk factor profile, given his previous mantle radiotherapy and the family history of coronary disease.

Focusing on the bleomycin lung, if the CT shows evidence of pneumonitis with a ground glass appearance of the lung parenchyma, high-dose corticosteroid therapy could be considered, to prevent further damage. But if it shows established fibrosis with the appearance of honeycombing, that will mean that irreversible damage has been done. He should be given pulmonary rehabilitation to optimise the function of the residual lung tissue.

It is important to assess the side effects he has suffered from corticosteroid therapy. I am interested in his fasting blood sugar levels and the bone densitometry results.

On achieving disease remission, long-term issues of management will become important. Regular clinical review with history and physical examination would suffice for the surveillance of recurrence. Due to his exposure to cytotoxic therapy, particularly with alkylating agents, he needs to be watched for the occurrence of acute myeloid leukaemia during the first 4 years. Non-Hodgkin's lymphoma becomes an issue after about 10 years and solid cancers after about 15 years.

The mantle radiation therapy he received more than 10 years ago has the potential to cause hypothyroidism, and this should be checked for.

To address the social problems I want to consult the hospital social worker first, to assess the degree of financial difficulty this man is currently facing. It is necessary to explore other possible sources of income, including income protection schemes and government welfare schemes.

Given his adverse prognostic outlook, the issue of possible death and dying as well as the care of his children in such an eventuality should be discussed with the patient, with the support of the social worker and a counsellor. Advance directives regarding his finances and assets, a living will and power of attorney, as well as a legal guardian for decisions regarding medical treatment in case of incapacity, should also be discussed.

Questions and answers

Q: How would you have managed this man when he presented with high fevers and a neutrophil count of 2×10^9/L one month ago?

A: This is a case of febrile neutropenia, and my management approach would be first to perform a comprehensive septic work-up. This would include a detailed history, a thorough physical examination aimed at finding a septic focus, and investigations in the form of three sets of both aerobic and anaerobic blood cultures taken from separate sites at different times (one set taken from the portacath), urine analysis followed by microscopy and culture, and a chest X-ray. I would commence this man on empirical antibiotic therapy pending the investigation results. The agents that I would use include two broad-spectrum agents that would cover Gram-positive organisms (most common causative organisms in the setting of neutropenia are Gram-positive) as well as Gram-negative organisms, including *Pseudomonas aeruginosa* (*Pseudomonas* causes most mortality). My choice would be ticarcillin with clavulanic acid or imipenem with cilastin together with an aminoglycoside (gentamicin 5 mg per kg daily with daily serum levels) given intravenously. If the patient does not defervesce within 24 hours of commencement of the above antibiotic regimen I would add vancomycin 1 g intravenously to cover for possible methicillin-resistant *Staphylococcus aureus*.

Q: What concerns would you have if he were to need intubation and ventilation?

A: Bleomycin lung is susceptible to oxygen toxicity, so I would be inclined to use the minimum amount of oxygen that would maintain arterial oxygen saturation above 95% for the minimum period necessary. In addition, it is important to guard against barotrauma to his diseased lungs from high inspiratory pressures.

Q: What other treatment options do you have for this man's malignancy?

A: Given the aggressive and resistant nature of his disease, he needs aggressive therapy to achieve complete remission. I would prefer autologous bone marrow transplantation following myeloablative chemotherapy.

Q: **What does he think about the possibility of dying and what plans does he have for the care of his children?**

A: This patient strongly believes that he will survive this illness. However, it is necessary to discuss this topic with the patient and cooperate with the social worker to formulate an action plan. This plan should initially include a conference with the participation of the patient, the social worker, his mother, who happens to be his main social support, and if possible his former wife.

Q: **Can you please describe this chest X-ray?**

A: The frontal view chest X-ray of RW taken on (insert date) shows diffuse non-confluent opacification of the lower zones of the pulmonary parenchyma bilaterally. This appearance is consistent with consolidation, acute pneumonitis, fibrosis or atelectasis. I would like to see the high-resolution CT of the chest for further clarification.

Q: **What do you think about this CT scan?**

A: There are changes seen in the lower zones, particularly in the lower lobes bilaterally extending from the peripheries. These are areas of honeycombing surrounding scattered islands of ground glass appearance. This picture is consistent with fibrosis of the lower lobes with areas of active pneumonitis scattered in between.

Q: **You said that he has lost weight. Do you think he is malnourished?**

A: Despite significant weight loss, this man still weighs 90 kg. He did not have clinical findings consistent with malnourishment and nutrient deficiency in the form of angular stomatitis, cheilosis, and atrophic glossitis or diffuse dermatitis. Although I did not measure his mid-arm circumference, I judged him to have satisfactory muscle bulk and power in that region. So this man is not malnourished currently.

Q: **Did he have any B symptoms when he initially presented 11 years ago?**

A: No, the diagnosis of Hodgkin's disease was incidental on that occasion.

Q: **What issues would you discuss with a young patient who was offered cytotoxic chemotherapy?**

A: Cytotoxic chemotherapy can lead to gonadal damage and infertility, particularly in the male patient. Therefore I would counsel the patient regarding this and offer sperm banking or ova banking if future reproduction was anticipated. I would also seek professional psychological counselling, if needed, for the patient and their partner.

16

Long case 2

Themes: thrombocytopenia,
acute myocardial infarction

INTRODUCTION

KG is a 64-year-old man awaiting splenectomy for symptomatic thrombocytopenia. His case is complicated by a recent myocardial infarction as well as the difficulties associated with being far from his home.

CASE IN DETAIL

KG presented to a rural base hospital 2 months ago with severe recurrent epistaxis associated with easy bruising of 3 weeks' duration. He denied any other mucosal bleeding or symptoms of anaemia. On investigation, he was diagnosed with idiopathic thrombocytopenic purpura (ITP) and initially treated with high-dose oral cortico-steroids for 2 weeks. Despite treatment, his platelet count failed to recover and his symptoms persisted. He denied any steroid-associated side effects such as weight gain, insomnia, mood swings or oral candidiasis during this period. He had further inves-tigations, including a bone marrow biopsy, and the diagnosis was not altered. He was then transferred to a hospital in the city for further treatment with intravenous normal immunoglobulin and plasmapheresis. The response to this treatment was suboptimal. At this point it was decided to carry out therapeutic splenectomy, which he is currently awaiting. Meanwhile he is managed on prednisolone 35 mg daily. He still experiences occasional epistaxis and skin bruising, but it is less severe than at presentation.

He had an acute myocardial infarction 3 months ago, from which he has made an uneventful recovery. Follow-up coronary angiography revealed the existence of double-vessel coronary disease and he is managed on medical anti-ischaemia therapy. He denies any ongoing angina or dyspnoea. He is currently on atenolol 50 mg daily, enalapril 10 mg mane and topical nitrate 25 mg 8 am to 8 pm daily. He denies any side effects associated with this therapy. He has the following risk factors for ischaemic heart disease: male sex, a past smoking history of 40 pack-years (he gave up smoking 4 weeks ago) and hypertension.

He was diagnosed with hypertension 9 years ago and has been managed on differ-ent medications. He is currently on amlodipine 5 mg twice daily and denies having any side effects associated with this medication. His general practitioner monitors his blood pressure, but not regularly. He has been told that his blood pressure is well controlled.

He denies any risk-prone behaviour for HIV infection.

His current medications in summary are atenolol, enalapril, nitrate patch, amlodipine and prednisolone. He is not on any therapeutic agent that is known to cause thrombocytopenia. He has no known allergies.

KG's family history is unremarkable for any significant medical condition. His father died at the age of 87 and mother at the age of 84, and he is not aware of the causes of their deaths. His brother, aged 57, is well.

He worked as a clerk and is currently retired on an age pension, which is barely adequate to meet his and his wife's needs.

KG is from a rural town more than 1000 km from the city, where he lives with his wife, aged 60. His wife is well. They have been married for 40 years and have two daughters, aged 37 and 40, both well, married, and living separately but still in the same town.

He is independent with his activities of daily living. He sees his GP only rarely. He lives in a house with two steps at the entrance and has no difficulty negotiating these.

The dietary history reveals satisfactory nutrition and he denies any problems with sleep. He consumes alcohol only on social occasions (less than 40 g per week).

While in hospital in the city for the past 2 weeks, only his wife has been visiting him. His wife stays at the accommodation facility provided by the hospital.

He has satisfactory insight into his condition.

ON EXAMINATION

KG is a moderately obese man. He was alert and cooperative. He was receiving normal saline through an intravenous cannula in his right forearm, the entry site of which appeared inflamed with surrounding erythema, warmth and tenderness.

His respiratory rate was 12 at rest, pulse rate 90 per minute. His blood pressure was 130/85 mmHg and he was afebrile. His estimated body mass index was 30 kg/m^3.

He had diffuse non-palpable purpura over the dorsal and ventral aspects of his lower limbs distally and proximally, bilaterally. There were several ecchymoses in the dorsal aspect of his thorax. There was no evidence of mucosal bleeding or conjunctival pallor. His per rectum examination showed no evidence of gastrointestinal bleeding. There was no lymphadenopathy or splenomegaly.

In the cardiovascular examination, the jugular venous pressure was not elevated. His apex beat was palpable in the fifth intercostal space in the mid-clavicular line. The heart sounds were dual and normal. All his peripheral pulses were clearly palpable.

The examination of the respiratory and neurological systems were unremarkable. Surprisingly, there was no proximal muscle weakness.

His abdomen was soft and non-tender and there were no organomegaly or masses. There was moderate abdominal obesity but no purple striae.

Musculoskeletal examination was unremarkable and there was no bony tenderness, including in the vertebral column.

In summary, my impression is of a 64-year-old man presenting with symptomatic idiopathic thrombocytopenic purpura resistant to steroid therapy and necessitating splenectomy. He also has a history of hypertension and his situation is complicated by a recent myocardial infarction.

The two main issues with this man are the risk of haemorrhage and the risk of sustaining a myocardial insult perioperatively during splenectomy.

In approaching the management of this man, I have identified an incidental urgent medical problem, two semi-urgent medical problems and one social problem.

- **Urgent medical problem**
  - He has an infection of the intravenous cannula site. I would immediately remove this cannula and send the tip for microscopy and culture. I would also like to see his temperature chart for the past 24 hours to see whether he has had any spikes of fever. Currently, even though he does not look septic, he has localised cellulitis and therefore I would treat him with oral flucloxacillin 500 mg twice a day for 1 week. He is immunosuppressed on systemic corticosteroids, and therefore runs the risk of serious infection.
- **Semi-urgent medical problems**
  1. Assessment of his cardiovascular tolerability to general anaesthesia and surgery and optimisation of the risks involved.
  2. Achieving sustained remission of his idiopathic thrombocytopenic purpura.
- **Social problem**
  - Addressing the issues of social isolation and support for his wife.

In approaching the management of these problems, first I would like to see his full blood count, to estimate the severity of the thrombocytopenia and to exclude any haematological malignancy. I would also like to see the results of the serology test for antiplatelet antibodies, and the recent bone marrow biopsy.

In addition, I would like to see the results of an autoimmune screen (antinuclear antibody and antibody to extractable nuclear antigen), rheumatoid factor level, thyroid function tests and antibody titres to common viral antigens.

Although he denies any risk-prone behaviour, given the resistant nature of his thrombocytopenia I would also consider testing him for HIV infection.

Questions and answers

Q: His platelet count is 20×10^9/L. Do you agree with the proposed therapeutic plan?

A: Despite treatment with high-dose systemic steroids, intravenous normal immunoglobulin and plasmaphaeresis, his platelet count still stands at 20. He also suffers from spontaneous bleeding. To prevent significant haemorrhage and spare him the adverse effects of steroid therapy, I believe that, although risky, splenectomy is highly indicated.

Q: Why do you ask for the antiplatelet antibody test, the autoimmune screen and the thyroid function test results?

A: The antiplatelet antibody test is not essential for the diagnosis of idiopathic thrombocytopenic purpura and only 60–70% of patients with the disease would actually test positive. But the presence of a positive result would help confirm the diagnosis, particularly in the setting of poor primary response to corticosteroids. Idiopathic thrombocytopenic purpura is essentially a diagnosis of exclusion.

Autoimmune thrombocytopenia can be associated with other autoimmune disorders, such as systemic lupus erythematosus and autoimmune thyroid disease. Another possible cause is a recent subclinical viral infection, which could have triggered the thrombocytopenia.

Q: Please interpret this bone marrow biopsy result.

A: There is megakaryocytosis, which is consistent with the current diagnosis of idiopathic thrombocytopenic purpura. The rest of the picture is normal and therefore the possibilities of bone marrow infiltration by a malignant process as well as marrow aplasia are excluded. This bone marrow picture can also suggest hypersplenism, but I did not find clinical splenomegaly and this man has no known history of chronic liver disease as a cause of splenomegaly.

Q: How would you manage this patient?

A: The initial management issue involves the diagnosis and, if possible, the control of the thrombocytopenia. Given the diagnosis of idiopathic thrombocytopenic purpura, I would initially try high-dose oral corticosteroids in the form of prednisolone 60 mg daily with daily platelet counts. The majority will respond initially, but only 20% of patients have a sustained response. If the response was poor with steroid treatment alone, as is the case with KG, I would arrange for splenectomy. Splenectomy will improve the chances of sustained remission to 60%. If the thrombocytopenia persists in spite of splenectomy, I would consider treatment with danazol or immunosuppression with azathioprine.

Q: How would you prepare this patient for splenectomy?

A: There are three main issues that concern me regarding this man undergoing splenectomy. First, his cardiovascular fitness to undergo general anaesthesia and a major surgical procedure, given his history of a recent myocardial infarction. He runs a significant risk of reinfarction and possible death, so I would further evaluate his risks in that regard and weigh them against the expected benefits. Second, his current platelet count, as he is significantly thrombocytopenic (20×10^9/L). I would consider intravenous normal immunoglobulin infusion with or without platelet transfusion immediately before surgery, for a rapid elevation of the platelet count. The third issue of concern is the infection risk associated with splenectomy.

Q: How would you address the septic risks associated with splenectomy?

A: Post splenectomy, this man is at risk of suffering from fulminant sepsis due to encapsulated organisms such as *Meningococcus, Streptococcus pneumoniae* and *Haemophilus influenzae,* so he needs to be vaccinated against these organisms. He should be administered pneumococcal vaccine 3 weeks prior to the operation and the vaccine should be repeated at 5-yearly intervals. He should also receive *H. influenzae* type B vaccine if he has not been immunised before. Meningococcal vaccination would be necessary only if he was travelling to an area where *Meningococcus* type A was endemic. Unfortunately, there is no vaccination available against type B, which is the prevalent form in the Western world.

Q: Would you advise the surgeons to operate on this man, and if so, when?

A: This man has an angiographic diagnosis of double-vessel disease and has been recommended medical therapy. But the more important risk is his recent acute myocardial infarction, which predisposes him to perioperative myocardial insult. During the first 3 months after an acute myocardial infarction, the risk of perioperative infarction is at its highest, at about 6%. This risk dwindles to 2.5% after 4 months. So before deciding on surgery for splenectomy it is important to weigh the benefits against the risks.

With the current level of thrombocytopenia he runs the significant risk of a major spontaneous bleed, with significant morbidity and possibly mortality. So it is important to attempt disease control with splenectomy.

As he had his infarction only 3 months ago, I would endeavour to postpone the operation by at least another month while closely monitoring his platelet count with maximum medical therapy. If the platelet count did not improve, I would go ahead with the splenectomy.

Q: **How would you manage the cardiac risk that this man has in association with an operation?**

A: This man's perioperative risk of a myocardial insult can be regarded as substantial but not extremely high, due to his stable functional capacity and the good symptom control afforded by his anti-ischaemia therapy.

I would formally evaluate his functional capacity by performing an exercise stress test, and if his functional capacity was more than 5 METs I would recommend surgery with less reservation. Perioperatively I would closely supervise his cardiac and haemodynamic function with systemic and pulmonary arterial monitoring. I would monitor his cardiac function intraoperatively and postoperatively with continuous electrocardiography. I would perform 6-hourly troponin I levels intraoperatively and postoperatively during the first 24 hours. It has been observed that most perioperative acute myocardial infarctions occur during the first few days postoperatively.

The fact that he is on a beta-blocker may offer further protection against a perioperative cardiac insult. I would ensure strict control of his blood pressure and heart rate during this period.

Q: **How would you plan to manage his social problems?**

A: He and his wife need better social support while in the city. I would get together with the social worker to formulate a plan to provide the necessary support. First I would look into the possibility of organising for the rest of his family from home to visit him. I would then see whether they had any relatives or friends in the city who might provide help and support. In addition, I would look into the services run by government and voluntary organisations (e.g. church groups, social service organisations) that might be of some help.

Q: **KG has a blood sugar level (BSL) of 11.1 mmol/L. What do you think of this blood test report?**

A: This result suggests hyperglycaemia consistent with a diagnosis of diabetes. I would repeat the test for confirmation and also check his glycosylated haemoglobin level, looking for an elevation. The most likely cause for this picture is his prednisolone therapy. But incidental diagnosis of latent chronic diabetes mellitus cannot be excluded.

It is important to control his blood sugar level well, given his existing coronary artery disease. First I would put him on a strict diabetic diet and monitor his blood sugar level. If the level remained significantly high, I would treat him with insulin until he had his splenectomy and the prednisolone was stopped. I would also check his fasting lipid profile, looking for hypercholesterolaemia, and perform a urinalysis, looking for proteinuria or microalbuminuria. I would commence him on a statin agent regardless of his cholesterol level, given that he has established coronary artery disease.

17

Long case 3

INTRODUCTION

DB is a 72-year-old obese woman with exertional angina and persistent dyspnoea presenting for coronary angioplasty and stenting on a background of triple-vessel coronary artery disease, a recent acute myocardial infarction, persistent diarrhoea, diabetes mellitus, hypertension, asthma, emphysema, osteoporosis, carcinoid tumour of the lung and depression.

CASE IN DETAIL

DB was diagnosed with acute myocardial infarction when she presented at hospital 3 months ago with a 2-day history of epigastric discomfort, nausea and general malaise. Her admission was further complicated by an episode of diabetic hyperosmolar coma, which was managed with hydration and parenteral insulin. She was discharged from hospital 9 weeks ago after a hospital stay of 3 weeks. Post discharge she experienced angina on exertion. She could walk 50 metres on flat ground before experiencing retrosternal chest discomfort. Subsequent coronary angiography revealed triple-vessel disease.

She was scheduled for revascularisation therapy through angioplasty and stenting 1 week ago. The treatment had to be postponed due to severe dyspnoea on second presentation. The dyspnoea was present at rest, with associated orthopnoea and episodes of paroxysmal nocturnal dyspnoea. These symptoms have been present in varying degrees of severity over the past 3 months. Currently her ischaemic heart disease is managed with isosorbide mononitrate 60 mg daily, quinapril 5 mg daily and aspirin 150 mg daily. She has a significant risk factor profile for coronary artery disease, which includes:

1 a family history of ischaemic heart disease, with her mother dying of an acute myocardial infarction at the age of 67 and father dying of the same at the age of 65
2 a smoking history of 50 pack-years. She stopped smoking 10 years ago.
3 hypercholesterolaemia managed with pravastatin 10 mg daily. The patient does not know her previous or current cholesterol levels.
4 hypertension diagnosed 1 year ago and managed with diltiazem 240 mg daily. She denies any side effects associated with this medication. The local pharmacist

monitors her blood pressure at monthly intervals. She cannot remember the most recent blood pressure reading.

5 diabetes mellitus, which was diagnosed 4 years ago. Initially she was managed on a diet and the oral hypoglycaemic agent metformin. But metformin was very soon stopped due to its adverse effects, including nausea, diarrhoea and rash. Subsequently she was commenced on gliclazide. Three months ago this was stopped due to erratic blood sugar control, and she was commenced on insulin therapy. She is currently maintained on the following insulin regimen:
   - 10 units of short-acting insulin before breakfast, 10 units before lunch and 6 units before dinner
   - 14 units of mixed short- and long-acting insulin 20/80 administered before dinner.

She monitors her blood sugar levels four times a day. She does not comply with the diabetic diet.

Usually her blood sugar levels fall between 8 and 10 mmol/L. She denies ever experiencing hypoglycaemic episodes and is unaware of the usual warning signs of hypoglycaemia.

She suffers from the multiple end-organ complications associated with diabetes:

1 Ocular complications—an ophthalmologist reviews her eyes every year. She has bilateral cataracts and is awaiting excision. She is unaware of any other ocular complication and denies any visual impairment.

2 Renal complications—she has her urine tested by her general practitioner every month and is currently unaware of any nephropathy. But she complains of recurrent polydipsia, polyuria and nocturia, symptoms that may suggest renal failure.

3 Macrovascular complications—she has peripheral vascular disease and has a claudication distance of 10 metres. She has never had a stroke.

4 She complains of postural dizziness, a symptom that may suggest autonomic neuropathy.

DB denies any paraesthesias or loss of peripheral sensation. She also denies any foot complications such as callosities, corns or ulcers.

She also suffers from asthma, which was diagnosed many years ago, and emphysema, diagnosed 8 years ago.

Her airway symptoms are worst in the winter. Perfumes and pollen are known precipitants of her asthma attacks. She denies nocturnal cough. She has never been admitted to hospital with exacerbation of airway disease. She monitors her peak flow weekly and it varies around 150–200 L/min. Her airway disease is currently managed with nebulised salbutamol and ipratropium bromide four times a day and salmeterol via a metered dose inhaler twice a day. She has been managed on variable doses of prednisolone previously, but she cannot recall the maximum or minimum doses that she has been on.

Prednisolone causes easy bruising but she denies any other side effects associated with this therapy, including pathological fractures and weight gain. She cannot remember whether she has had her bone density assessed.

She was diagnosed with carcinoid tumour of the left lung 8 years ago when she presented with resistant wheezing, dyspnoea and cyanotic spells. She denies any facial flushing or diarrhoea during that presentation. The diagnosis was made after imaging studies followed by bronchoscopy and biopsy. She is managed with regular endobronchial laser therapy at 2-yearly intervals and her last treatment episode was 1 year ago.

She has had persistent diarrhoea for 3 months. On average she has 6–10 bowel movements a day. The diarrhoea is watery in nature and she denies any associated blood loss. She denies any abdominal pain, nausea, vomiting or anorexia. She has previously tried several antidiarrhoeal agents without much success.

She also suffers from painful muscle cramps occasionally, which are treated with quinine bisulfate as required.

Her current medications in summary are diltiazem, isosorbide mononitrate, pravastatin, insulin, salbutamol, ipratropium bromide, salmeterol and quinine bisulfate.

This woman's allergies include metformin and penicillin, both of which cause rash.

Her family history also includes one brother aged 81 suffering from Alzheimer's disease and one sister aged 69 suffering from rheumatoid arthritis and breast cancer.

She has previously worked as a chef and is currently on a pension. She finds this income barely enough to meet her needs.

She consumes alcohol only very occasionally.

She has been married for 51 years and her husband, aged 74, is well and supportive. She is usually independent with activities of self-care, but has been experiencing difficulties lately due to the dyspnoea. She lives in a house where there are no steps to negotiate. She has been driving until about 3 weeks ago.

She has a son aged 47 and a daughter aged 44 years; both are well, married and living apart from their parents, and she has four grandchildren. She has regular contact with them.

The dietary history I obtained suggests satisfactory nutrition but with inappropriately high joule and lipid intake.

She has poor sleep hygiene, with initial and terminal insomnia. She has about 5 hours of sleep each day but denies daytime somnolence.

She has had the occasional feeling of depression but has never sought medical help and denies any current depressive feelings.

At home she spends most of her spare time knitting.

I felt that she had very poor insight into the multiple disease conditions that she suffers from.

ON EXAMINATION

DB was alert and cooperative. She had an estimated body mass index of 30. Her cognitive function was well preserved, with a Mini-Mental State score of 29/30. She was breathing oxygen via nasal prongs at a rate of 2 L per minute.

Her blood pressure was 148/68 mmHg and there were postural drops of 20 mmHg systolic and 20 mmHg diastolic. Her respiratory rate was 20 at rest. She was afebrile.

Examination of the cardiovascular system showed a jugular venous pressure elevation to a level 5 cm above the angle of Louis. Her apex beat was not palpable. There were two heart sounds and both were normal with no added sounds. There was bilateral pitting ankle oedema to the level of the knee.

In the examination of her respiratory system I noticed a moist cough, but no sputum was available for inspection. She was using accessory muscles of respiration. She had oropharyngeal crowding. The percussion note was resonant throughout and the breath sounds were vesicular, with polymorphic wheezes audible in the lower zones bilaterally. In addition there were coarse inspiratory crepitations in the lung bases bilaterally. The forced expiratory timing was prolonged to 7 seconds.

Gastrointestinal examination showed no oral candidiasis. Her abdomen was obese and soft, and there was no organomegaly or masses. Bowel sounds were well audible.

Neurological examination showed a visual acuity of 6/9 in the right side and 6/24 in the left with correction. Fundoscopy showed multiple flame-shaped bleeds with cottonwool spots and increased tortuosity of the retinal vasculature. The rest of the cranial nerve examination was unremarkable.

Upper limb examination showed normal tone, power, reflexes and coordination bilaterally. There was diminished pinprick sensation in the periphery up to the level of the wrist. Other sensory modalities were normal.

Lower limb examination showed normal motor function and coordination, with impaired pinprick sensation up to the level of the knees bilaterally. Other sensory modalities were preserved. The plantar response was flexor bilaterally and Romberg's test was negative.

Musculoskeletal examination was unremarkable and there were no areas of bony tenderness.

There was no lymphadenopathy. The diabetic foot examination was unremarkable except for the abovementioned sensory impairment.

In summary, this is a 72-year-old obese woman with triple-vessel coronary artery disease, multiple coronary risk factors and a recent myocardial infarction, presenting for angioplasty and stenting of the coronary stenoses. This admission has been complicated by recalcitrant dyspnoea. She also suffers from persisting diarrhoea, diabetes mellitus with end-organ damage, hypertension, hyperlipidaemia, carcinoid tumour of the lung, asthma, emphysema and occasional depression.

Currently her major problems are dyspnoea and coronary ischaemia.

In approaching her management I have identified four problems that need initial attention:

1 Diagnosis and management of the dyspnoea
2 Coronary revascularisation and optimising of the control of her coronary risk factor profile
3 Review of the management of her diabetes
4 Restoration of mobility, control of the diarrhoea and improvement of her overall quality of life.

I believe this woman's dyspnoea to be multifactorial. The possible differential diagnoses include pulmonary oedema, pulmonary sepsis, infective exacerbation of her airway disease, poorly controlled asthma, carcinoid syndrome and pulmonary embolus. To exclude the above causes I would like to see the results of the following investigations:

1 Chest X-ray, looking for pulmonary congestion, consolidation, hyperinflation and/or cardiomegaly
2 Arterial blood gases, looking for hypoxia and carbon dioxide retention
3 Full blood count, to exclude anaemia or leucocytosis
4 Lung function studies in the form of a flow–volume loop or spirometry, to ascertain the presence of obstructive or restrictive lung pathology
5 Echocardiogram, looking for evidence of ventricular hypokinesis or left ventricular hypertrophy as well as right-sided valvular lesions secondary to the carcinoid tumour

6 If the above investigations are not diagnostic, a ventilation-perfusion scan is indicated, to look for areas of mismatch.

To treat her symptoms I would first optimise her airway therapy and stabilise her airway function. I would administer a short course of systemic steroid therapy, starting with 25 mg prednisolone daily to achieve early control of her airway inflammation. I would also commence regular inhaled steroids in the form of fluticasone via an Accuhaler device at a dose of 500 mg twice daily. I would stop the long-acting bronchodilator and manage her with regular nebulised salbutamol and ipratropium bromide administered 4–6 times a day. I would monitor her serial spirometry results while in hospital and stop the systemic steroid therapy as soon as possible once airway stability was achieved, because of her diabetes and obesity. While she was on systemic steroids I would closely monitor her blood sugar level four times a day and step up her diabetic therapy according to need.

I would also optimise her left ventricular function and relieve pulmonary congestion with regular diuretic therapy in the form of frusemide and ACE inhibitor therapy, the diuretic dose to be titrated according to the response. I would monitor her potassium level closely. I would continue her ACE inhibitor therapy and consider increasing the dose of quinapril to 10 mg daily while closely observing the renal function indices.

If there was evidence to suggest infection, I would commence antibiotic therapy as guided by the chest X-ray and sputum microscopy and culture.

Questions and answers

Q: **Would you please interpret this chest X-ray?**

A: This is a frontal projection, posteroanterior view chest X-ray of DB done on (insert date). It shows diaphragmatic flattening suggesting pulmonary hyperinflation, which is characteristic of emphysema. It also shows increased translucency in the peripheral lung fields, further confirming emphysema. She has an increased cardiothoracic ratio, estimated at about 60–70%, together with prominent hilar shadows suggesting congested main pulmonary vessels and a diffuse, patchy infiltrate, all features suggesting pulmonary congestion secondary to left heart failure.

I would like to look at her lateral-view chest X-ray, results of a recent echocardiogram and results of the lung function tests to confirm my findings.

Q: **She has been treated with high-dose frusemide therapy, 120 mg mane and 80 mg nocte, but she is still symptomatic. What would you do now?**

A: She remains in symptomatic cardiac failure despite being managed with high-dose diuretic and ACE inhibitor therapy. To augment the diuretic treatment, I would add a thiazide diuretic to her regimen, commencing while she is still in hospital, and place her on a fluid restriction of 1 L/day and a low-salt diet. I would follow her up with observation for clinical improvement of her symptoms and signs, monitoring the urine output and daily weighing.

I would expedite coronary revascularisation once her clinical status was stable, because with the restored blood flow the hypoperfused 'hibernating' myocardium could be brought in to augment the ventricular contraction.

If her clinical status deteriorates, she might benefit from a short course of intravenous inotropic therapy, given via a centrally placed venous catheter. The agent I would use is dobutamine.

Q: Would you please interpret these lung function test results?

A: This lung function test report shows severe obstructive airway disease with impaired gas exchange. This confirms the clinical and radiological findings of emphysema. I would like to test further for reversibility of airway obstruction with a bronchodilator challenge, and perform arterial blood gases, looking for hypoxia and carbon dioxide retention.

Q: What do you think about the choice of angioplasty for coronary revascularisation in this woman?

A: This woman has triple-vessel coronary artery stenosis, cardiac failure and diabetes mellitus. I would like to see the angiogram to ascertain the severity of the coronary disease and to see whether there is significant disease in the left main coronary artery. Her prognosis is guarded by the fact that she has cardiac failure as well as diabetes mellitus. The best modality of coronary revascularisation for this patient is coronary artery bypass grafting. But given her severe airway disease, obesity, diabetes and poor functional status, it is doubtful whether she would survive general anaesthesia and major surgery. Therefore I would attempt to treat her with coronary angioplasty. But diabetic patients usually have low rates of maintenance of coronary patency after angioplasty. Stenting the treated stenosis will help maintain its patency for a longer period of time. Best medical therapy (see box) is another option I would consider in this case. However, adding further agents to her list of medications may lead to polypharmacy and associated issues with poor compliance.

Antiangina medical therapy
- Beta-blockers
- ACE inhibitors
- Calcium channel blockers
- Nitrates (topical or oral)

For resistant cases, consider adding the following:
- Nicorandil
- Perhexiline
- Ivabradine (those not tolerant to beta-blockers)

Q: How would you optimise her coronary risk factor profile?

A: First I would like to reassess her coronary risk factor profile. She was marginally hypertensive at the time of my examination. But she is already on considerably high doses of antihypertensive agents. I would continue to monitor her blood pressure while she was in hospital before altering her antihypertension therapy. To evaluate her usual blood sugar control, I would like to see her glycosylated haemoglobin level done during this admission. Guided by this measure and the recent blood sugar levels, I would optimise her insulin regimen to strictly control her blood sugar level. I would like to know her fasting serum lipid profile to see whether she would need review of her anticholesterol therapy.

Significant weight reduction would certainly improve this woman's overall prognosis, but it would be a serious challenge!

Q: Her latest serum total cholesterol level is 6.1 mmol/L and triglyceride level 2 mmol/L. Would you change her therapy?

A: Because of her existing ischaemic heart disease I would like to have her total cholesterol level maintained below 4.5 mmol/L. I would provide her with further advice on lipid-lowering dietary habits, encourage her to engage in low-impact physical exercise and also increase the dose of pravastatin to 20 mg/day.

Q: How would you manage her diarrhoea?

A: Initially I would like to ascertain the exact cause of this woman's diarrhoea. The differential diagnoses I would consider are as follows:

1   Infectious causes such as *Campylobacter, Salmonella, E. coli* or parasitic agents such as *Giardia*
2   Medication-induced diarrhoea (excessive diuretics)
3   Osmotic diarrhoea due to lactose/disaccharide intolerance. I would fast her for 12 hours to see whether the diarrhoea settled, as is the case with osmotic diarrhoea.
4   Endocrine or metabolic causes, such as diabetic autonomic neuropathy, hyperthyroidism and carcinoid syndrome
5   Inflammatory causes, such as ulcerative colitis or collagenous colitis
6   Malabsorption syndrome or chronic bacterial overgrowth
7   Villous adenoma.

If all the above were excluded, it could be considered irritable bowel syndrome. To evaluate the exact cause I would like to see the results of the following investigations:

1   Microscopy and culture of stool, looking for leucocytes, pathogenic bacteria, parasites, ova and cysts
2   Stool test for *Clostridium difficile* toxin
3   Stool electrolytes and pH and osmolality. An acidic pH may suggest carbohydrate malabsorption and an osmotic gap of > 50 mOsm/L might confirm this finding.
4   If the above tests were unrevealing I would like to perform faecal fat quantification, looking for evidence of malabsorption
5   Colonoscopy and biopsy to exclude malignancies, inflammatory bowel disease and microscopic colitis. This should be done after her having had coronary revascularisation.

6   I would further like to ascertain the level of activity of this patient's carcinoid syndrome by performing a 24-hour urinary quantification of 5-hydroxyindole acetic acid (5-HIAA) and look for any hyperthyroidism by performing thyroid function tests.

Q: **All the above tests were non-diagnostic. What would you do?**

A: Diabetic autonomic neuropathy or irritable bowel syndrome are the likely diagnoses in this case, and I would start treating her with a trial of antidiarrhoeal therapy in the form of loperamide chloride or diphenoxylate.

Q: **How would you manage her steroid-related complications?**

A: This woman has diabetes mellitus, of which the control is complicated by steroid therapy. I would endeavour to minimise the duration of systemic steroid therapy. I would also perform bone densitometry, looking for evidence of osteoporosis. I would vaccinate this woman against the influenza virus every year and against *Pneumococcus* every 5 years.

Q: **Please interpret this bone densitometry report.**

A: It shows a Z score of −2.7 and a T score of −2. This is highly suggestive of osteoporosis. I would treat this woman with calcium supplements in the form of calcium carbonate or caltrate, vitamin D supplements in the form of calcitriol, and bisphosphonate therapy in the form of daily oral etidronate or monthly intravenous pamidronate. I would warn the patient about the erosive oesophagitis that etidronate can cause and advise her to take the medication before breakfast every day and not to lie supine for at least half an hour after ingestion of the drug.

Q: **Do you think her carcinoid syndrome is well managed?**

A: Her 5-HIAA level is normal, and therefore it is likely that she currently has no carcinoid syndrome.

Q: **If this woman were to develop symptomatic carcinoid syndrome, how would you manage it?**

A: Carcinoid syndrome usually presents with facial flushing, dyspnoea, wheezing, weight loss and persistent diarrhoea. I would check her serum serotonin level and also do a hepatic ultrasound scan, looking for hepatic metastases, to determine the level of disease activity. Symptomatic management is achieved with the use of antiserotonin agents such as cyproheptadine. If the symptoms were severe, I would use octreotide to treat her. Definitive therapy involves removal of the tumour bulk. As this woman has been satisfactorily managed with laser therapy in the past, I would use further laser therapy to reduce the bulk of the tumour.

Q: **How are you going to improve this woman's quality of life?**

A: Adequate control of the airway disease and coronary revascularisation will most definitely improve her symptoms and will also improve her exercise tolerance. I would commence her on a cardiorespiratory rehabilitation program with regular physiotherapy to expedite her recovery. I would formulate a program of weight loss with the help of the dietitian. I would consult the occupational therapist with a view to assessing her functional capacity and providing necessary support.

INTRODUCTION

LS is a renal transplant patient on immunosuppressive therapy who presents with recurrent pneumonia, anaemia and occasional depression. She also suffers from hypertension and recurrent cutaneous malignancy.

CASE IN DETAIL

LS is a 45-year-old woman who presented 3 weeks ago with fevers, rigors and drenching sweats of 4 days' duration. She also had a productive cough with green, rusty sputum and pleuritic chest pain in the left subscapular region. She was subsequently diagnosed with pneumonia and treated with intravenous antibiotics until 2 weeks ago. Her symptoms settled on this treatment. This was her third admission for pneumonia within the past 5 months.

During this admission she was also diagnosed with significant anaemia. However, she could not remember her haemoglobin level at the time of diagnosis. She denied any symptoms suggestive of anaemia prior to presentation. She was investigated thoroughly with multiple blood tests, upper and lower gastrointestinal endoscopy and a bone marrow biopsy. She was not aware of the outcomes of any of the above investigations. She was treated with the transfusion of two units of packed cells and discharged from hospital 10 days ago. She denies any known source of bleeding. She is currently stable but feels very lethargic.

LS was diagnosed with end-stage renal failure 5 years ago when she presented with frank haematuria, bipedal pitting oedema, dyspnoea at rest, persistent nausea and vomiting. She had multiple investigations including a renal biopsy. A diagnosis of end-stage renal failure secondary to IgA nephropathy was established. Almost immediately she was commenced on haemodialysis. She was dialysed for 2 years, initially at the hospital and then at home until 3 years ago, when she received a cadaveric renal allograft. Three months later she developed severe rejection non-responsive to pulse methylprednisolone therapy and she was recommenced on dialysis. Two years ago she received her second cadaveric allograft, which has been functioning well to date.

She has been treated with multiple immunosuppressant medications, including prednisone at various doses, azathioprine and cyclosporin, for 3 years.

She has received oral prednisolone as well as parenteral pulsed methylprednisolone at different times. The maximum dose has been 500 mg methylprednisolone intravenously for 3 days during the rejection episode of her first allograft. The minimum is 10 mg oral prednisolone, which is her current maintenance dose. She denies any adverse effects associated with her corticosteroid therapy, but she has never had her bone densitometry measured.

She also takes 150 mg cyclosporin twice daily. With her cyclosporin therapy she has experienced side effects of gum hypertrophy, hypertension and recurrent gouty arthritis. The first gout attack was 1 year ago. On controlling the acute gout attack with colchicine and local corticosteroid injection, she was commenced on allopurinol maintenance therapy, and the azathioprine she was on was replaced with mycophenolate mofetil. Since the commencement of maintenance therapy with allopurinol, she has not suffered from any acute exacerbations of gouty arthritis. Her cyclosporin level is monitored at the local hospital's renal clinic at 2-weekly intervals and the most recent trough level has been 175 ng/L. Her cyclosporin-induced hypertension is managed with long-acting nifedipine 30 mg daily and she denies any side effects associated with this therapy. Her blood pressure is monitored at the local renal clinic every second week and has been well controlled at around 130/85 mmHg.

She is currently managed on 1 g mycophenolate mofetil twice a day. She denies any side effects associated with this therapy.

She has had multiple skin malignancies associated with her immunosuppression, excised over the past 3 years by her general practitioner and a plastic surgeon. The most recent was a squamous cell carcinoma removed from her forehead 2 months ago.

In summary, her medications are: cyclosporin-A, mycophenolate mofetil, prednisolone, nifedipine and allopurinol. She denies any allergy.

LS's mother is 68 years old and suffers from emphysema and diabetes mellitus. Her father is 70 years old and has ischaemic heart disease. She is an only child.

She lives with her partner, aged 47, who is well and supportive. She has one daughter, aged 12, who is well. She lives in a farmhouse with only one step at the entrance. There are many animals living on the farm, including swine, cattle and various birds. She is independent with activities of daily living.

She gave up smoking 4 years ago, but prior to that she had a significant smoking history of 30 pack-years. She smokes marijuana once a month and consumes alcohol only very rarely.

She works as a gardener at a local nursery and has prolonged periods of sun exposure.

My dietary history of LS suggests satisfactory nutrition. She denies any significant weight loss in the recent past. She has no problems with sleep.

She had an episode of depression about 4 months ago, due to a dispute with her partner. She believes that he is getting tired of all her medical problems. She is also anxious about the current developments with her medical condition. She denies any vegetative symptoms of depression or anxiety.

ON EXAMINATION

LS was alert and cooperative. She had a clinically functioning arteriovenous fistula in her right forearm. There were multiple healed scars of previously excised cutaneous malignancies in her left forehead, left cheek and over the right shoulder. There was an ulcerative lesion in her left thigh of 1.5 cm diameter with a hard, everted edge and a dry, erythematous base. There was no evidence of any granulation tissue. This lesion was not tender and the features were very suggestive of a squamous cell skin malignancy.

Her pulse rate was 50 beats per minute, regular in rhythm and normal in character. Her blood pressure was 140/95 mmHg and there was no postural drop. Her respiratory rate was 10 per minute. The estimated body mass index was 20. She was afebrile and her cognition was preserved.

Respiratory tract examination showed normal chest expansion, in both the apical and basal regions. There was no area of dullness to percussion, and breath sounds were vesicular throughout. There were fine crepitations in the right lung base. There was no sputum mug available for inspection.

Cardiovascular system examination showed no palmar crease or conjunctival pallor. Her heart sounds were dual and normal in character and there was no murmur. There was no peripheral oedema.

In the gastrointestinal system examination, her abdomen was not distended or tender. There was a longitudinal scar of 4 cm in the left lower quadrant, underneath which a non-tender, firm mass suggestive of the renal transplant was palpable. There was no organomegaly and the rest of the abdominal examination was unremarkable.

Neurological examination showed an unremarkable cranial nerve examination. Her visual acuity was preserved at 6/6 without correction. Fundoscopy showed silver wiring of the arteries and arteriovenous nipping with no haemorrhage or exudates. Fundoscopic findings suggest grade 2 hypertensive changes according to the Keith-Wagener-Barker classification.

Upper and lower limb examinations showed normal tone, power, reflexes and coordination with an unremarkable sensory examination. Importantly, there was no proximal muscle wasting or weakness noticed.

Her rheumatological examination was unremarkable and there was no lymphadenopathy.

In summary, LS is a 45-year-old renal transplant patient with a recent diagnosis of anaemia. She is on multiple immunosuppressive medications with associated complications of hypertension, gout, recurrent infections and cutaneous malignancy. She suffers from occasional depression and anxiety. She also has the important problem of hazardous occupational sun exposure.

The main problem with this woman is the management of immunosuppression appropriately so as to minimise complications and maximise graft survival and function.

In approaching the management of this patient, I have identified the following five problems:

1 Diagnosis of the aetiology of this woman's anaemia and the treatment of same
2 Ascertaining the cause of her recurrent pneumonia and taking appropriate preventive measures
3 Reviewing her immunosuppressive medication regimen and optimising efficacy while minimising the complications
4 Tackling the issue of her skin malignancies and protection from further sun exposure
5 Addressing her current state of anxiety and helping the family with effective coping strategies.

First I would address the problem of anaemia. The first differential diagnosis I would consider is bone marrow suppression associated with immunosuppressive therapy. Other differential diagnoses that I would consider in this situation are:

1 Iron deficiency anaemia due to gastrointestinal bleeding
2 Anaemia of chronic disease
3 Anaemia due to chronic renal failure, if the graft is failing
4 Anaemia due to bone marrow infiltration by malignancy
5 Haemolytic anaemia
6 Myelodysplastic syndrome
7 Myelofibrosis or aplastic anaemia.

To ascertain the severity of the anaemia and to exclude the above differential diagnoses, I would like to see the results of the following investigations:

1 Full blood count, looking at the haemoglobin levels. I would like to see both the current haemoglobin level and the haemoglobin level on presentation.
2 Blood film, looking at red cell morphology and reticulocyte count
3 Iron studies in the form of serum iron, serum ferritin and serum transferrin levels, together with the serum vitamin B_{12} level and red cell and serum folate levels
4 Results of the recent endoscopic procedures, gastroscopy results looking at peptic ulcer disease or gastritis, and colonoscopy result looking for colonic mass lesions
5 Results of the recent bone marrow biopsy, looking for marrow suppression showing hypocellularity, marrow infiltration or ring sideroblasts
6 A haemolytic screen: the blood film, looking for spherocytes, red cell fragments and reticulocytes, together with the serum haptoglobin, serum bilirubin and serum lactate dehydrogenase levels
7 Urine analysis, looking for haematuria to exclude glomerulonephritis, recurrent IgA nephropathy, uroepithelial malignancy and paroxysmal nocturnal haemoglobinuria.

Management of this patient's anaemia will be guided by the results of the above tests. Depending on the haemoglobin level and the clinical symptoms, I would decide on the need for blood transfusion.

Questions and answers

Q: Please interpret this full blood count and the blood film report of this patient on presentation:

- Hb—7.9 g/dL
- White cell count—4 × 109
- Platelet count—50 × 109
- Blood film morphology of normochromic, normocytic anaemia with reticulocyte count of 1%.

A: There is significant anaemia together with thrombocytopenia. The severity of the anaemia warrants blood transfusion, and I would transfuse this woman with three units of packed cells. I would use leucocyte-filtered blood for the purpose of transfusion in order to prevent immune sensitisation, which might preclude future transplant prospects if needed. The suboptimal reticulocyte count suggests inadequate bone marrow response to the anaemia, and I would be keen to follow this up with the bone marrow biopsy, looking at both the aspirate and the trephine pictures.

Cytomegalovirus disease is another possibility with anaemia and thrombocytopenia. Although this tends to be more common in the early post-transplant period, I would like to rule it out with CMV PCR.

Q: **The bone marrow biopsy shows hypocellularity. How does this finding influence your management plan for this woman?**

A: I believe that the anaemia is likely to be due to bone marrow suppression associated with the immunosuppressive therapy. However, to exclude aplastic anaemia and myelofibrosis, I would like to see whether there was any evidence of cellular atypia. Cyclosporin or corticosteroids are not known to cause bone marrow suppression, as would azathioprine and mycophenolate mofetil. In this situation the likely drug is mycophenolate. I would do further research into the adverse effects of this drug. I would cut her current dose of mycophenolate mofetil to 500 mg twice daily and increase her prednisolone to 15 mg daily to compensate.

Q: **What options do you have if the proposed dose reduction does not work?**

A: In such a situation I would consider withdrawing mycophenolate and replacing it with an alternative agent, such as sirolimus or tacrolimus. Unfortunately, the full side-effect profiles of these drugs have not yet been described. Therefore it would be a decision that I would take after extensive consultation with colleagues who have practical experience with the use of these agents.

Q: **Please interpret the electrolyte profile of this patient:**
- Na—136 mmol/L
- K—4.3 mmol/L
- Cl—100 mmol/L
- HCO_3—21 mmol/L
- Urea—9.3 mmol/L
- Creatinine—220 mmol/L.

A: This picture is consistent with moderate renal failure. I would like to see some previous figures to see whether this is acute or chronic renal failure, and, if it is chronic, to see whether it is progressive.

Q: **Six months ago her urea level was 7.1 mmol/L and creatinine level was 180 mmol/L.**

A: There is chronic renal failure and it is progressive. The possible differential diagnoses are chronic allograft nephropathy, recurrent glomerulonephritis or viral infections of graft due to CMV or BK virus. I would also do an ultrasound of graft and, if it is normal, I would proceed with a renal biopsy for a definitive diagnosis.

Q: **The renal biopsy done 2 weeks ago shows striped fibrosis and evidence of chronic rejection. How would you approach this?**

A: This pathology report suggests cyclosporin toxicity as evidenced by striped fibrosis in combination with chronic rejection. Cyclosporin toxicity should be addressed with dose reduction, which is possible with either the addition of an agent like sirolimus or substitution of cyclosporin with sirolimus. Sirolimus is known to have a synergic effect with cyclosporin.

To address the issue of rejection, there is a need to increase immunosuppression. It is difficult to increase mycophenolate mofetil in this case due to the anaemia it has possibly caused. Therefore I would increase the prednisolone dose while introducing sirolimus to the regimen, as I described before.

Q: What is the haemolytic screen?

A: Haemolytic screen includes blood film, serum bilirubin (particularly the unconjugated fraction), reticulocyte count, serum haptoglobulin level, Coombs' test and cryoglobulins. Urine should be tested for bilirubin, haemosiderin and urobilinogen levels.

Q: Why do you suspect bone marrow infiltration?

A: With her current immunosuppressed status, she is susceptible to various malignancies. She has already been diagnosed with cutaneous malignancies, and therefore bone marrow metastases with an occult or inadequately excised squamous cell carcinoma or a melanoma should be considered high on the list of differential diagnoses. Immunosuppressed individuals also tend to suffer from a high incidence of lymphomas and epithelial malignancies, so I believe malignant infiltration of the bone marrow needs to be excluded.

Q: How would you approach the management of her recurrent chest infections?

A: I would consider the following differential diagnoses:

1 Recurrent community-acquired pneumonia associated with immunosuppression
2 Recurrent exacerbation of chronic airway limitation, considering her significant past smoking history
3 Atypical pneumonitis due to avian exposure in the form of psittacosis or bird fancier's lung
4 *Neumocystis carinii* (PCP) pneumonia associated with immunosuppression.

I would like to see the results of the following investigations to formulate my approach to the management of her recurrent chest infections:

1 Chest X-rays—both the current film and one taken during the recent infective episode
2 Formal lung function studies, looking for an obstructive flow–volume curve
3 Blood cultures, sputum cultures, and acute and convalescent sera for atypical organisms
4 Avian precipitins.

Whatever the diagnosis, I would regularly immunise this woman against *Pneumococcus pneumoniae*.

Q: What do you know about transplant rejection?

A: There are three types of transplant rejection: hyperacute, acute and chronic. Hyperacute rejection happens immediately after transplantation, is not treatable, and the prognosis is grave. This form of rejection is mediated by preformed HLA antibodies against the HLA antigens of the donor. Management is immediate transplant nephrectomy. Another early form of rejection mediated by preformed antibodies is accelerated acute rejection. This takes place over the first few weeks post transplantation.

Acute rejection can be classified into acute cellular rejection or acute humoral (antibody-mediated) rejection. Acute cellular rejection is characterised by tubulitis and interstitial infiltration with mononuclear cells, whereas humoral rejection shows vascular changes. The former has a better prognosis if treated promptly with immunosuppressive agents, such as high-dose corticosteroids or anti-thymocyte globulin (ATG). Vascular rejection in the form of intimal arteritis or transmural arteritis has a poor prognosis. The most common form of chronic graft failure is chronic allograft nephropathy, which is due to a combination of previous episodes of rejection, calcineurin inhibitor toxicity, hypertension and dyslipidaemia.

Q: **Would ongoing sun exposure associated with her occupation put her at risk of further cutaneous malignancy?**

A: She suffers from recurrent skin malignancies. This may be significantly contributed to by previous prolonged sun exposure. It is the sun exposure during the first two decades of life that places later immunosuppressed transplant recipients at risk of skin malignancy. Therefore I would not advise her to change her job, but I would definitely advise her to wear sunscreen and adequate protection against the sun's radiation. I would also prescribe retinoids, which have some proven efficacy in treating skin cancers in transplant patients.

Q: **How would you propose to manage her depression and anxiety?**

A: This woman suffers from anxiety and occasional depression. She denies vegetative symptoms of anxiety or depression, but I feel that she is distressed and needs therapy to preserve the quality of her life. Also, given the significant complications associated with the medical condition she suffers from at present, and the potential for deterioration of the disease in the future, she needs treatment before she develops significant depression. I would commence her on a selective serotonin reuptake inhibitor agent such as fluoxetine 30 mg daily. I would advise her that it takes about a week for the agent to start acting and warn her of the possible side effects, such as agitation and insomnia.

In addition I would consult the social worker to assess her home situation and the family's ability to cope with her problems. I would like to investigate the level of support that is available to her. I would also refer the patient to a counsellor or a psychologist with expertise in the field of renal disease, to help her with advice and reassurance. Her partner's coping strategies need to be improved, and a group therapy approach with the attendance of the patient, her partner and other close family or friends would be helpful in this regard.

INTRODUCTION

DP is a 61-year-old morbidly obese diabetic woman who presents for optimisation of her disease control. In her background she has multiple medical problems, including symptoms of ischaemic heart disease, hypertension, osteoarthritis, obstructive sleep apnoea, reflux oesophagitis, asthma and hypothyroidism.

CASE IN DETAIL

DP was admitted to hospital 1 day ago by her physician to optimise her blood sugar control. The blood sugar levels have varied between 16 and 28 mmol/L for about 6 months. She has also complained of polyuria, polydipsia, nocturia and lethargy associated with a weight gain of 7 kg in 3 months.

DP's diabetes was diagnosed 22 years ago when she presented with polyuria, polydipsia and lethargy. Initially she was treated with oral hypoglycaemic agents, namely metformin and glibenclamide. She is currently on metformin 500 mg three times daily. Fourteen years ago glibenclamide was replaced by regular insulin.

Her insulin regimen includes subcutaneous rapid-acting insulin 30 units given before meals three times daily and long-acting insulin 50 units given before dinner. She self-injects these. She monitors her blood sugar levels only occasionally. She regularly experiences mild episodes of hypoglycaemia, which manifest as lethargy and intense hunger, but has never had seizures or loss of consciousness. She has multiple complications associated with diabetes mellitus:

1　She suffers from recurrent urinary tract infections, for which she has had multiple hospital admissions in the past at irregular intervals, and the last admission was 3 months ago. She is currently managed with prophylactic antibiotic therapy with nitrofurantoin 50 mg daily. She denies any urethral symptoms currently and any side effects associated with this therapy.

2　She had bilateral cataracts extracted 6 months ago. She has not been diagnosed with diabetic retinopathy and she denies any current visual symptoms. She visits the ophthalmologist every year.

3 She was diagnosed with early diabetic nephropathy 3 years ago on detection of proteinuria by her diabetician. She is unaware of her current level of renal function. She suffers from early-morning headaches and bilateral ankle oedema, symptoms suggestive of possible renal failure. The ankle oedema is treated with indapamide hemihydrate 5 mg every morning with good effect. She denies nausea, pruritus or any other symptom of uraemia.

4 She suffers from postural dizziness and chronic diarrhoea, symptoms suggestive of diabetic autonomic neuropathy, but no formal diagnosis has yet been made. She has had watery diarrhoea 7–8 times a day for many years with occasional abdominal discomfort and bloating. Despite multiple investigations including colonoscopy, no diagnosis has been made. Her bloating is treated with cisapride 10 mg daily, with some relief.

5 She has paraesthesias in the feet bilaterally but denies any loss of sensation or chronic superficial pain. She has never had nerve conduction studies performed.

6 She suffers from ischaemic heart disease and experiences frequent unstable angina, almost daily. She also suffers from dyspnoea on minimal exertion, orthopnoea and paroxysmal nocturnal dyspnoea. She has been investigated with exercise stress testing and nuclear imaging within the past 3 months, but surprisingly she is not on any anti-ischaemia therapy.

She denies ever having had a stroke or leg claudication.

She was diagnosed with hypercholesterolaemia 6 months ago, and is treated with simvastatin 40 mg daily. Her latest blood cholesterol level was 4 mmol/L. She denies any side effects associated with this treatment.

She was diagnosed with hypertension 3 years ago and is currently managed with verapamil one tablet daily. She denies any side effects associated with this therapy. Her GP monitors her blood pressure every 2 weeks, and lately the readings have been around 160/90 mmHg.

Her risk factor profile for coronary artery disease, in addition to diabetes mellitus, hypertension and hypercholesterolaemia, includes physical inactivity, obesity and a positive family history. Her mother had an acute myocardial infarction at age 55 and she has a brother aged 63 who suffers from ischaemic heart disease.

She has hypothyroidism, diagnosed many years ago when she presented with lethargy and cold intolerance. She is currently treated with thyroxine 100 μg daily. She does not know the causative pathology behind her hypothyroidism and denies any symptoms suggestive of ongoing thyroid disease.

She has had osteoarthritis involving the distal and proximal interphalangeal joints bilaterally, the lower cervical spine and the lumbar spine, for many years. She experiences frequent pain and impairment of mobility due to stiffness, particularly at night. However, she is not on any treatment.

She has had asthma for almost 20 years. She is currently managed with salbutamol via a metered dose inhaler as needed. Currently she uses it on average four times a week. She has previously been treated with inhaled steroids but the treatment was stopped due to the side effect of persistent cough. She has never been treated with systemic steroids. Five years ago she had an admission to hospital with exacerbation of asthma. She has not had any other hospital admissions for asthma. She has recurrent nocturnal cough. She does not monitor her peak flow. The only trigger factor for exacerbations she has identified is exercise, and she has not noticed any seasonal variation of her asthma symptoms.

She has glaucoma in both eyes, diagnosed 12 years ago. She has previously been treated with laser iridotomy bilaterally and is currently on topical pilocarpine therapy twice daily and topical acetazolamide twice daily.

She was diagnosed with reflux oesophagitis 10 years ago when she presented with burning epigastric pain. She was investigated with upper gastrointestinal endoscopy. She is being treated with omeprazole 10 mg twice daily but still suffers from dyspeptic symptoms.

She was diagnosed with Ménière's disease 5 years ago. Although she experiences the symptoms of tinnitus and vertigo very often she is not on any treatment. She denies deafness.

She was diagnosed with obstructive sleep apnoea 2 years ago and is managed with nocturnal nasal continuous positive airway pressure; however, she still has daytime somnolence and early-morning headaches.

She started gaining weight after commencing insulin therapy 15 years ago. She has previously attempted to lose weight, particularly through dieting, without much success. She has never attempted regular exercise.

Her medications in summary are metformin, insulin, nitrofurantoin, indapamide, cisapride, verapamil, salbutamol and thyroxine. She claims appropriate compliance with all her medications.

She is intolerant to sulfur-containing medications, which cause 'dizziness', the description of which suggests presyncope rather than vertigo.

She has never smoked. She was a heavy alcohol consumer 15 years ago when she drank 50 g/day of whisky for almost 2 years. She now consumes alcohol only on social occasions.

She lives with a female friend. She has been married three times before and the last partner she divorced 10 years ago. She has one daughter, aged 27, from her first marriage. She keeps in regular contact with her daughter, who is well and lives separately.

She is independent with the activities of self-care but requires assistance with shopping and housekeeping. Her friend provides help with these.

She lives in a villa with five steps at the entrance, which she finds difficult to negotiate due to her back pain and dyspnoea.

She works part-time as a social worker in the community. She does not drive and travels by public transport.

The dietary history I obtained suggests excessive joule intake in the form of lipids and carbohydrates, and she admits that she is not compliant with the diabetic dietary recommendations.

She also complains of depression and the associated vegetative symptom of initial insomnia, but denies any loss of appetite.

ON EXAMINATION

DP was alert and cooperative. She was obese, with an estimated body mass index of 35. Her blood pressure was 140/95 mmHg and there was a postural drop of 30 mmHg systolic and 10 mmHg diastolic. Her pulse was 90 beats per minute, and it was normal in rhythm, rate and character. There was no postural change in the pulse rate. Her respiratory rate was 30 per minute.

Cardiovascular examination showed no jugular venous pressure elevation. Her apex beat was not palpable. There were two heart sounds, which were normal, and there was mild pitting oedema bipedally.

Respiratory tract examination showed oropharyngeal crowding. There was decreased chest expansion bilaterally in the lower zones. Breath sounds were vesicular with bibasal crepitations.

Gastrointestinal examination showed abdominal obesity, with multiple injection scars and lipodystrophy in the abdominal wall. The abdomen was soft and non-tender. There was non-tender hepatomegaly with a smooth and regular edge. Bowel sounds were present.

In the neurological examination, the cranial nerve examination was unremarkable. Fundoscopy was difficult to perform due to bilateral pupillary meiosis secondary to topical meiotic therapy.

Motor and sensory examination of the upper limbs was normal.

Motor examination of the lower limbs was normal but there was impairment of all modalities of sensation to the level of the knee bilaterally. Coordination was normal bilaterally, in both the upper and lower limbs. Plantar response was flexor bilaterally.

Her gait examination showed excessive lumbar lordosis, and the Romberg's test was positive.

Musculoskeletal examination showed nodal osteoarthritis of both hands, with Bouchard's nodes and Heberden's nodes present in the interphalangeal joints of all fingers bilaterally. There was no warmness to touch, tenderness or impairment of movement. Hand function was well preserved. There was midline tenderness to palpation in the lower cervical spine and the lumbar spine. Spinal mobility, however, was preserved.

Diabetic foot examination was unremarkable for any corns, callosities, ulcers or Charcot's joints.

In summary, this is a 61-year-old, obese, diabetic woman presenting with dyspnoea and chest pain on a background of poor diabetic control, multiple complications of diabetes as well as hypertension, osteoarthritis, obstructive sleep apnoea, reflux oesophagitis, asthma, Ménière's disease and hypothyroidism.

This woman's main problem is her obesity. However, diagnosis and treatment of her coronary symptoms are of primary importance.

The other issues with this woman include coronary risk factor modification, better control of diabetes and the management of respiratory causes of dyspnoea.

She suffers from chest pain, with features highly suggestive of cardiac ischaemia. Also her dyspnoea and associated symptoms can suggest congestive cardiac failure. She runs the risk of having an acute myocardial infarction; therefore, her chest pain should be investigated and managed first.

First, I would like to see the result of a recent electrocardiogram, looking for evidence of cardiac ischaemia and left ventricular hypertrophy. I would like to see a recent chest X-ray, looking for evidence of pulmonary congestion and cardiomegaly. In addition I would like to see the results of a recent full blood count, looking for anaemia that can contribute to dyspnoea, a coagulation profile and the electrolyte profile, and renal function indices, looking for any renal failure.

Questions and answers

Q: Please interpret this electrocardiogram and describe this chest X-ray.

A: This ECG of DP done on (insert date) shows sinus rhythm with a left-axis deviation. There is a left bundle branch block and, in light of that, it is impossible to further interpret this ECG for any cardiac ischaemia. I would like to see previous ECGs to ascertain how recently this bundle branch block has developed.

This frontal-projection, posteroanterior view chest X-ray of DP done on (insert date) shows poor chest expansion, increased cardiothoracic ratio suggesting cardiomegaly, and increased vascular markings in the upper zones suggesting left ventricular failure and upper lobe diversion. I would like to follow up this X-ray with a nuclear medicine gated heart pool scan to ascertain left ventricular ejection fraction, and formal lung function tests to assess her lung physiology.

Q: Why do you want a gated heart pool scan?

A: Due to this woman's body habitus, a transthoracic echocardiogram would not be very accurate in interpreting the ventricular function. I consider a gated heart pool scan to be more accurate and suitable in this setting.

Q: How would you approach the management of her ischaemic heart disease?

A: It is questionable whether this woman has been conclusively diagnosed with ischaemic heart disease, given that she is not on any anti-ischaemia therapy. But she is at extremely high risk of ischaemic heart disease considering her current symptomatology and the risk-factor profile. So I would like to perform a pharmacological stress-perfusion scan in the form of a dipyridamole-sestamibi scan to look for any coronary flow reserve.

Meanwhile, I would commence her on regular low-dose aspirin therapy and sublingual nitrate therapy, as needed, for her chest pain.

If the investigations prove the presence of reversible cardiac ischaemia, I would follow her up with coronary angiography in order to define coronary anatomy and decide on definitive revascularisation therapy.

Coronary reperfusion will considerably improve her cardiac function. But for now I will treat her with a diuretic such as frusemide and an angiotensin receptor inhibitor. An ACE inhibitor will help control her hypertension and protect her from progressive diabetic nephropathy. I would be cautious with using beta-blocker agents in this woman due to her history of asthma.

Then I would review her cardiac risk-factor profile with a view to optimising control. For this purpose I would check her fasting cholesterol profile, and if she has hypercholesterolaemia I would consider appropriate therapy.

Q: She has presented for optimisation of her blood sugar control. How would you go about doing that?

A: She needs better control of her diabetes as well as management of end-organ complications. Initially I would like to see her glycosylated haemoglobin level to ascertain her level of control of the blood sugar over the past 6 weeks. Lack of compliance with diabetic medications as well as the diabetic diet is a major cause for suboptimal control in the majority of patients. Therefore I would ensure regular medication and strict compliance with the diabetic diet while she is in hospital. I would initially observe her for 3 days to see whether her blood sugar control improved. If there was no significant improvement I would change her insulin regimen to a twice-daily dose of a combination long- and short-acting insulin to be given 15 minutes prior to the two main meals. I would commence her on a long- and short-acting 30/70 mixture given subcutaneously twice daily, with 30 units given before breakfast and 15 units before dinner. I would increase the metformin dose to 1 g three times daily. I would educate her on the diabetic diet in consultation with the diabetic educator and a specialist dietitian. I would encourage her to do low-impact exercise, such as walking or wading in a pool, for about half an hour each day.

Q: **What is the rationale behind your therapeutic plan?**

A: High doses of insulin can lead to further weight gain and worsening of insulin resistance. My objective is to break this vicious cycle by managing her on the lowest possible insulin regimen while increasing metformin, which is an agent that improves peripheral insulin sensitivity and is beneficial to the obese. Weight loss is of major importance in the management of diabetes in this woman, so I would initiate a definite plan of action with a view to losing 5–10 kg of body weight over a period of 3–6 months. If successful, this amount of weight reduction will help improve her blood sugar control too.

Q: **How would you plan the weight reduction program? How easy or difficult do you think it will be?**

A: It is certainly not going to be easy, but I am keen on trying it because she has not previously tried such a program. I would obtain a detailed dietary history to calculate her current level of joule intake and make necessary arrangements to restrict the amount of joules she consumes. I would plan a diet aimed at weight reduction in consultation with the dietitian. This diet would be rich in complex carbohydrates with a low glycaemic index and deficient in simple sugars and saturated fats. I would educate the patient in joule counting and encourage her to keep a record of her food intake. The diet will comprise 15% protein, 15% lipids (mainly in the form of mono- and polyunsaturated fats) and 70% carbohydrates. In addition, I would encourage her to take up regular low-impact exercise, such as walking or wading in a swimming pool, to be done for about half an hour each day. I would advise the patient's GP to monitor her progress at regular intervals of 2 weeks.

Given her history of hypothyroidism, I would check her serum thyroid-stimulating hormone level and free T4 and T3 indices to exclude persistent hypothyroidism, which could very well contribute to her obesity.

If she failed to achieve substantial weight loss goals through conservative measures, I would commence her on orlistat, a gastrointestinal lipase inhibitor, and warn her of the possible side effects of greasy stool, diarrhoea, flatulence and abdominal discomfort.

Q: **What are your goals in treating this woman's diabetes?**

A: I would aim to maintain her fasting blood sugar levels below 6.1 mmol/L and postprandial blood sugar levels below 7.8 mmol/L. I would aim at keeping her HbA1c level below 7%. To monitor this I would initially advise her to check her blood sugar level immediately before and 2 hours after each main meal.

Q: **How would you monitor her for end-organ complications?**

A: To evaluate the degree of renal involvement, I would like to see the latest renal function indices in the form of the blood urea and serum creatinine levels. In addition, I would like to see the results of a recent urinalysis, looking for proteinuria, and a spot urine test to calculate the albumin-to-creatinine ratio, looking for evidence of microalbuminuria. If there was frank proteinuria, I would proceed with a 24-hour urine collection for the purpose of quantification.

I would also perform a renal ultrasound scan, looking for diminished renal size.

Q: **Her albumin to creatinine ratio is 3.6. How does this affect the management of this patient?**

A: This signifies the presence of microalbuminuria and she is at very high risk of cardiovascular events such as myocardial infarction and stroke. I would repeat the test on two more occasions at 3-monthly intervals to confirm microalbuminuria. Meanwhile I would control her blood pressure at a level below 130/80 mmHg and ensure strict glycaemic control. Commencement of ACE inhibitor therapy would benefit her kidneys. I would commence her on a cholesterol-lowering statin agent regardless of her cholesterol level.

Q: **If she has diabetic nephropathy with proteinuria, how would you manage her?**

A: I would ensure strict control of her blood pressure and also place her on a protein restriction of 0.8 g/kg per day. I would ensure adequate hydration at all times and stop all potentially nephrotoxic drugs. I would ensure strict glycaemic control as much as possible. I would continue to monitor her renal function indices to ascertain the rate of progression and plan renal replacement therapy if indicated.

Q: **What do you think her dyspnoea is due to?**

A: Her dyspnoea could be multifactorial. It is possibly due to a combination of left heart failure due to ischaemia and hypertension, poorly controlled asthma and restrictive ventilatory defect secondary to obesity. Pulmonary embolisation is another contributory factor that should be considered. Pleural effusion associated with hypothyroidism is also a remote possibility. To further investigate this, I would like to see the results of arterial blood gases on room air, looking for hypoxia and hypercapnoea, and formal lung function studies, looking for a combination of obstructive and restrictive patterns together with impaired gas exchange. If there was significant hypoxia in the blood gas result I would also perform a ventilation-perfusion scan, looking for mismatch defects that would suggest pulmonary embolism.

Q: Why is she still complaining of daytime somnolence despite the treatment of her sleep apnoea?

A: She has multiple risk factors that contribute to obstructive sleep apnoea, including morbid obesity, oropharyngeal crowding and possible hypothyroidism. On the other hand, obstructive sleep apnoea can be contributing to many of the medical problems she currently suffers from, including poorly controlled hypertension, dyspnoea, depression and early-morning headaches. The persistence of daytime symptoms including somnolence despite nocturnal nasal continuous positive airway pressure may be due to poor technique, but I would like to confirm the diagnosis of obstructive sleep apnoea conclusively. She needs a repeat sleep study and assessment of her technique with the nocturnal continuous positive airway pressure machine. Once again, achievement of weight loss goals will certainly improve her prognosis in this respect.

Q: How would you manage hypercholesterolaemia that is not responding to the maximum available dose of the statin medication you have commenced?

A: If the fasting total cholesterol level remains above 4.0 mmol/L despite statin therapy at 40 mg/day for more than 3 months, I would add ezetimibe 10 mg to the regimen. This agent is known to reduce the cholesterol level by a further 15% over what is achieved with the maximal statin dose.

INTRODUCTION

SF is a 38-year-old man with decompensated cirrhosis due to alcohol abuse and chronic hepatitis C infection, now presenting with severe abdominal pain and gastrointestinal bleeding.

CASE IN DETAIL

SF's current problems started with the gradual onset of lower abdominal pain 1 week ago. This was accompanied by abdominal distension. His pain gradually progressed in intensity and became generalised. The pain was dull and constant in nature and he could not identify any precipitating or relieving factors. Associated with these symptoms he developed anorexia and nausea, but did not vomit. This was followed by black, tarry bowel motions, which he first noticed 3 days ago. He presented to the emergency department of the hospital 1 day ago, where he was investigated with multiple blood tests, abdominal ultrasonography and upper gastrointestinal endoscopy. He was significantly anaemic and was transfused with 4 units of packed red cells. He was also commenced on an octreotide infusion and kept nil by mouth. On endoscopic examination he was diagnosed with bleeding varices as well as erosive gastritis. He was treated with banding of the varices and high-dose intravenous omeprazole therapy at 20 mg twice daily. He was also commenced on lactulose 10 mL three times daily for the prevention of hepatic encephalopathy. With this therapy he experienced diarrhoea with liquid motions on average five times a day. He underwent a diagnostic paracentesis and was subsequently commenced on intravenous ceftriaxone 1 g daily. However, he denied any fevers, rigors or drenching sweats.

SF was diagnosed with hepatic cirrhosis 1 year ago when he presented with abdominal distension and haematemesis. He was also noted to be hepatitis C antibody-positive on this presentation. He admitted having had body piercing and tattoos as a possible risk factor but denied any previous blood transfusions or intravenous drug use. Subsequent upper gastrointestinal endoscopy showed oesophageal varices, which were managed with banding. During the same admission he was commenced on a low-salt diet and advised against further alcohol consumption, but he did not comply with either instruction. He was followed up on discharge with four more 3-weekly endoscopic bandings.

Eight months ago he was readmitted with severe abdominal distension, dyspnoea and ascites, which was treated with abdominal paracentesis. He was then commenced on spironolactone 100 mg daily and propranolol 40 mg daily. Subsequently he has presented on three more occasions with tense abdominal distension for paracentesis, and the last episode was 6 weeks ago. He is currently on spironolactone 200 mg daily and frusemide 40 mg daily.

He was diagnosed with a duodenal ulcer 2 years ago when he presented with severe epigastric pain, nausea and vomiting. Diagnosis was made on gastroscopy. He was commenced on ranitidine 150 mg twice daily. Five months ago his symptoms recurred and his general practitioner changed his treatment to omeprazole 20 mg daily. He denies any knowledge of his *Helicobacter pylori* status and denies ever having been treated for *H. pylori*.

In summary, his current medications are frusemide, spironolactone, omeprazole, propranolol, lactulose and ceftriaxone.

He denies any allergies.

His family history is significant, with his father dying of bowel carcinoma at the age of 52. His mother is alive at the age of 65 and is well. He has three brothers: the oldest, aged 44, suffers from alcoholic cirrhosis and the second brother, aged 42, was operated on this year for bowel carcinoma; his youngest brother, aged 36, is well.

He lives by himself in a local hotel and has a flight of 10 steps to negotiate to get to his room. He is independent with the activities of daily living. He was married once but he divorced his wife 5 years ago. He has two daughters, aged 10 and 8, both of whom are well and living with his former wife. He rarely sees his daughters, and the last time was 3 years ago. His main social support is a group of friends that he meets in the pub. He does not visit his GP regularly. He spends most of the day in the pub, with his friends.

He worked as a seaman and a waterfront labourer before retiring 5 years ago after a back injury. But he denies any symptoms associated with it currently. He survives on a disability pension and claims it is adequate for his survival.

He smokes approximately one packet of cigarettes a day and has a history of 30 pack-years. He consumes in excess of 100 g alcohol a day in the form of cheap wine or rum. My directed assessment (CAGE questionnaire) confirmed that he is alcohol dependent. He has tried giving up drinking on previous occasions without any success. He has not undergone alcohol detoxification previously. He had his last drink prior to hospitalisation, 1 week ago. He denies any other previous or current recreational drug use.

My nutritional history suggests inadequate nutrition. He usually has his meals at the local fast-food outlet and often neglects his main meals.

He demonstrates very poor insight into his medical and social conditions. He has suffered from depression in the past and has been treated medically. He denies any ongoing vegetative symptoms of depression and is currently not on any antidepressant medication.

He complains of daytime somnolence and nocturnal insomnia.

ON EXAMINATION

SF was drowsy but rousable and cooperative. He appeared cachectic and had mild scleral icterus. He had tattoos on the ventral and dorsal aspects of his thorax and an intravenous cannula in the dorsal aspect of his right hand; the cannula site was not inflamed. He had multiple ecchymoses in the forearms bilaterally and in the forehead.

His pulse rate was 90 beats per minute and respiratory rate 20 per minute. He was afebrile, and his blood pressure was 130/95 mmHg with no postural drop.

His estimated body mass index was 20. His cognitive function was preserved, with a Mini-Mental State score of 28/30.

In the gastrointestinal examination there was no clubbing of the fingers, but there was palmar erythema bilaterally and a Dupuytren's contracture in the left palm. There was a mild hepatic flap. He had parotidomegaly but no fetor hepaticus. His oral hygiene was poor. There were multiple blistering lesions in the perioral region, some filled with clear fluid and some crusted. There were multiple spider naevi in the upper thorax, both anteriorly and posteriorly. There was gynaecomastia. He had generalised abdominal distension without superficial venous dilatation. There were multiple scars in the left lateral aspect of the abdomen—possible evidence of previous paracentesis. On palpation the abdomen was firm and non-tender. There was firm-to-hard, non-tender hepatomegaly with an irregular edge. The hepatic span was 19 cm along the right anterior clavicular line. His spleen was just tippable in the left upper quadrant. There was a positive fluid thrill and a shifting dullness of 3 cm in the flanks. The kidneys were not ballotable and his bowel sounds were positive and normal.

There was evidence of testicular atrophy, and I would like to confirm this with formal orchidometry.

His cardiovascular examination demonstrated a parasternal heave and two heart sounds. The pulmonary component of the second sound was louder. Jugular venous pressure was not elevated but was visible 3 cm above the angle of Louis. There was bilateral pitting ankle oedema up to a level midway from the ankle. All peripheral pulses were well palpable.

Respiratory system examination showed normal lung expansion bilaterally, and there was no dullness to percussion. There were medium coarse crepitations in both bases and the breath sounds were vesicular.

Neurological examination showed normal cranial nerve examination, with preserved visual acuity of 6/6 bilaterally without correction. Fundoscopy was normal. In the upper limbs, motor function was preserved and the coordination was normal. But there was impaired proprioception, soft touch and pinprick sensation in the hands in a glove distribution to the level of the wrists bilaterally. Otherwise, the sensory examination was unremarkable.

In the lower limb examination, his gait was wide-based with bilateral foot drop. He demonstrated a positive Romberg's test. There was significant wasting of the musculature distal to the knee bilaterally but without pes cavus. The tone was normal. There was significant weakness at the level of ankle bilaterally in all directions of movement. There was sensory impairment to vibration, joint position, soft touch and pinprick sensation bilaterally in a stocking distribution to a level just above the ankles. The deep tendon reflexes and coordination were preserved. He demonstrated flexor plantar response bilaterally.

His rheumatological examination was unremarkable and there was no lymphadenopathy.

I would like to see the result of his per rectum examination.

In summary, this is a 38-year-old man presenting with decompensated cirrhosis of the liver with portal hypertension, associated with chronic alcoholism and hepatitis C infection on a background of peptic ulcer disease, depression and peripheral neuropathy. He also has the significant problems of alcohol dependency, poor compliance, poor social support and a family history of carcinoma of the bowel.

His main problem currently is the management of multiple acute complications of cirrhosis, namely gastrointestinal bleeding, portal hypertension, sepsis and hepatic encephalopathy.

In addition to the above, I have identified four medical problems and a social problem:

1 Further investigation of his firm/hard irregular hepatomegaly
2 Investigation and management of the peripheral neuropathy
3 Establishment and maintenance of alcohol abstinence
4 Poor compliance with medical management
5 Lack of adequate social support, and self-neglect.

Approaching the management of this man's main acute problem of decompensated cirrhosis, I would like to see the results of the following investigations:

1 Full blood count, looking for leucocytosis, anaemia with macrocytosis, and thrombocytopenia
2 His temperature chart, looking for recent fevers
3 Coagulation profile, looking for a high international normalised ratio
4 Electrolyte profile, looking for hyponatraemia, hyperkalaemia and renal failure, and the liver function indices, looking for abnormalities
5 Microscopy and culture of ascitic fluid, and the serum-to-fluid albumin ratio
6 Serum ammonia level.

Questions and answers

Q: How would you manage this patient when he initially presents?

A: The immediate objective in the management of this patient is to control the gastrointestinal bleeding and achieve haemodynamic stability. I would quickly assess the patient's haemodynamic status by looking at the oral mucosa and skin turgor to assess the level of hydration, and check the arterial pulse and the blood pressure and look for any postural drop in blood pressure. Then I would insert large-bore cannulae in two large peripheral veins (e.g. the cubital fossa) and perform urgent blood tests for the haemoglobin level, haematocrit, and coagulation and electrolyte profiles. I would cross-match six units of blood and platelets and commence an intravenous infusion of colloids or crystalloids to maintain vascular volume. Given his history of bleeding varices and duodenal ulcer disease, I would start intravenous infusions of octreotide as well as omeprazole. I would keep the patient nil by mouth, organise urgent gastroscopy and also notify the general surgeon.

Q: He has been afebrile. Do you still think that he has spontaneous bacterial peritonitis?

A: Yes, it is still possible, because these patients may not have the classic manifestations of sepsis, and therefore I would like to see microbiological tests done on his ascitic fluid and to commence him on empirical antibiotic therapy.

Q: **How would you manage spontaneous bacterial peritonitis?**

A: I would perform a diagnostic paracentesis for microscopy and culture and assess the pH of the ascitic fluid. Even if microbiological tests were unyielding, an acidic pH would suggest infection. The most likely organism is *E. coli,* so I would commence this man on 1 g daily intravenous ceftriaxone. On recovery I would maintain him on long-term prophylactic antibiotic therapy with norfloxacin.

Q: **Would you give him gentamicin?**

A: No, I would not. Gentamicin has the potential to cause renal damage and in this setting it can lead to hepatorenal syndrome.

Q: **How would you manage his encephalopathy?**

A: He is drowsy and has a hepatic flap, so he has grade 1 hepatic encephalopathy. First I would address the possible precipitating causes— control and treat gastrointestinal bleeding and treat spontaneous bacterial peritonitis. I would give him oral lactulose, commencing with a dose of 30 mL twice daily and gradually increasing the dose so as to cause diarrhoea at least four times a day. I would also put the patient on a low-protein diet. If these measures did not achieve adequate control of the encephalopathy, I would commence the patient on oral neomycin.

Q: **Why did you say that you wanted to further investigate his hepatomegaly?**

A: This man has known cirrhosis of the liver, and usually cirrhosis causes shrinkage of the liver, so it is not usual to present with hepatomegaly in the clinical setting of hepatic cirrhosis. This man runs the risk of developing a hepatocellular carcinoma in the cirrhotic liver, which could very well lead to decompensation of his cirrhosis. Also, with his significant family history of large bowel carcinoma, there is an indication to exclude metastatic bowel cancer. To approach this issue I would first like to check his serum alpha-fetoprotein levels and the results of an ultrasound scan of his liver. If there was a mass lesion I would proceed with a liver biopsy once the patient was haemodynamically stable and his coagulopathy treated.

Q: **How would you manage this man if he has a hepatocellular carcinoma?**

A: If there was a biopsy-proven hepatoma, my approach to its management would be first to stage the disease. Staging would be done with following investigations:

1   Chest X-ray
2   CT scan of the abdomen
3   A three-phase bone scan
4   CT scan of the head.

   If the patient has a tumour confined to one lobe of the liver, he should be considered for hepatectomy and liver transplantation in consultation with a liver transplant unit. But given his decompensated condition, his prospects of being a candidate for liver transplantation are grim. Depending on the stage, the other therapeutic options include alcohol injection, intraarterial chemoembolisation or intraarterial chemotherapy. If he has disseminated disease, the management option would be palliative.

Q: **If endoscopy shows a duodenal ulcer, how would you manage it?**

A: If there is a duodenal ulcer I would like to know whether there is evidence of recent bleeding in the ulcer and also features that would suggest a high likelihood of a rebleed, such as a visible vessel in the ulcer base or a blood clot. If there is evident bleeding, it should be treated with adrenaline injection or electrocautery.

On securing haemostasis, I would perform a rapid urease test and a biopsy to ascertain the *H. pylori* status of the patient. If the patient was positive for *H. pylori* I would treat him with a 10-day course of triple therapy, consisting of omeprazole 20 mg twice daily, amoxycillin 500 mg twice daily and clarithromycin 100 mg twice daily. I would follow the patient up 4 weeks later with a urease breath test to confirm eradication of the organism. If the patient tested negative for *H. pylori* I would treat him with oral omeprazole 20 mg daily.

Q: **What do you think about this patient's peripheral neuropathy?**

A: His neuropathy is most likely to be due to the chronic alcoholism. The other differential diagnoses that should be entertained are vitamin B_{12} deficiency and peripheral neuropathy, possibly associated with as yet undiagnosed diabetes or mononeuritis multiplex due to hepatitis-C-induced cryoglobulinaemia. To approach the management of this neuropathy, I would like to perform nerve conduction studies to ascertain the exact nature of the neuropathy and perform blood tests looking for vitamin B_{12} deficiency, hyperglycaemia (fasting blood sugar levels) and cryoglobulins. I would also refer the patient to a podiatrist for foot care and for foot orthotics to facilitate safe mobilisation. I would educate the patient in the implications of the peripheral neuropathy, the dangers involved, and stress the need for good foot care for the prevention of complications such as burns, pressure ulcers and Charcot's joints.

It is likely that this neuropathy is irreversible, but progression can be controlled by addressing the causative factor, if possible, once definitively diagnosed.

Q: **What are you going to do about this man's alcoholism?**

A: My objective is to achieve full abstinence. To arrive at this goal I would formulate a plan of action in collaboration with the drug and alcohol facility of the hospital, the social worker and the patient's GP. First I would educate the patient in the absolute need for abstinence and inform the patient of the various supportive facilities available to people with problems associated with alcohol. I would refer the patient to the local drug and alcohol outpatients clinic and, if the patient was interested, to organisations that help people overcome alcohol abuse, such as the Salvation Army and Alcoholics Anonymous. If the patient cannot maintain the detoxification achieved during this admission to hospital, consideration may be given to anti-craving medications such as acamprosate in collaboration with the alcohol or liver clinic.

Q: **What would you do to optimise his social support network?**

A: I would assess his home situation and the support available in collaboration with the social worker. I would also call a family conference to explain the patient's situation and to ascertain what level of care the family can provide. He may need community resources, such as home care and the community nursing sister. I would also formulate a shared-care program for the ongoing medical management of the patient with his GP.

Q: **Would you continue to treat his hepatitis C infection?**

A: No, not at this stage. He would not tolerate interferon alpha treatment because of decompensated cirrhosis. A further deterrent to antihepatitis C therapy is his continued alcohol abuse.

Q: **Is this man a candidate for liver transplantation?**

A: No. He has to be abstinent prior to being considered for transplantation. Therefore, once he was stable I would first refer him for psychological assessment and counselling.

Q: **What else would you want to do for this man?**

A: I would strongly advise him on lifestyle measures, to curb the spread of his hepatitis C infection to others. Advice would be given not to share razors etc. I would educate him in the need for proper compliance with medical therapy and in proper nutrition with the help of the dietitian. I would also commence him on regular oral thiamine supplements.

21
Long case 7
Themes: rheumatoid arthritis, osteoporosis,
chronic airways disease

INTRODUCTION

NV is a 65-year-old woman who presents with fever, dyspnoea, weight loss and malaise on a background of severe generalised rheumatoid arthritis, diabetes mellitus, osteoporosis and chronic airflow limitation.

CASE IN DETAIL

For 2 months now, NV has noticed a weight loss of 5 kg, with associated severe lethargy and progressive exertional dyspnoea. On presentation she could not walk more than 10 metres on flat ground. However, she denied any associated orthopnoea or paroxysmal nocturnal dyspnoea. Two weeks ago she developed a cough, which soon became productive with yellow-green sputum. She also had intermittent fevers at irregular intervals, with associated chills and rigors. She denied any chest pain. Five days ago her family doctor prescribed her an antibiotic, which did not cause any improvement in her symptoms despite good compliance. She presented to the hospital 2 days ago, and after multiple investigations a diagnosis of pneumonia was established and she was commenced on an intravenous antibiotic. She has not experienced any fever since commencement of the current medication, and she believes that her cough is improving.

She has had generalised rheumatoid arthritis for the past 10 years. Involved joints include hand and wrist joints, elbows, shoulders, knees, ankles and toes bilaterally together with the left hip joint. Five years ago she had a prosthetic hip replacement in the left side and her left ankle fused. Three years ago she had her right knee replaced too. She also has cervical spinal involvement, but with no neurological deficit.

She experiences joint stiffness in the morning, particularly in the hands, shoulders, neck and feet, which lasts about 2 hours and improves with activity. She is dependent in most activities of daily living but is able to feed herself. She usually cannot walk more than 50 metres due to joint and limb pain, and on such occasions she uses a wheelchair. Her daughter is her main carer.

She has been managed on variable doses of prednisone over the past 10 years, the maximum dose being 50 mg daily and the minimum 5 mg daily. She currently takes 7.5 mg prednisone daily. She has experienced multiple side effects associated with the chronic steroid treatment, including weight gain, acne, easy bruising, osteoporosis and diabetes mellitus.

She has also been treated with multiple other medications over the years, including diclofenac sodium, sulfasalazine and parenteral gold. Diclofenac therapy was stopped due to gastritis and sulfasalazine was stopped due to a rash. Gold therapy was stopped due to proteinuria. Currently she is managed on methotrexate 7.5 mg twice weekly together with celecoxib 200 mg twice daily. Both medications were commenced 8 months ago. She also takes folic acid 5 mg daily. She denies any known side effects associated with this treatment so far.

Her symptoms have never been completely controlled by any of the medications she has been treated with and she has experienced progressive deformity of both hands and feet over the years. The current level of control is the best she has ever achieved.

She denies any eye complaints, oral symptoms, vasculitic symptoms or sicca symptoms associated with her rheumatoid arthritis.

She was diagnosed with gastritis 8 years ago when she presented with epigastric pain. She denies any gastrointestinal bleeding, and the diagnosis of gastritis was established on gastroscopy. Subsequently the diclofenac therapy was stopped, and she was commenced on ranitidine 150 mg twice daily and has been symptom-free ever since. She does not know her *Helicobacter pylori* status and denies ever having been treated with the triple-therapy combination.

She was incidentally diagnosed with diabetes mellitus 6 years ago. She denied any symptoms of polyuria, polydipsia or weight loss on presentation. She was initially treated with dietary modifications and exercise alone. She was commenced on metformin 2 years ago. Currently she is managed on 500 mg metformin three times daily. She denies any side effects associated with this therapy. Her GP monitors her blood sugar level every 2 weeks and currently it averages around 6–10 mmol/L. She has seen an ophthalmologist on only one occasion, about 2 years ago. She was not diagnosed with any ocular complications. She denies any current ocular symptoms. She denies any known diabetic nephropathy. She has had proteinuria on only one occasion previously, which was attributed to the gold therapy. It resolved on stopping the drug. Her GP checks her urine every 6 months. She has never seen a podiatrist and denies any symptoms in her feet.

She denies ischaemic heart disease, stroke or calf claudication. She denies any neurological symptoms associated with diabetes.

She was diagnosed with osteoporosis 1 year ago when her rheumatologist ordered bone densitometry, but she denies any fractures. Her osteoporosis is treated with monthly pamidronate injections, which she has had for the past 6 months without any side effects. She also takes calcium carbonate 1500 mg daily together with calcitriol 0.5 mg twice daily.

She was diagnosed with chronic airflow limitation 1 year ago when she was investigated for progressive exertional dyspnoea. She is treated with salbutamol and ipratropium bromide via a metered dose inhaler two puffs twice daily. She was hospitalised for 3 days, 7 months ago, with infective exacerbation of chronic airflow limitation, which was treated with intravenous antibiotics.

Her current medications include prednisone, celecoxib, methotrexate, metformin, pamidronate, calcium carbonate, calcitriol, salbutamol and ipratropium bromide.

She gave up smoking 1 year ago, prior to which she had a smoking history of 20 pack-years. She consumes alcohol only very rarely, on social occasions.

She denies any known allergies.

She has been a divorcee for the past 15 years. She was married only once and has two adult daughters. She lives with her older daughter, who is 42 years old and is well. The second daughter is 38 years old, is married and lives separately but in the same city. She has two grandchildren. She has regular contact with her second daughter too. She is dependent on her daughter for assistance in all activities of daily living except feeding. She lives on the ground floor of a two-storey house. She has no steps to negotiate. Her house was modified previously under an occupational therapist's recommendations to accommodate her needs. Her usual pastimes are watching television and listening to radio.

Her dietary history reveals adequate nutrition but no compliance with the diabetic diet.

She denies any sleep problems and she has never been depressed, despite her multiple significant medical problems.

Her family history is significant, in that her mother suffered from severe rheumatoid arthritis. She died at the age of 75 from an unknown cause. Her father died of an acute myocardial infarction at the age of 60. She has no brothers or sisters.

She worked as a clerk typist before retiring 20 years ago. She is on a disability pension, which is just adequate for her living. The daughter who lives with her is employed part-time as a nanny.

Her insight into her multiple medical problems seems satisfactory.

ON EXAMINATION

NV was alert, oriented and cooperative. She appeared cachectic and unwell. Her pulse rate was 72 beats per minute and respiratory rate 24 per minute. Her blood pressure was 110/60 mmHg without postural drop, and she was afebrile. Her estimated body mass index was about 20.

She had an intravenous cannula in the dorsum of her left hand and its insertion site was not inflamed. There were multiple ecchymoses in the dorsal aspect of her hands and forearm bilaterally.

She was using accessory muscles of inspiration and demonstrated pursed-lip breathing. Chest expansion was reduced in the upper and lower zones bilaterally and there was no dullness on percussion. Breath sounds were vesicular in the upper zone but there were crepitations in the mid- and lower zones bilaterally. Vocal resonance was not increased. The sputum mug contained yellow-green sputum.

Rheumatological examination showed bilateral symmetrical arthropathy of the hands and wrists with ulnar deviation at the metacarpophalangeal joints, 'Z' deformity of both thumbs, swan-neck deformity of the left index and right ring fingers and boutonnière deformity of the right middle finger. There was subluxation of the wrist joints bilaterally. There was wasting of the intrinsic musculature of the hands. These joints were oedematous but not tender or warm to touch. There was severe restriction of movement in all directions in the metacarpophalangeal joints, proximal interphalangeal joints and wrist joints bilaterally due to swelling, stiffness and deformity. Her hand power was severely restricted and functionality significantly compromised, with inability to unbutton, pick up a pen and write, or hold a cup.

There were non-tender, firm nodules of 2 cm diameter in the dorsal aspect of her elbows bilaterally.

There was tenderness in the anterior aspect of the left shoulder joint together with restriction of abduction to 60°, flexion to 90°, internal rotation and external rotation to 10° in each direction, bilaterally, due to stiffness.

There was tenderness over the C2, C3, C6 and C7 vertebrae, with severe restriction of neck flexion, extension and rotation.

There was tenderness over the temporomandibular joint bilaterally.

There was valgus deformity and medial joint line tenderness, together with crepitus on flexion, in the knee joints bilaterally. There was no Baker's cyst.

There was hallux valgus deformity bilaterally in the feet with subluxation of all metatarsophalangeal joints. There was no tenderness or warmth to touch. Severe wasting of the intrinsic musculature of the feet was present.

Cardiovascular examination was unremarkable, with dual and normal heart sounds and the presence of all peripheral pulses.

Neurological examination showed a visual acuity of 6/24 with correction bilaterally. Fundoscopy showed multiple hard and soft exudates in the macular region bilaterally. The rest of the cranial nerve examination was unremarkable.

Upper limb examination showed profound weakness bilaterally in the intrinsic musculature of the hand and on shoulder abduction. Power was preserved at the other levels together with tone, reflexes, coordination and sensation.

Lower limb examination showed moderate proximal weakness with 3/5 power, bilaterally, on hip flexion, extension, abduction and adduction. Otherwise the lower limb neurological examination was unremarkable. The plantar response was flexor bilaterally.

She had difficulty with mobilisation due to weakness and a waddling gait.

Gastrointestinal examination was unremarkable. There was no organomegaly.

She had no lymphadenopathy.

Diabetic foot examination did not show any painful callosities, corns or ulcers.

In summary, this is a 65-year-old woman with severe rheumatoid arthritis presenting with a history of progressive dyspnoea and fevers on a background of diabetes mellitus, osteoporosis and chronic airway limitation. Her independence is severely compromised.

I have identified one acute problem and two main long-term problems that need addressing:

- The acute problem is the definitive diagnosis and treatment of her lung pathology. The possible differential diagnoses include pneumonia secondary to infective exacerbation of chronic airway limitation, or pulmonary sepsis secondary to relative immunocompromisation due to multiple causes, which include diabetes mellitus, chronic corticosteroid use and myelosuppression associated with methotrexate therapy. Pulmonary fibrosis secondary to rheumatoid arthritis or methotrexate therapy should also be considered.
- Long-term problems include optimal management of the rheumatoid arthritis so as to achieve maximum disease control, at the same time as minimising therapy-related complications, restoring mobility and planning discharge with maximum supportive services.

To address the issue of pulmonary disease, I would like to see:

1 The latest full blood count, looking for leucocytosis or leucopenia with associated anaemia
2 Arterial blood gases done on room air, looking for hypoxia or hypercapnoea

3   A recent chest X-ray, looking for consolidation, hyperexpansion or lung fibrosis
4   The results of formal lung function studies, looking for a mixed obstructive and restrictive pattern. In addition I would like to see the blood culture results if she was febrile on presentation, and the sputum microbiological test results.

Questions and answers

Q: How would you interpret this full blood count and what would you do about it?

- Hb—9.9 g/dL
- MCV—85 fL
- WCC—5.00
- Neutrophils—2.5

A: This result shows a normocytic, normochromic anaemia. The possible causes include mixed haematinic deficiency secondary to chronic gastrointestinal bleeding and malnutrition, anaemia of chronic disease and myelosuppression due to methotrexate therapy. I would like to follow these results up with a blood film, iron studies, B_{12} and red cell and serum folate levels, and a bone marrow biopsy. There is leucopenia with a neutropenia and mild thrombocytopenia. These results collectively suggest myelosuppression, and the bone marrow biopsy will further clarify this.

I would stop the methotrexate therapy immediately but continue with the folic acid replacement. I would commence parenteral folinic acid rescue therapy to facilitate marrow recovery. I would maintain disease control by increasing the prednisolone dose to 10 mg daily. I would also commence antibiotic therapy against community-acquired organisms with intravenous ceftriaxone 1 g daily and oral roxithromycin 150 mg twice daily. I would closely monitor her temperature and the white cell count.

Q: What do you think about this chest X-ray?

A: This frontal-projection, posteroanterior view chest X-ray of NV done on (insert date) shows patchy opacifications diffusely distributed in the mid- to lower zones of the lung fields bilaterally. I cannot see air bronchograms. There is flattening of the diaphragmatic shadow, hyperinflation of the lungs and osteoporosis of the skeletal structures. The lateral projection shows similar diffuse patchy opacifications in the right middle lobe and the lower lobe and in the left lower lobe. I would like to further correlate this chest X-ray with high-resolution CT of the chest, looking for a ground glass appearance in the mid- to lower zones of the lung fields.

Q: What would you look for in the CT scan?

A: The patchy changes may signify consolidation due to pneumonia or areas of interstitial pneumonitis or areas of fibrosis. She has two risk factors that can cause pulmonary fibrosis. First is her severe rheumatoid arthritis. Second is the methotrexate use. A ground glass appearance may suggest active pneumonitis. In that case, stopping methotrexate and increasing the corticosteroid dose may help prevent progression of the pneumonitis and arrest progression to fibrosis.

Q: **How active do you think this woman's arthritis is currently?**

A: I believe this woman's rheumatoid arthritis is currently clinically active. The clinical markers of disease activity are: 1) duration of joint stiffness, and 2) swollen joint count. This woman experiences about 2 hours of joint stiffness in the morning and her swollen joint count exceeds 12—these findings indicate active disease. I would like to confirm my clinical findings by looking at the most recent erythrocyte sedimentation rate and serum C-reactive protein level.

Q: **Well, her ESR is 80 mm/h and CRP is 105 mg/L. If you were to stop methotrexate, given the severity and the resistant nature of this woman's disease, how would you propose to manage her rheumatoid arthritis?**

A: My plan of action for the management of her rheumatoid arthritis has two arms. One is the use of disease-modifying drugs to control disease progression and antiinflammatory medications to control inflammation and related symptoms. The second arm is physical therapy to preserve/restore joint mobility and rehabilitation.

On stopping methotrexate I would consider commencing this woman on leflunomide. Until the leflunomide started acting I would maintain this woman on a tapering course of oral corticosteroid therapy. I would plan to maintain her at the lowest prednisolone dose possible and stop completely when the disease-modifying agent started to take effect, after about 2–3 months. For antiinflammatory therapy I would continue the cyclo-oxygenase-2 inhibitor celecoxib at the current dose. Other options that I might consider include infliximab or etanercept.

I would refer her to a physiotherapist for light mobilisation exercises and hydrotherapy.

Q: **If leflunomide fails to control her disease, are there any other therapeutic options that you could consider?**

A: In the event of disease progressing in spite of maximum-dose leflunomide therapy, I would consider novel therapeutic agents (such as infliximab, which is a monoclonal antibody against TNF-alpha or etanercept, which is a soluble TNF receptor), according to their availability. Another agent I would consider in case of resistant disease is cyclosporin.

Q: **How would you administer infliximab or etanercept?**

A: Infliximab is given intravenously once every 2 months and etanercept is given subcutaneously twice a week. Therefore I would educate the patient's daughter in injection techniques or organise the therapy to be administered by her GP or at the infusion centre of the local hospital.

Q: **Please interpret these liver function test results. What do you think is the problem?**

- AST—557 mU/L
- ALT—768 mU/L
- ALP—110 mU/L
- Bilirubin—35 mg/L
- Albumin—23 g/L

A: These liver function indices show a moderate hepatitic picture with significant elevation of the AST and ALT levels disproportionate to the ALP elevation. There is also hyperbilirubinaemia and a low serum albumin level. I consider methotrexate-induced liver toxicity as my top differential diagnosis. Other possible differential diagnoses are chronic active hepatitis due to hepatitis B or hepatitis C, autoimmune hepatitis and diabetic fatty liver.

I would image her liver with CT or MRI looking for parenchymal or anatomical changes, and check hepatitis B, hepatitis C and autoimmune serology (antinuclear antibody, anti-liver-kidney microsomal antibody type 1 and antibodies to soluble liver antigen) to further clarify the diagnosis.

I would follow up her liver function tests, looking for improvement on stopping methotrexate.

Q: **How would you manage her chronic airways disease?**

A: The oral steroids prescribed for her rheumatoid arthritis will help improve airway inflammation too. I would advise the patient to use the short-acting bronchodilator medication only when symptomatic with wheezing or dyspnoea. I would maintain her on regular twice-daily inhaled corticosteroid therapy with fluticasone 500 mg via the Accuhaler device, given its efficacy of drug delivery and convenience of use. After 4 weeks, if there was no significant improvement in disease control, I would add a long-acting inhaled bronchodilator to the therapeutic regimen.

Q: **How would you plan her discharge?**

A: On resolution of her symptoms I would plan her discharge in association with the physiotherapist, occupational therapist, social worker and her daughter. I would consult the occupational therapist regarding assessing and optimising her functional status. I would obtain their assessment and recommendations on safety and comfort in the patient's home environment.

I would initiate a program of rehabilitation with the physiotherapist and plan continuation of this on discharge, either at a local facility or at the outpatients physiotherapy department.

In association with the social worker I would assess how her daughter was coping and organise necessary assistance and support.

INTRODUCTION

SL is a 44-year-old man with HIV infection presenting with progressive lethargy, weight loss, fevers, night sweats and epistaxis on a background of poor compliance with antiretroviral therapy.

CASE IN DETAIL

SL has been experiencing progressive lethargy over the past 2 months. His lethargy is so severe that he feels exhausted even on minimal exertion. Over this period he has noticed weight loss of about 10 kg despite a well-preserved appetite, and watery diarrhoea without associated abdominal pain, vomiting or nausea. Over the past 2 months he has been suffering from occasional epistaxis that spontaneously resolves. This has gradually progressed in frequency and on presentation he was experiencing epistaxis about four times a week. Each episode settles spontaneously and he loses about 20 mL blood. He denies any bleeding from other mucosal surfaces and denies frequent bruising.

He started to develop high fevers up to 39°C and drenching night sweats 1 month ago. For the past week he has been experiencing night sweats almost every night. He denies any cough, headache or urinary symptoms. He did not seek medical help until 3 days ago, when he presented to the HIV outpatients clinic for his 3-monthly follow-up. On assessment, he was referred for hospital admission for further investigation and management. Since admission he has had multiple blood tests and imaging studies, including CT scans of the head, chest and abdomen, a gallium scan, testing of urine and stool samples and a bone marrow biopsy.

SL was diagnosed with HIV infection 5 years ago when he presented with progressive dyspnoea, significant weight loss and seborrhoeic dermatitis. He was diagnosed with *Pneumocystis carinii* pneumonia on this presentation, and treated with intravenous and oral trimethoprim and sulfamethoxazole together with oral prednisolone. Since his recovery from the acute episode he has been maintained on trimethoprim and sulfamethoxazole 160/800 mg, one tablet daily, for secondary prophylaxis. He claims good compliance with this treatment and denies any side effects. On recovery from the *P. carinii* pneumonia he was commenced on antiretroviral therapy with zidovudine. He tolerated this agent well. Three years ago zalcitabine and indinavir were added to the regimen due to viral count rebound.

He experienced severe ureteric colic due to nepholithiasis after the commencement of this combination. Indinavir was ceased immediately. He was maintained on zidovudine and zalcitabine until 1 year ago when saquinavir was added to the regimen after a progressive decline in the CD4 count was noted. He did not experience any distressing side effects with these medications. Six months ago he voluntarily stopped all antiretroviral therapy because he found consuming so many tablets a tremendous inconvenience.

When his HIV infection was first diagnosed, his CD4 count was 0 and the viral load 230 000 HIV RNA copies/mL. His most recent CD4 count taken 3 days ago when he presented at hospital was 100/mL and the viral load was 20 000 HIV RNA copies/mL.

He was diagnosed with cytomegalovirus retinitis one year ago when he presented with blurred vision and occasional floaters in the left eye. He was treated with intravenous ganciclovir for a period of 3 weeks and then changed to oral ganciclovir. He is currently maintained on 2 g ganciclovir three times a day. He denies any side effects associated with this therapy. He has follow-up with the ophthalmologist every 3 months and claims that he is compliant with the therapy.

He has experienced oral candidiasis twice in the past, the first time 4 years ago and then again 5 months ago. He was treated with oral fluconazole on both occasions. He is maintained on 150 mg fluconazole daily. He has not experienced any side effects with this treatment.

He denies any other opportunistic infections in the past.

He was diagnosed with diabetes mellitus 10 years ago when he presented with polyuria and polydipsia. The diabetes was considered to be a complication of the haemochromatosis, which was diagnosed subsequently. His diabetes was treated with combination insulin initially and he is now on twice-daily rapid-acting insulin, 40 units in the morning and 25 units at night before meals. He monitors his blood sugar levels twice daily and the recent readings have been between 6 and 8 mmol/L. He is compliant with the diabetic diet. He has never experienced hypoglycaemic episodes or suffered from diabetic ketoacidosis.

His general practitioner has investigated him for diabetic nephropathy with spot urine tests. The last test was done about 6 months ago and he was informed that he had no protein in his urine. He has never performed a 24-hour urine collection for testing. He denies any symptoms of chronic renal insufficiency. He sees his ophthalmologist every 3 months and has not been told of any diabetic retinopathy or cataract formation. He denies any visual symptoms currently. He has never seen a podiatrist. He has experienced paraesthesias of the distal extremities in both the upper and lower limbs, but has never had formal nerve conduction studies performed. He denies postural dizziness or impotence.

His haemochromatosis was diagnosed 10 years ago when his diabetes was investigated. He was initially treated with two 3-monthly desferrioxamine infusions followed by 6-monthly infusions for 2 years. He has not had any therapy for haemochromatosis for 8 years. His GP monitors his serum iron levels every 6 months. He denies any known hepatic involvement or any other complications of haemochromatosis.

In summary, his current medications are trimethoprim-sulfamethoxazole, ganciclovir, fluconazole and insulin.

He denies any allergies to medications.

He is an adopted child and therefore does not know whether there is any significant medical history in the family. He has never known his biological family.

He lives on the sixth floor of an apartment block with his partner. He has lived with two other partners previously and his first partner died of an AIDS-related illness. This was a traumatic experience for SL, even though he was separated from the man at the time of his demise. His second partner is also HIV-positive. He has been living with his current partner for the past 3 years and he is HIV-negative. Prior to meeting his first steady partner and after the two previous separations, he had unprotected sexual intercourse with multiple other partners on a casual basis. He has never suffered from any other sexually transmissible disease. He has been vaccinated against hepatitis B and hepatitis A in the past.

His current partner is very sympathetic and supportive. SL does not have any children.

He uses the lift to get to his apartment, and he has two steps inside his apartment that he negotiates without any difficulty.

He smokes 30 cigarettes a day and has a smoking history of 60 pack-years. He rarely, if ever, consumes alcohol. He smokes marijuana regularly at weekly intervals and rolls his own joints. He denies any other recreational drug use.

SL denies any sleep problems and has a satisfactory appetite. He has felt depressed at various times but has never sought medical help for this. He denies any current feeling of depression or suicidal ideation. He worked as a business consultant until 3 years ago when he decided to stop work due to lack of motivation. Currently he survives on sickness benefits, which he finds inadequate to support his lifestyle.

ON EXAMINATION

SL appeared cachectic. He had a depressive affect. His estimated body mass index was about 20. His pulse rate was 70 beats per minute, and it was regular in rhythm and normal in character. With the adoption of an upright posture his pulse rate rose to 90. His blood pressure was 110/70 mmHg without a postural drop and he was afebrile. His respiratory rate was 16 per minute at rest. He was alert and very cooperative. His cognitive function was intact, with a Mini-Mental State score of 30/30.

He had an intravenous cannula in his right forearm and the cannula site was not inflamed. He was not receiving any intravenous therapy at the time of examination. There was seborrhoeic dermatitis on the forehead and the nose as well as in the ventral aspect of the left forearm. No other cutaneous lesions were observed.

Gastrointestinal system examination showed no peripheral stigmata of chronic liver disease. There was oral candidiasis but there were no lesions in the perioral region. His abdomen was soft and non-tender. There was no palpable organomegaly or mass lesion. Bowel sounds were present. I was informed that the per rectum examination was unremarkable.

The respiratory system examination was unremarkable. Chest expansion was symmetrical with vesicular breath sounds.

Cardiovascular examination showed no elevation of the jugular venous pressure or peripheral oedema. He had two heart sounds, which were normal in character.

In the neurological examination his visual acuity in the left eye was 6/6 and in the right eye 8/6 without correction. Pupils were reactive and regular bilaterally. Fundoscopy showed a large cream-white patch immediately inferior to the macula in the left eye. Surprisingly, his visual fields were preserved, with intact extraocular movements. The remainder of the cranial nerve examination was unremarkable.

Upper limb examination showed generalised muscle wasting, with normal tone and reduced power of 4/5 at all levels bilaterally. Reflexes and coordination were normal. There was impaired pinprick sensation in a glove distribution bilaterally, with other modalities of sensation preserved. Sensory impairment extended to the level of the wrist bilaterally.

Lower limb examination showed generalised muscle wasting, with normal tone and impaired power of 4/5 at all levels bilaterally. Reflexes and coordination were preserved. Plantar response was flexor bilaterally. Pinprick sensation, joint position sensation and proprioception were impaired bilaterally to the level of the ankle in a stocking distribution. His gait was unremarkable.

There was no lymphadenopathy or bony tenderness.

His rheumatological examination was unremarkable.

In summary, this is a 44-year-old man with HIV infection presenting with constitutional symptoms on a background of poor compliance with antiretroviral therapy. He also suffers from haemochromatosis and diabetes mellitus.

The main problem with this man is non-compliance with antiretroviral therapy.

In addition I have identified four other medical problems and one social problem that need addressing.

The immediate medical problems are:

1   To diagnose the cause for his current symptoms
2   To assess the current status of his HIV infection
3   To assess the level of activity of different opportunistic infections in this man
4   To assess the level of activity of his haemochromatosis and associated complications.

The possible differential diagnoses for his presenting picture include:

1   End-stage acquired immunodeficiency syndrome (HIV wasting syndrome)
2   An opportunistic infection such as disseminated *Mycobacterium avium* complex
3   Human immunodeficiency virus-associated non-Hodgkin's lymphoma
4   Disseminated cytomegalovirus infection
5   Bacterial infection, such as *Salmonella septicaemia*
6   Cirrhosis with the development of a hepatoma.

The management objectives for this man are:

1   Treat the current clinical problem
2   Formulate the optimal antiretroviral regimen for his maintenance.

To start with, I would like to see the results of the following investigations:

1   Full blood count, looking for anaemia, leucocytosis, lymphopenia and thrombocytopenia
2   Blood cultures, including acid-fast cultures, that have been performed
3   Coagulation profile, looking for a coagulopathy
4   Current viral load and the CD4 lymphocyte subset count, to assess the activity of his HIV infection and the degree of CD4 subset lymphopenia
5   CT scan of the head, looking for ring-enhancing lesions, of the chest, looking for changes in the lung parenchyma and mediastinum for mass lesions, and of the abdomen, looking for organomegaly, lymphadenopathy and evidence of metastatic disease.
6   Gallium scan, looking for multiple foci of activity that may suggest lymphoma or disseminated sepsis.
7   Bone marrow biopsy, for the diagnosis of infiltrative lymphoma or infection with *M. avium* complex.

Questions and answers

Q: **What is the antiretroviral therapy combination that you would recommend for this man?**

A: The issues that need consideration in the recommencement of an antiretroviral regimen in this man are the need to overcome the viral resistance that may have developed to the formerly used agents, and formulation of a combination with a minimal side effect profile. Because he has been off antiretroviral therapy for almost 6 months it is likely that the virus will have reverted to wild type. I would consider commencing a new combination, comprising combivir and nevirapine. Combivir is a single tablet made with a combination of zidovudine and lamivudine, and can be given as two tablets twice daily. The combination of two agents in one tablet will reduce the number of tablets he has to take and thus improve compliance. This combination has a minimal side effect profile and, in particular, no neurotoxicity. I would not use any agent with the potential for neurotoxicity in this man due to his peripheral neuropathy.

Q: **Would you exercise any caution in introducing nevirapine?**

A: Yes, nevirapine can cause a severe rash. Therefore I would initially introduce it as two tablets once daily for about 2 weeks while observing for any rash. Then I would progress to the full dose of two tablets twice daily.

I chose nevirapine because it has been shown to have synergistic antiretroviral activity when combined with zidovudine and lamivudine.

Q: **Interpret the following full blood count and tell us what you would do about it.**

- Hb—8.01 g/dL
- WCC—4.1×10^9/mL
- Platelet count—21×10^9/mL

A: There is moderate anaemia and a significant thrombocytopenia. The anaemia is likely to be multifactorial. The likely contributors are chronic blood loss, anaemia of chronic disease, autoimmune haemolytic anaemia, *M. avium* complex sepsis and infiltrative lymphoma.

The other main abnormality in this blood picture is the profound thrombocytopenia, which may be the main contributing factor to his recurrent epistaxis. Thrombocytopenia may be due to bone marrow infiltration by lymphoma or *M. avium* complex or thrombocytopenia of the HIV infection itself.

To investigate his anaemia further, I would like to have a look at his blood film to ascertain the exact morphology of his red blood cells. In addition, I would like to know the results of the following investigations: serum creatinine and blood urea levels, looking for renal failure, reticulocyte count, serum iron studies, serum B_{12} and folate levels, and a haemolytic screen.

To treat this man I would transfuse him with two units of packed cells. Definitive management would depend on the results of the above investigations. But I believe diagnosis and treatment of his presenting condition and the recommencement of antiretroviral therapy would help improve both the anaemia and the thrombocytopenia.

Q: **His liver function test results are as follows. What do you think is going on?**

- AST—56 mU/L
- ALT—40 mU/L
- ALP—750 mU/L
- Bilirubin—10 mg/L
- Albumin—21 g/L

A: This man has a significant and dissociative elevation of serum alkaline phosphatase. AST and ALT are elevated only marginally. This picture fits disseminated *M. avium* complex (MAC) infection rather than hepatic infiltration with a lymphoma, hepatoma or cirrhosis due to haemochromatosis. I would pursue the diagnosis of disseminated *M. avium* complex infection.

Q: **How would you diagnose *M. avium* complex infection?**

A: I would perform multiple blood cultures taken at different times at least 12 hours apart. In total I would like to have four blood cultures done. I would request the cultures to be done using the BACTEC culture system, as this is the quickest and most reliable way of detecting MAC in the blood. I would also test bone marrow for acid-fast bacilli.

Q: **Microscopic examination of the bone marrow aspiration biopsy showed acid-fast bacilli. How would you approach the management of this patient?**

A: The diagnosis of *M. avium* complex is very likely, according to the clinical picture and also the investigational markers. I would commence treating him with a combination of clarithromycin 500 mg twice daily, rifabutin 300 mg daily and ethambutol 15 mg/kg daily. I would observe the patient for 2–6 weeks for any improvement in the clinical picture.

I am conscious of the fact that rifabutin is an inducer of the hepatic microsomal enzyme system and may decrease the serum levels of other drugs that this man takes. Therefore some of those drugs may need a dose increment.

Q: **How long would you treat this man for the MAC infection?**

A: I would treat him with this initial regimen for 12 weeks. Thereafter I would commence him on a suppressive regimen made up of the two agents azithromycin given at weekly intervals and rifabutin given daily. This therapy is given lifelong. Prior to the commencement of ethambutol therapy I would obtain an ophthalmology review for the patient and follow him up with ophthalmology reviews at regular intervals.

Q: **What do you think is the cause of his thrombocytopenia and how would you manage it?**

A: This is highly likely to be thrombocytopenia of HIV infection, which is an autoimmune phenomenon akin to idiopathic thrombocytopenic purpura. In addition, the infiltration of megakaryocytes by the virus can lead to a thrombocytopenia. The best treatment for the thrombocytopenia is to recommence antiretroviral therapy.

Q: What do you think is his likely prognosis?

A: His prognosis is extremely poor, but I would still actively treat his MAC infection and continue antiretroviral therapy, given his young age and previously good functional state.

Q: Could he have a lymphoma?

A: Non-Hodgkin's lymphoma can occur at any stage of HIV infection. Given his significant immunosuppression, he is highly susceptible to the development of lymphoma.

His initial clinical presentation is consistent with the usual presentation of HIV-associated non-Hodgkin's lymphoma, but he did not have any lymphadenopathy, mass lesions or organomegaly, which are the expected signs in lymphoma. I would like to see the results of bone marrow biopsy, looking for lymphoma cells; results of the CT scans of head, chest, abdomen and pelvis, looking for lymphadenopathy and organ involvement; serum lactate dehydrogenase level, for an elevation; and a gallium scan, looking for 'hot spots'.

Q: What else would you want to do for this man?

A: Another major cluster of problems that this man suffers from is weight loss, lethargy and anorexia. I believe these problems may resolve to a large extent with the treatment of his MAC infection and the HIV infection. It can be addressed further by treating him with agents such as megestrol acetate, dronabinol or the anabolic steroid nandrolone decanoate. Further to this I would recommend a high-protein, high-energy diet in consultation with a dietitian with expertise in dealing with patients with HIV.

His persistent diarrhoea should be investigated and treated appropriately. The likely contributing factors include MAC infection, HIV wasting disease, salmonellosis and infestation with parasites such as *Cryptosporidium*, *Microsporidium* and *Isospora belli*. I would test his stool samples for parasites, parasitic ova and cysts.

This man has significant social and psychological problems, warranting specialised care. Depression or dysthymia may contribute to his non-compliance with the antiretroviral therapy. To cope with his current physical debility, he may need psychological support. I would organise a review of his situation by a psychologist for evaluation and therapy. He also needs specialised counselling and further education, stressing the importance of antiretroviral therapy and compliance with it. He should be reassured that HIV is a chronic disorder that needs ongoing suppressive therapy and that modern medications are very successful in improving overall prognosis and quality of life. I would organise the hospital social worker to assess his financial status and the level of support available for him in the community.

Q: How would you manage his neuropathy?

A: His neuropathy is multifactorial. The main differential diagnoses are antiretroviral therapy toxicity and diabetic peripheral neuropathy. Antiretroviral drugs such as stavudine, didanosine and zalcitabine can cause a peripheral neuropathy, and this man was on zalcitabine previously. His neuropathy seems to persist despite stopping zalcitabine 6 months ago, and therefore the chance of its contributing significantly is low. A change of antiretroviral therapy to agents with no known neurotoxicity and strict blood sugar control are the remedies I would consider.

Q: **How would you manage his haemochromatosis?**

A: I would like to see the results of his recent iron studies. The parameters I want are: 1) serum ferritin, 2) transferrin saturations, and 3) serum iron. Any evidence of iron overload would warrant therapy with desferrioxamine rather than phlebotomy, given his anaemia on presentation.

The previously shown liver function profile does not exclude hepatic involvement of haemochromatosis and cirrhosis. Therefore I would follow him up with an MRI of the liver.

The main objective of discharge planning is to ensure that the patient is released to a safe, supportive and accessible environment. Another objective is to prevent recurrent admission to hospital. The candidate should demonstrate an astute knowledge of the community resources available to the patient and the modalities of establishing appropriate coordination among the different service providers concerned. Social workers and occupational therapists should be involved early in the discharge planning process. If relevant, disease-specific educators and a clinical nurse consultant with expertise in the area should be made available for the purposes of patient education, reassurance and support. A family conference and consultation with the patient's family practitioner should then be carried out. Remember to mention an action plan focused on the principle of shared care with the family doctor. Mention the other community resources that you would involve, such as the community aged care package, community nursing sister, home care service and meals on wheels.

Remember to be ready to talk about topics of current interest and the latest in evidence-based medicine.

Appendix B
Internet directory of internal medicine

Cardiology
http://www.heart.org
http://www.americanheart.org
http://www.acc.org
http://www.theheart.org

Hypertension
http://www.ash-us.org

Haematology
http://www.hematology.org

Nephrology
http://www.nephrologychannel.com
http://www.hdcn.com

Geriatrics
http://www.americangeriatrics.org
http://www.healthandage.com

Respiratory medicine
http://www.ajrccm.org
http://www.njc.org

Gastroenterology
http://www.gastro.com
http://www.gastro.org

Rheumatology
http://rheumatology.org
http://www.rheumatologyweb.com

Infectious diseases
http://www.idlinks.com
http://www.idsociety.org

HIV medicine
http://sis.nlm.nih.gov/HIV/HIVMain.html
http://www.aidsmap.com

Neurology
http://www.neuroguide.com

Endocrinology
http://www.endocrinology.com
http://www.endocrinology.org

Oncology
http://www.cancer.org
http://www.asco.org

General medicine
http://www.medscape.com
http://www.medicalnews.com
http://www.prous.com/ttm
http://www.mednets.com
http://webmd.com

Index

➡

Page references followed by 'f' denote figures; those followed by 'b' denote boxes.

Troglitazone, 135
Trust, 5
Tuberculosis, 232

U

Ulcerative colitis
approach to, 176–8
corticosteroid-resistant, 180
investigations for, 178–9, 179f
management of, 179–80
remission of, 180
Ulcerative proctitis, 179
Ultrasound
abdominal, 232
intracardiac, 242
intracoronary, 242
Upper limbs, 8f, 9
Urea breath test, 175
Urge incontinence, 80
Urinary analysis, 71
Urine analysis
cardiac failure evaluations, 37
hypertension evaluations, 27
rheumatoid arthritis evaluations, 191
systemic lupus erythematosus evaluations, 200

V

Vaccinations
in heart transplant patients, 50
Pneumococcus, 41
Varenicline, 59

Vasodilators, 29, 229
Ventilation-perfusion scan, 227
Ventricular fibrillation, post-infarct, 34
Ventricular tachycardia, 212, 214f
Vertigo, 21
Villous atrophy, 184, 185f
Vitamin B complex, 165
Vitamin D supplementation, 140

W

Waldenström's macroglobulinaemia, 113, 117
Warfarin, 42
Watershed infarction, 239f
Weight reduction, in diabetes mellitus patients, 136
Weight reduction program, 287
Wenckebach phenomenon, 212
Western blot test, 157
Wide-based gait, 10b
Wilson's disease, 169b
Wolff-Parkinson-White syndrome, 213, 215f

X

X-rays
abdominal, 232
chest. *See* Chest X-rays

Z

Zalcitabine, 160–1
Zidovudine, 160–1